TREATMENT IN PSYCHIATRY

TREATMENT IN PSYCHIATRY

Second Edition

By

OSKAR DIETHELM, M.D.

Professor of Psychiatry
Cornell University Medical College
Psychiatrist-in-Chief, The New York Hospital
(Payne Whitney Psychiatric Clinic)

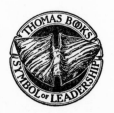

CHARLES C THOMAS · PUBLISHER
Springfield · Illinois · U.S.A.

CHARLES C THOMAS • PUBLISHER
BANNERSTONE HOUSE
301-327 EAST LAWRENCE AVENUE • SPRINGFIELD • ILLINOIS • U.S A.

Published simultaneously in The British Commonwealth of Nations by
BLACKWELL SCIENTIFIC PUBLICATIONS, LTD., OXFORD, ENGLAND

Published simultaneously in Canada by
THE RYERSON PRESS, TORONTO

Copyright, 1936, by Charles C Thomas
Copyright, 1950, by CHARLES C THOMAS • PUBLISHER

First Edition, 1936
Second Edition, 1950

Printed in the United States of America

PREFACE TO THE SECOND EDITION

PROGRESS in psychiatric treatment during the last twelve years has been marked along several lines. Somatic procedures have become well established. Advances in psychotherapeutic methods in adults and children have been valuable. It has become generally accepted that therapy frequently must be directed toward the individual members of the patient's family as well as toward the patient himself. A closer relationship with the other medical disciplines, especially with internal medicine and pediatrics, has been mutually fruitful. This evolution of treatment has necessitated considerable changes in this new edition.

The psychobiologic and psychopathologic basis for treatment is discussed in the introduction. The concept of personality as a psychobiologic unit is now so universally accepted in treatment that it seems sufficient to present the theory in the introduction and to omit reference to it in the succeeding discussions.

Treatment in psychiatry must be broad and inclusive and cannot be presented from the point of view of any special school.

In the rewriting of this book I have been much influenced and helped by the members of the staff of the Payne Whitney Psychiatric Clinic and of Cornell University Medical College. I wish to acknowledge especially the aid and criticism of the following staff members in the preparation of the topics indicated: Dr. Sara A. Bonnett, psychoanalytic procedures; Drs. Ade T. Milhorat and Harold G. Wolff, internal medicine and neurology; Dr. Fred V. Rockwell, convulsive therapy; Dr. Helen E. Daniells, sodium amytal treatment; Dr. Edwin J. Doty, general paresis; Dr. Thomas A. C. Rennie, teaching of psychiatric treatment. I am greatly indebted to my secretary, Miss Ethel Hammer, for her help in the editing of the manuscript.

I wish also to express my appreciation to the following publishers and journals for permission to quote material originally published by them: Baillière, Tindall and Cox, The Hogarth Press, W. W. Norton and Company, Charles C Thomas • Publisher, American Journal of Psychiatry, and the North Carolina Medical Journal.

O. D.

PREFACE TO THE FIRST EDITION

WITH THE development of dynamic psychiatry, the physician found it necessary to concern himself not only with the disease pattern of a case but also with the personality in which it appeared. Although a beginning has been made, much remains to be done to bring about a satisfactory union of both methods of approach. Both the teacher and the practicing physician have a tendency to stress one or the other mode of procedure. Books, too, rarely deal with the whole range of therapeutic possibilities. It would seem, therefore, that there is room for an attempt to outline clearly a theory of therapeutic procedure which combines both points, and which regards such procedure as teachable. It must be acknowledged that many physicians, and even some quacks and mental healers, possess great skill in the treatment of disorders of the personality. Instead of designating such ability as solely intuitive, and the treatment as an art essentially unteachable, the scientific physician will analyze these procedures most carefully to determine the helpful principles involved and to formulate them so that they may be taught to others. The assertion that psychiatric treatment depends to a large extent upon common sense and the ability to take advantage of opportunities as they present themselves must, for the sake of accuracy, be restated: Psychiatrically trained common sense allows the physician to see and create therapeutic opportunities and deal with them constructively.

Since the province of psychiatry covers all disorder and malfunctioning of the personality, this book deals not only with the treatment of the major illnesses designated as psychoses and neuroses, but also with the minor personality reactions of everyday life and with reactions to physical illnesses and handicaps. In the first six chapters the general principles of treatment and various methods are outlined; in the remaining eleven chapters, the treatment of specific reaction patterns, grouped more from a therapeutically practical than a nosologic point of view. At the beginning of several of the chapters a brief discussion of the psychopathology is offered, as a necessary theoretical basis for the treatment outlined afterwards.

[vii]

This presentation of psychiatric treatment is the result of ten years of association with Dr. Adolf Meyer, the Psychiatrist-in-Chief of the Johns Hopkins Hospital. On his advice I began in 1926 to formulate the main principles of psychiatric treatment in lectures delivered to the students of the Johns Hopkins Medical School. Although I have been stimulated by my reading and by my many contacts with psychiatrists of different training and ideas, it is nevertheless correct to state that this whole book is based on the teaching and methods of treatment of Dr. Adolf Meyer.

O. D.

INTRODUCTION

THIS BOOK attempts to do justice to the principle that we need to treat the patient suffering from a disease and not the disease-entity. It is important, of course, to determine the illness from which the patient suffers, but it is no less vital to understand how the patient, as a personality, reacts to his illness, for the study of the personality always opens up new avenues of procedure. No opportunity to influence the patient beneficially should be neglected. Although, to be sure, the fundamental factors involved must be treated first, yet there are times when symptomatic treament may be of genuine value.

Psychiatric treatment, i.e., the treatment of personality disorders, does not confine itself to psychotherapeutic measures only. The physician should strive to correct anything that may be in need of correction, whether the difficulty lies in the psychologic or the somatic field or in the patient's environment. Psychiatric treatment works with facts. It is therefore concrete and tangible and not dependent on intuition. The physician should proceed only after careful deliberation, planning his treatment, if necessary, in minute detail but with a constant alertness to such unforeseen opportunities as may present themselves and to such unforeseen obstacles as may arise. The emergence of either opportunities or obstacles, or both, may change his therapeutic course temporarily or even permanently. Plasticity — a willingness to be guided by facts, by constructive imagination, and by a self-critical optimism — is characteristic of the therapeutically successful physician. The fatalism of the older schools, which were interested mainly in the nosology of disease and in explanations in terms of histology, physiology, and heredity, has led to considerable therapeutic nihilism.

All kinds of disorders of the personality are subject to psychiatric treatment. A treatise of this type should be so broadly conceived that it offers the physician an outline for the study and treatment of the emotional influences which affect a person's well-being and successful functioning. In this book, treatment is presented in a form which considers the individual personality and the psychopathologic facts present. It is not the outgrowth of a special school of therapy but endeavors to utilize whatever has been found valuable in research carried out from different points of view. References are offered for those who may be interested in the use of various special methods and procedures. It is the chief purpose of the introduction to give a compact statement relative to the concept of psychobiology and to the evaluation of psychopathologic observations.

Present-day psychiatry is on a psychobiologic basis in the sense that it proceeds on the hypothesis that matter and its function belong inseparably together, forming a unit, functioning as a unit. A brief elucidation of the basic theory is therefore desirable. Theories which are related to special procedures are discussed in connection with them.

Psychobiologic thinking is the outgrowth of the biologic and physiologic development of the latter part of the 19th century. Its outstanding exponent in psychiatry was Adolf Meyer, who, by using the principle of integration, helped greatly in freeing psychiatry from the traditional dualism of body and mind and from the difficulties which spring from this dualism in the understanding and treatment of psychogenic influences. In the study of any biologic unit made up of several cells, one cannot consider this unit as the result of a mere summation of the individual constituent cells. The several cells are in constant interrelation, so that some functions are modified and new functions, the functions of the unit, emerge. Physicians are acquainted with the concept of integration in neurology and in physiology. Psychobiology bases its understanding of personality on the same principle of the ceaseless interplay and interrelation of structure (matter) and of function.

Any kind of treatment in the entire field of medicine must recognize that there is no separation of physiologic functions and those of the whole personality. The human personality is a highly complicated, integrated unit. Its complexity necessitates the consideration and study of this unit with its specific qualities and functions as well as its parts, each with its own properties and functions. In this analysis, however, one must not forget that in the living person each unit, e.g., the anatomic or physiochemical unit, is integrated in itself as well as in the total personality. All integrated units have functions which are determined by the inter-relations existing among all its parts as well as by its integration with other units. Although scientific investigation will lead to a constant further analysis, it is not conceivable that a final analysis can be reached. Each new step in analysis demonstrates the fact of integration.

The physician does not work with a psyche but rather with functions which have been integrated into a psychologic unit. By way of illustration: a physiologic reflex preparation which has been separated from the organism for the study of the knee-jerk may be considered from the point of view of stimulus and reaction; in such a study no personality function can intrude. However, when the same apparatus functions as part of the total living organism, as in the act of walking or dancing, for instance, then, among other things, memories and anticipations enter into the reaction. The function is that of a specific unit which is called the personality. To be able to function with the help of sensations, conceptions, emotions, and planning, an integrated organism with a sufficiently developed brain is necessary. This specifically integrated unit, with its function of consciousness and its other specific functions, and its biography, is the personality. The most essential characteristic of this psychobiologic personality is that it makes use — with the aid of symbols — of reality and imagination, past, present, and future, personal and general, as if everything were here right now and only with this subject.

This psychobiologic formulation of the personality and its functions is the necessary result of the logical development of the principle of integration. "Mind" must be perceived in a dynamic way, i.e., as function. It may serve to avoid misunderstanding if instead of "mind" one used the term, "mentation," referring to functions which form the process of mentation rather than of "faculties." The latter term has been used to designate the units of a static mind.

Careful observation and interpretation of the experiments which nature offers in pathologic reactions have destroyed the naïve conception of a variety of faculties localized in different parts of the brain. The localization theory, while not entirely in error, was based on observations which were uncritically used and from which therefore certain erroneous conclusions were drawn. These considerations are especially important if one must evaluate the results of surgical operations on the brain and if one wishes to incorporate specific brain operations in psychiatric treatment.

At this point, the consideration of the concept of personality is indicated. Personality is the name given to individuation of the highest biologic development — the human being. Individuation can be recognized throughout the biologic scale — even in the non-biologic world, as, for instance, physico-chemical unit formation. The first step in biologic individuation is seen in the vegetative integration of simple cells, cell colonies, and the more highly specialized species of plants. The next step in biologic individuation is the zoologic type, with motion as a leading characteristic. Beginning with this group, mental functions become demonstrable. In human beings, the consciousness of oneself as a separate unit is highly developed. Everyone considers himself distinct from others, as an individual. Every personality relates occurrences to itself as the center or subject. I do not wish to discuss here the definition of the concept of subject. This belongs to philosophy. Each of us knows that "I am I," but we cannot explain how this becomes known to us. Ever since mankind has existed this must have been one of the chief topics of philosophic contemplation. "Ego" and "self" are terms which are used for it, with varying meaning, in psychology. It will be wiser and not binding to use the term, "subject."

The principle of symbolization, which means the working with symbols, is of great importance in psychobiologic integration. Symbols are functions which serve as signs with meaning. They may be pictorial (images caused by sensory stimuli and memory of previous experiences) although in man they are predominantly verbal. Thinking in symbols enables us to economize and to use various functions in an abbreviated form. Symbolization forms what one calls imagination, i.e., the picturing of situations. Imagination may be constructive and deal with reality or it may be of a more autistic type. Imagination which is not subjected to the test of reality may lead to psychopathologic difficulties and also strengthen hallucinatory experiences.

Mental functions have an inherent tendency to form associations. This characteristic is of fundamental importance and has been clearly recognized since Aristotle. Since Hume it has been studied especially in the English psychologic school. Unfortunately, it was later regarded as the most characteristic feature and used to explain all mental processes in one way or another. At present, psychiatry in many countries still holds to this theory which has greatly affected therapeutic methods. One should use associative tendencies as a valuable therapeutic agency, but guard against making it the exclusive basis of investigation and treatment.

Psychobiologic integration takes into consideration that an individual can bring his relationships to reality and fancy, to past, to present, and to future events on the same level, including personal and social functions as if all these matters were all present here and now and with that one subject. Essential privacy is obtained as well as a remarkable range of fusion and differentiation. One should not intrude into this personal life without a careful evaluation of the meaning to the person.

Psychobiology, as presented here, can be accepted by any philosophic trend. It is a formulation of the personality which is based on present knowledge of the life processes, and does not attempt to offer a solution to philosophic problems. It does not restrict scientific curiosity and investigation, but stimulates them, showing us the narrow field of our knowledge and the possibilities for further search in the immense field of the unknown. It is a science which allows us to deal with people as we find them in life and offers us a basis for possible modes of modification of the personality. Psychobiology should not prevent the use of any of the theories which are current in psychiatric treatment, if one is willing to accept the unit of the life-grown personality and its integration in the environment.

The psychobiologic approach forces us to study both the overt and the implicit performances of a person. The overt is the objectively observable performance, which may be expressive or effective. Both activities are always integrated by mental functions, which constitute the implicit performance. This is a highly subjective and individual activity, known to us as perception, fancy, thought, and inference. We can deduce from the overt some of the implicit activities, and with the help of questions we are able to get a more or less clear picture of them.

Some space should be delegated to a discussion of the concept of consciousness. Its definition belongs to metaphysics — we are interested only in its working as a function. Everyone can easily observe that there are different stages of consciousness, best described by "more or less." Since Leibnitz, many attempts have been made to show the existence of unconscious mental functions. This is a purely philosophic question, and hypotheses which are based on it must be considered problematic. We do not deal with unconscious thinking but with mental functions of which the subject is not aware because of his attention's being directed elsewhere. This occurs in various degrees and has led to the division into unconscious and subconscious. The psychologists who accept this division define unconscious as designating a kind of mental functioning which corresponds in many ways to our involved and elaborate conscious thinking, but which is not open to the observation of the conscious personality. Subconscious mental activity differs from conscious activity merely by not being in the realm of awareness, but it is available to the subject by directing his attention to it. The concepts of integration and subject-organization explain the varying degrees of consciousness, allowing a far-reaching degree of coordinated mental functioning of which we are not aware and which often is not available to the person because of dissociation. Emotional factors may interfere with the associative tendencies and prevent the person from becoming aware of certain impulses and mental activities.

Many experiences called into consciousness by various searching methods of personality analysis are supposed to be the expression of unconscious mental activity and to offer proof for the existence of unconscious thinking. The setting in which those experiences occurred in the biographic development of the individual can never be completely reconstructed. Furthermore, these experiences existed in the person in a highly abbreviated form through the economizing functions of symbolization. When these experiences are remembered, as a result of the working of their associative tendencies, they contain many facts which originally had little or no relation to them.

Dreams are a kind of mental activity which is not under the influence of attention. Tendencies which are not allowed to come out into the open in a state of awareness work freely in dreams, and their analysis is therefore of considerable therapeutic value. In dreams the same economizing principle is at work which may be observed in the thinking of daily life. Instead of the formation of highly verbal symbols and abstract concepts, primary symbols (images) are fused and composite primary symbols developed. It is unfortunate that in psychiatry the word "symbol" is used in various different ways and almost entirely for the higher pictorial composites. Little is known yet in what way dreams are influenced by the psychobiologic setting in the first few years of childhood and in the advanced aging period, and by the different psychopathologic settings.

Any kind of psychiatric treatment must be based on a clear recognition of the psychopathologic facts present and must be guided by them. The understanding of these facts, which is limited to a varying degree in each patient, will increase with the progression of treatment and constantly influence the therapeutic plan. The psychopathologic findings will force modification of the therapeutic procedures and influence the physician's conception of the goal.

Psychopathology includes the subjective, objective, and psychodynamic aspects of each individual person. Through Kraepelin, experimental procedures and clear description of the phenomena observed were brought to psychopathology; through Freud, a psychodynamic-genetic approach; and through A. Meyer, the relationship to environment and physiologic manifestation. Modern psychopathology combines these three historical contributions and offers a sound basis for the treatment of all types and intensities of personality disorders.

BIBLIOGRAPHY

MUNCIE, W.: *Psychobiology and Psychiatry* (2nd ed.). C. V. Mosby Company, St. Louis, 1947. (The most inclusive treatise of A. Meyer's Teaching.)

CONTENTS

TREATMENT IN PSYCHIATRY

Chapter I

STUDY OF PERSONALITY

IN THE STUDY of human beings and their reactions, one must always consider the whole individual personality. One cannot observe an isolated reaction of a patient and analyze it into its elements without also considering it as the reaction of the total personality. Psychobiology, which is the science of the functions of the personality, emphasizes the inseparable unity of structure and function, of physical and mental. The concept of personality as a unit replaces the psychophysical parallelism of Wundt, which postulates that parallel to psychic phenomena occur physiologic processes, and insists on a division of mental and physical. This parallelistic separation has influenced the conceptions of most psychiatrists of modern times and has interfered with therapeutic progress. Through the development of the psychobiologic attitude, a dynamic and analytic-synthetic approach to personality difficulties and disturbances has been made possible, and the basis has been laid for an active and individually modifiable treatment. The main psychobiologic concepts, which form the basis for the treatment of personality disorders, have been formulated in the introduction. In this chapter the practical issues referring to treatment are presented. Current psychologic theories which have exerted an influence on therapeutic procedures are briefly mentioned. They are more fully discussed in the various chapters on psychotherapy. The second part of the chapter offers a guide for the study of personality, and the third part presents practical suggestions for keeping a person functioning well.

Of fundamental importance for the understanding of the working of a personality, and therefore, the basis for treatment, are the concepts of integration and individuation. These concepts have been discussed fully in the introduction. It may therefore suffice to state that psychobiologic integration means that the functions of the personality which one studies and tries to correct in a person are the expression of the personality working as a whole. Physical and mental are inseparably linked together. It is essential that the person be studied and understood in the setting of his development, but living at the present time and having his characteristic attitude and anticipation to the future. All these factors, the present personality with the biographic development and the attitude to the future, must be considered and evaluated carefully. Whatever can be modified, whether it deals with the personality functions in a narrower sense or with the somatic condition, with work or environmental factors, should be utilized therapeutically.

Each person is organized as a unit which refers everything to itself as the center (the I, or self). Each individual is different from every other individual. The different individual personality setting colors the psychopathologic reaction, and many different reactions result which, however, can be grouped into the reaction-sets, the various types of illnesses. In treatment, justice should be done to individual differences. Many illnesses which are not directly influenced by treatment nevertheless offer therapeutic possibilities if one knows how to ultilize the individual personality factors involved. This therapeutic procedure differs from mere symptomatic treatment inasmuch as it is not directed to the removal of symptoms but at the modification of personality factors which are recognized as important. On the other hand, symptomatic treatment may also be considered indicated if it leads to the modification or removal of symptoms which impede the treatment or which are especially painful or difficult for the patient. Therapeutic attention to symptoms should always be judged from the point of view of the psychopathologic picture.

Psychiatry based on the principle of integration cannot be merely a science of abnormal "mental functions." The whole personality, with due attention to physical and mental aspects, has to be considered if one wants to understand and treat these disturbances. One therefore should not consider psychotherapy the sole method of psychiatric treatment. It will frequently be necessary to try to effect physiologic changes, even in disturbances which are primarily psychogenic. The physician should not hesitate to treat chemically what is accessible or to use procedures which attack physiologic factors, if these methods are indicated. Of course, such psychiatric treatment has to be based on careful investigation of the personality and cannot be outlined in a dogmatic form. On the other hand, one should not neglect the influences of other levels of integration in the study and treatment of specific organic illnesses. Any disturbance in any integrated unit results in a disturbance of the total organism. However, these disturbances may be so small or so localized that one will not be able to observe them or that one can neglect them for practical reasons. The conclusion which is to be drawn from these considerations is fundamental:

In any disturbance, whether it be physiologic, structural, or psychologic in nature, one must examine carefully all these aspects and consider possible interrelations and influences. In other words, one always has to consider the total organism.

One of the characteristic features of mental functions is the inherent tendency to form associations. Many psychiatrists still hold to the theory that this feature is more important than many other personality functions and use it to explain all mental processes in one way or another. This overevaluation has influenced current therapeutic methods greatly. It is important that one use associative tendencies as a valuable therapeutic agency, but one should guard against making this factor the exclusive basis for every method of investigation and treatment.

The subject or personality reacts differently from moment to moment. The facts which are presented at the time to the sense organs bring perceptive and presentative functions into activity. Ideas and material representative of things and facts beyond the senses, as well as memories of past experience, are utilized through a more or less constructive imagination. By means of this function they are brought into interrelation through associative assets which are knit together in more or less focused attention. Emotions and effects are the regulative tendencies in the integrated psychodynamic process. They are the finest reagents and indicators of the personality. On the interrelations of all these functions inference and reasoning, planning and choice, action tendencies and actions are based. The result is seen in expressive and effective overt acts. The process of symbolization, with its highly developed possibilities for economizing, enables the organism to react from moment to moment with this complicated process.

In looking at a personality in this way one does justice to all its possibilities as a unit. There is no artificial division into cognition, affects, and volition, and one is therefore not afraid of accepting interrelations which disturb these unities. The processes of discrimination and fusion, orientative and constructive functions are accepted and understood. There is no need for different faculties. One realizes that one deals with psychodynamic processes which are far beyond the structural organism. What one observes at any given time is part of the stream of psychobiologic processes of the observed personality, open to study as behavior and mental functions.

Man's grasp of space and time is limited. Therefore, when studying a person, one's investigations are restricted to a time period or to a special task. One must realize that one is dealing with an artificial and relative unit, a cross-section in a continuous development. Only through a study of the past and of the attitude to the future can one obtain a correct understanding of the person who is the object of the study; therapeutic investigations should not be limited to a special period.

From a practical point of view, it is desirable to single out phases in the development of each personality (phases, in this connection, refers to the successive modes of behavior). One is apt to talk of the change of a personality during adolescence, but there are also distinct changes later in life. Features which have heretofore been dominant become less important, and less obvious features take a leading role. Childhood and adolescence offer an understanding of the increasing organization of personality functions. An illness, also, is only a phase in a person's life, and in the development and process of the illness various phases can also be distinguished. Such a discrimination, while it may seem arbitrary to the untrained mind, offers itself quite naturally. The analysis of the various phases of an illness permits one to get closer to the dynamic factors. These phases have further to be considered in their interrelations with each other, forming the unit which one calls the illness with its place in the setting and development of the whole personality.

The personality itself is not an absolute unit in space. We live in our surroundings and there are constant social interrelations. Treatment must consider social functions and attempt to achieve an adjustment to the group. It can therefore never be individualistic in the sense of treating only the individual as if he were detached from his environment.

We exist in the midst of the cosmos, the eternity of space and time. In studying a person one must therefore include interrelations which belong to a suprabiologic integration, the investigation and explanation of which are beyond the realm of psychology. Philosophy offers gratification to such questions and needs. In treatment this aspect cannot be neglected and it is important that the person's attitude to these problems be studied.

Treatment is based on the study of the overt and implicit performances of a person. Introspection is an amplification of one's study, but one should realize that it is uncritical and often erroneous and one ought to be careful to restrict its use. The subject can never make himself the object of study as someone else can. Self-analysis is frequently more destructive than constructive and often interferes with treatment. Therapeutic interviews should be brief, lasting no longer than an hour. It is best if they can be ended with a constructive understanding on the patient's part that the rest of the day the patient should lead an active life which will allow the material which has been brought to the surface to settle down and to become a part of the person. The patient should learn to utilize and practice what he has learned in the interview.

In the introduction I discussed the concept of consciousness. It is important that one realize where one deals with facts and where theories are the guiding principle. Attention should be paid to the dynamic tendencies of which the patient is not aware. When opportunity arises, dreams and symbolic acts should be studied constructively.

In every action and reaction of the patient one should study the contributing factors, the ramifications and their modes of working. Practically, one should make it a rule in formulating the problem to consider first the simplest integration, emphasizing adjustments where opportunities for correction of physico-chemico, exogenic, physiologic, and neuro-biologic factors have been found inadequate.

In the study of a personality one should investigate behavior by direct observation and by inquiry into the life history. Thus one deals with longitudinal sections (life history) and cross-sections (at any given time). One must be objective, using observation and experiment, and not merely deduction based on hypothesis. To know what a person is, one must observe him, his actions and reactions, his behavior. One will then be able to decide what can be predicted and prevented. Isolated reactions may have to be studied, but such a study is incomplete and fallacious if one does not determine the influence of the total reaction. The therapeutic approach should be selected according to the needs of the individual case. Psychobiology permits a broadminded attitude, using the method which will promise the best results with regard to modification and readjustment of personality difficulties.

The basis for treatment is the understanding of the patient's personality. The physician should choose the method of treatment according to the patient's make-up, his assets and liabilities and their modifiability, and try to formulate to himself what might be reasonably expected. Each individual is different from any other individual, but all have certain traits in common. Such traits can be singled out and grouped to form types in which personalities are classified. The selection of such traits and the formation of corresponding types naturally depends on the investigator's point of view. Some classify according to the possibilities and needs for social adjustment; others give more consideration to emotional aspects and temperament; others stress ethical attitudes; and a large group tries to link certain personality features with the physical make-up. However useful these types may be from a special point of view, their value for the therapeutic approach is negligible. The physician should be prepared to investigate the individual patient and should not depend on the short-cuts which are provided by typology.

It is desirable to be acquainted with a methodical approach to personality investigation. One should learn to study the patient's behavior and draw conclusions from it, but the greater part of one's knowledge must still be obtained through direct questioning. Questions should not present mere adjectives to the patient, from which he can choose what seems to him the most suitable. One should ask him to relate the traits mentioned to situations which seem characteristic and then analyze them in that setting. In such a way one considers the performance of a person, whether actually observed by the physician, or described by the patient or by outsiders (relatives, friends, employers).

It is important that one try to separate constitutional endowment and development from changes in the personality which are due to illness. In both normal and pathologically changed personalities, one must determine to what extent some traits are modifiable or whether they are so ingrained that a change is impossible. One should evaluate the assets of the personality and then determine how they can be utilized for correction or neutralization of undesirable features. It is essential not to be satisfied with the manifest traits, but also to consider possible latent tendencies which need to be treated or utilized. It is difficult to determine the actual constitutional endowment; that is, what is present at birth; but it is practically unimportant to distinguish between constitutional traits and traits belonging to the earliest development, as these traits are so ingrained that they form an unchangeable part of the personality.

The personality investigation deals not only with a cross-section at the time of treatment but also includes the historical development of the individual and his attitude to the future. One needs to know the family setting into which the patient was born, his individual development from infancy to the time he became a patient, and the outstanding formative factors which seem to have played a role. An understanding of hereditary tendencies makes one aware of the personality traits which are so ingrained that they cannot be modified.

Every feature has a double aspect and the physician therefore not only has to consider obvious tendencies but must also look for the possibilities of the other aspect. A person may, for instance, be sensitive to certain types of criticism. This may be a handicap, but its asset is that this person will avoid such criticism of others. Often the patient is only aware of one aspect and the corresponding feature will then have to be developed therapeutically. The best technique in such investigations is to be guided by the principle that each feature is connected with its counterpart. By always keeping opposites in mind the physician will be prevented from arriving at erroneous conclusions, and where contradictions actually exist they will reveal disharmonious and antagonistic strivings which need to be adjusted. Any personality analysis should be considered from the point of view of the integrated whole. Such an analysis does not lead to an accumulation of descriptive adjectives, but to a dynamic formulation in which all possible interrelations are considered and justifiable inferences drawn by which we may arrive at new characteristics.

There are no tests which will offer a thorough understanding of the personality. There are certain tests with which one can investigate, for instance, the intellectual resources. The result, however, should not be taken in a mathematical sense. One should pay attention to the failures as well as to the correct answers and evaluate both in the setting of the whole personality. Studies of handwriting and the interpretation of ink-blots (the method of Rorschach) are very helpful, but can never take completely the role of a direct examination.

Every physician should know how to obtain an understanding of the personality through careful questioning of the patient and of the persons who know him. It is important that one ask for examples of situations in which certain personality traits show themselves. These situations can be used for a constructive discussion in which the reaction is studied from the point of view of personality setting and in which possibilities for modification and correction are determined. These discussions may be brief as, e.g., in diagnostic and other consultations, or they may develop into prolonged therapeutic personality studies.

METHOD OF STUDY

With increasing experience one will develop his own individual method of studying personality. The outline which is given below need not be used rigidly, but the main points which are mentioned should be considered even in the briefest study. The sub-divisions are selected from a practical point of view; they are artificial and overlap at some points. Different or additional sub-divisions may be found more practical by others.

The sub-divisions are:

1. Intellectual resources
2. Emotional tendencies and temperament
3. Volitional and action tendencies, interests, and strivings
4. Standards
5. Attitude to one's body and to the instinctive desires
6. Attitude to material needs
7. Attitude to oneself and ability to deal with oneself
8. Social needs and adustment to the group
9. Assets and handicaps and personality synthesis

1. INTELLECTUAL RESOURCES

Under this heading one studies the resources for new acquirements and the adaptability to new problems and conditions of life — with a utilization of the past and the possibility of evaluating future needs.

One should distinguish between knowledge and a person's ability to make use of it. An evaluation of the patient's knowledge allows one to arrive at certain deductions. In this way one can see his attitude in learning and his appreciation of manual and mental activities. One needs to investigate his ability to record and retain. Some persons have more talent for the retention of objects. In this group may be distinguished the retaining of digits, stories, visual objects, details or totality with neglect of details, names, concepts. Others are more inclined to retain personal experiences. Memory shows a different degree of clearness and vividness. Imagination may be rich, using pictorial or verbal symbols, dealing more or less with reality or with phantasies. The symbols show a different degree of vividness. Often people who believe that they have a wealth of imagination have only a superficial type of imagination, sticking close to reality and making little use of symbols.

One may deal with wealth or poverty of ideas. Ideas may be clear-cut or have a tendency to haziness. Speed of thinking can be fast or slow, or there may be a tendency to rambling. One distinguishes between the logical-discriminative and associative abilities. Some individuals are analytical in their procedure, others more synthetic, while a third group is inclined to take situations as a whole. This is closely related to intuitive appreciation (without need for analysis and proof). Many people are alert and have a keen ability to observe while others are more inclined to be daydreamers. There are concrete and abstract thinkers. Persons with marked perceptual ability turn more to the outer world, those with more conceptual ability to the inner world. Many are unable to take an impartial view and easily become biased, while others are more objective. This is not quite the same as being personal or impersonal. Thinking can be orderly or careless, and one finds various degrees of ability for systematization.

It is important that one understand the person's clearness in thinking, his ability to deal with complexities, and his method of planning. The investigation of special talents and outstanding abilities reveals to what extent they have been cultivated or even recognized. Creative abilities can be developed, but only according to a person's constitutional endowment. Closely related to early intellectual resources is the ability to pay attention without getting too easily distracted, yet without becoming too completely absorbed for any length of time. There are many degrees of persistence or, on the other hand, fatigability of attention. It should be realized that the possibility of utilizing one's intellectual resources depends on attention, the interest involved, the mood at the time, and volitional capacities.

2. EMOTIONAL TENDENCIES AND TEMPERAMENT

Every person has a basic mood, which may be cheerful or gloomy, even and with little variation, or with marked fluctuations. Changes in mood may be impossible to account for, or they may be reactive. Some people are easily aroused emotionally while others are rather stolid. The reactive mood may be superficial or far-reaching and the reaction may occur suddenly or be delayed. In some it is of brief duration; in others more lasting. Besides the pure moods of happiness and sadness, one reacts with irritability, annoyance, anger, resentment, hate, anxiety, discouragement, and fear, according to one's make-up and the specific situation.

The temperament indicates the mode of emotional reaction. One no longer speaks of sanguine and phlegmatic temperaments. These concepts were much too general and brought together various features which have to be differentiated. Temperament may be characterized by slow or quick action, restlessness, or indolent behavior. Activity is not always combined with joy in doing things. I shall refer to features of temperament again when I discuss the personality in action.

Emotional attitude to the future is characterized by optimism or pessimism — frequently by anticipation, anxiety, or fearfulness. Some people have a considerable amount of ease in the display of emotion while others are unable to express their emotions or have a need for constant self-restraint. Many respond easily to the emotions of others or to situational factors. Some are able to arouse emotions in others easily. The ability to experience sympathy and to display sympathy varies and these two features do not always go parallel.

Each person has a characteristic type of humor, which may be good natured, employed at the expense of others, or sarcastic.

It will become obvious later how all these factors are related to the use of the intellectual capacities, general behavior, and social adjustment.

3. VOLITIONAL AND ACTION TENDENCIES, INTERESTS, AND STRIVINGS

This sub-division is closely related to the preceding one because behavior is greatly influenced by mood and temperament, and strivings produce different emotions.

One should always study the general behavior of a person while talking to him. Much can be learned from his way of entering the room, shaking hands, talking, and from his facial expression, gestures, and posture. In general, one may distinguish persons who are active from those who are quiet. Active persons may react easily with fatigue or, on the other hand, may not be aware of it at all and therefore neglect rest. Many are fast but accurate in their actions, while others are more hasty and inaccurate or impulsive. The person who is slow in action frequently has difficulty in getting started, but such people are sometimes active in pursuing a goal. These concepts need not cover industriousness and laziness. A person may be active in making decisions and in dealing with obstacles — that is, decide and act quickly with energy, forcing his will. The passive type reacts with hidden or open resistance to interference, frequently combined with a non-relenting and persistent attitude. A third type of person expresses volitional features not in passive stubbornness but in reactive behavior in which he is stubborn and unwilling to bend. This is an active type of stubbornness. It is again important to consider the opposites of these features, deciding whether a person vacillates and is easily influenced in his decisions, showing a lack of resistance and giving in to difficulties. Many people are cautious in making decisions or even procrastinate, while others rush headlong. One can be orderly in action, even to the extent of being pedantic, or one may be careless. One may be to the point, or circumstantial, or constantly missing the essentials. Some people always feel ready for effort and enjoy difficulties in which decisions have to be made; others try to avoid them.

Emotions are the regulative functions of our personality and are therefore closely related to the behavior of the person in action. Underlying strivings naturally influence emotional and volitional expressions. Because of the strength of the underlying desire, one person may utilize his volitional capacities to the utmost and try to achieve his desire caused by the emotional influence, while the absence of such strivings or the presence of contradictory strivings may make it impossible for another person to use his natural resources. The various strivings are discussed under various headings and special attention must therefore be paid in this connection to standards, to the attitude to the body and the instinctive desires, to material things, to oneself, and to the group.

4. STANDARDS

Under this heading should be considered the ideals and higher needs of a person and his reaction to them. It therefore refers to ethical, aesthetic, and material needs. Everyone has definite ethical goals, of which, however, he is frequently unaware. Our attitude to ourselves, and similarly to others, may be tolerant or intolerant. Many persons are merely indifferent, while others are definitely frivolous. This latter type is in contrast to the person who is conscientious and has a high sense of duty. The concept of duty is peculiar to the individual. It may have to do with personal affairs or with the group (personal and social conscience). Some are labile in their ethical ideals, while others are more stable and live up to their ideals with much energy. One always has to decide whether there is a tendency to overevaluate (for instance, a tendency to hobbies or to fanaticism). Some may be extremists, others are inclined to be melioristic. This does not necessarily correspond to the desire to stick to the old (conservatism) or the need for change. The need for order and regulation should be investigated.

Honesty to oneself and to others plays an important role. Self-deceit is an important factor in many patients and one usually rationalized by them. In this connection, the tendency to exaggeration, dramatization, or hyprocrisy should be investigated.

People can be saving in various degrees or wasteful. An important feature is the tendency to envy and the inability to be satisfied with what one has. The need for pleasure of all kinds stands in contrast to an ascetic attitude. In many, there is a great need for justice, which allows them to forget humanitarian tendencies. Criticism can be given in a destructive or a constructive way and is frequently related either to a tendency to be deprecatory or to the ability to appreciate the value of others.

A person's aesthetic need should be considered. It may be a love of land and the need to be close to it and enjoy its beauty, or an appreciation of beauty in art or literature. These tendencies are complex, because our appreciation of beauty depends to a large extent on the content, which, naturally, is frequently of a symbolic nature, and on the emotions which it stirs up in us. In order to understand a person's standards we must know his attitude to religion, his mystical concepts, and his philosophy.

5. ATTITUDE TO ONE'S BODY AND TO THE INSTINCTIVE DESIRES

Many persons show little interest in their bodies or may even neglect them, while others are constantly concerned about them and compensate their shortcomings in various ways. This is not the same as physical courage or lack of it. The physical fitness of each person shows a wide range of fluctuation. The need for sleep and the type of sleep vary greatly, according to the time and depth of sleep. Dreams are more frequent at certain times. The state of general health also shows fluctuations. In women it is frequently related to menses, and in both sexes to climacteric changes. When one speaks of physical strength or weakness one should state whether this refers to general body conditions or more specifically to certain organs or activities. The type of fatigue should be studied and the way it affects a person physically and psychobiologically, his need for rest and physical exercise.

The instinctive desires, their quantity and strength, and how the person deals with them are of great importance. Hunger can usually

be satisfied without great difficulty, but some persons are not able to
overcome a craving for certain food or a tendency to excessive eating. These disorders of food intake are highly complex and must
be analyzed carefully. It is also worth while to investigate idiosyncrasies of various types. Thirst presents a problem mostly from
the point of view of craving for alcohol and will therefore be dealt
with in detail in Chapter XVIII. The sexual instincts present difficulties at one time or another in everybody's life. It is important that
one determine the amount of individual passion and the possibilities
of restraint, both well recognized in periods of continence, and
whole-hearted efforts at control, the physical and psychobiologic
sexual development, the ethical attitude to sex and its broader aspect — family formation (see Chapter XVII). One must know how
sex information was first obtained. Each person has his individual
tension curve, which is characterized by general and local tension
feelings, sexual preoccupations, and physiologic relief in dreams,
with or without discharge. One should study what other means of
relief a person has and what attempts at control have been made.
It is necessary to know by what situations a person gets easily stirred
sexually. This problem is discussed more in detail in the chapter on
sexual difficulties. An estimate of the patient's cravings and his
way of dealing with them should be obtained. This refers not only
to alcohol and drugs but also to tobacco and coffee.

The reaction to pain shows marked individual differences. There
may be a lack of sensitiveness to pain or a hypersensitiveness, an
unwillingness to show emotions, with or without an ease of control.
Similar factors play a role in the attitude to illness and physical
suffering; in addition, anticipation and strong emotional factors
should be evaluated as well as the possibility of the influence of
material and other personality needs.

6. ATTITUDE TO MATERIAL NEEDS

Material needs and attitudes vary greatly. Some persons have
a need for varying degrees of wealth for the sake of security, others
to satisfy the craving for a luxurious life. The need for the acquisition of wealth may also be based on a desire for power. Last,
there is a miserly type who loves wealth for its own sake. To some,
wealth means financial power, others have a desire for the ac-

quisition of land, clothes, etc., while still a third group is mostly interested in acquiring rare pieces (collector's type). A person's attitude to his position can be greatly influenced by his need for material security or by the ambition for power, social standing, etc. One should investigate the person's attitude to social standing. There are great differences in the material mode of living, from the ascetic to the modest to the luxurious.

7. ATTITUDE TO ONESELF AND ABILITY
TO DEAL WITH ONESELF

Everyone has a certain interest in himself, expressing it either by self-analysis, which may be self-critical, or by a self-contented attitude. One's estimate of oneself should be compared with what one would like to be. Many are not willing to face themselves and shrink from discussions concerning themselves. The capacity for self-denial is of great importance in the control of desires and cravings. One should determine on what these desires depend and whether there is any definite periodicity. An analysis of prevailing trends and habits, strivings, and aversions is necessary and an evaluation of the person's ability to deal with them. According to the make-up and occasion, gratification or suppression will be chosen and achieved with more or less success.

Not everyone achieves self-dependence and self-reliance. Many who have it on the surface lack confidence in themselves underneath. Self-restraint and self-indulgence are important factors. The role of impulse and circumstances, volitional resources, and emotional reactions has to be considered. Some individuals shrink from responsibility, some are actually unable to carry it, and others may enjoy it. A person should understand his amount of energy and endurance, to what extent he needs help, and to what extent he can be pushed. He has to know his need for recreation and vacation, his ability to deal with finances and social difficulties. One has to distinguish pride from haughtiness and dignity and to determine whether one deals with genuine modesty or whether it is the expression of a certain type of vanity or conceit. Every person has a certain sense of honor and need for self-respect. Vanity may show in behavior and need for personal attention and may lead to bragging or displaying one's assets, often with pretentiousness. The person who lacks a need for attention and is not concerned about the impression he makes on others is careless in his personal habits and does not fit in well socially.

One should study the person's attitude to the needs and tendencies which have been obtained under the previous headings.

The concept of freedom varies greatly from marked individualism to the desire to be led and guided by others and absorbed in a group. Some have a definite need for originality. The need for independence may refer to ethical as well as financial or social factors. Spontaneity should be cultivated, but can function well only if the person is able to be responsible for his actions. Feeling inadequate or insecure leads to the suppression of healthy spontaneity.

8. SOCIAL NEEDS AND ADJUSTMENT TO THE GROUP

A person may often feel isolated in the group, but he only develops a constant feeling of loneliness if he has at the same time a definite need to belong to the group. Another type feels that he belongs to the group and is an inherent part of it. This leads to the distinction of the socially dependent and the self-sufficient person. Persons who are concerned about the impression they make on others easily feel ill at ease and self-conscious and may refer remarks and actions to themselves. In this connection, I wish to stress the frequent discrepancy which exists between the impression which one believes one makes on others, and the actual impression. The self-assertive person shows this trait in aggressiveness and arrogant, domineering behavior. The submissive type, who wants to be led, can easily be stubborn and show a tendency to be quarrelsome. These traits do not coincide with the desire to be a leader.

Many persons are frank or have a need to confide in others, while some are very reserved. These tendencies may be confined to certain groups only, and one needs to consider this reaction with regard to family, a few friends, and to the group in general. The attitude to one's family is characterized by varying degrees of devotion with little or great emancipation, leading to an extreme or moderate amount of interest in one's family or to neglect. The attitude to one's wife is guided by similar tendencies. A study of the person's attitude to his friends reveals his need for social contacts and the type of devotion and allegiance which he has been able to develop. Many are exclusive in their friendships, while others have many but only superficial friends. Sympathy and thoughtfulness play a role and are often combined with the need for receiving sympathy. Its absence may be seen in envy, cruelty, and a lack of feeling for others. These tendencies are often combined with a need for receiving and giving affection or its absence. All these tendencies show in the attitude to the larger group. A person may react to various influences with submission or refusal. Some are able to take advice and criticism while others resent it. There are various tendencies to bear grudges and to be revengeful. The ability to be conciliatory and generous is an asset or a handicap, according to the degree in which it is developed. One may have the ability to affect others or one may be easily influenced by others (suggestibility). Thinking about one's impression on others may lead to dramatization and acting, also frequently expressed in a desire to pose. Others shrink and are shy. One should then investigate to what situations or persons they are especially sensitive. The diffident person has a lack of curiosity with regard to others. Sensitiveness is a general term and refers to a variety of trends. It is therefore necessary to determine the type as well as the degree of sensitiveness. Caution is an asset but frequently develops into suspiciousness, which stands in contrast to the trusting individual with his unsuspecting and naïve attitude. Some people are liked by others because of an innate charm, in spite of undesirable personality features. Some are genuinely kind, while others have a malicious streak. This again may only show with regard to certain situations. Many easily acquire politeness in behavior; to others this may be a difficult task. The tendency to be lenient or strict may influence our social conduct. One has to study a person's attitude to authority. He may have a need for it, respect, or believe in it, or may be antagonistic and averse to it.

9. ASSETS, HANDICAPS, AND PERSONALITY SYNTHESIS

During the whole outline I have stressed the need for keeping the total personality in mind and for evaluating the personality features obtained in relation to each other and to the setting in the integrated whole. In the final synthesis one must try to harmonize the various strivings and tendencies and consider whether they may coexist in a personality or whether they disturb or exclude each other, and with what result. This reveals the degree of stability or lability, incongruity or uniformity, maturity or immaturity of the personality.

By keeping in mind that each personality feature may have two aspects, two reaction tendencies in diametrically opposite directions, a feature and a counterpart, one is helped in clarifying the strength of negative aspects and their influence on other strivings and on the whole personality.

Considering not only one aspect of the personality but the inter-relations of all the features, further possibilities arise and can be utilized. Only by exact comparison of the disparate aspects of the personality and by a sizing-up of qualities which have been found to be present, by considering the effects that would be produced by the absence of those qualities, one will be able to avoid mistakes.

From a practical and therapeutic point of view, the physician should know the handicaps which brought the patient to him, frequently expressed in the form of complaints, and also the assets with which he will be able to work. Every person has his handicaps and assets in the various aspects of his personality that are frequently recognized as difficulties, and one needs to know how the person was able to deal with them spontaneously. It is always important that one consider the underlying drive and the possible resistance, as well as the reaction to outside obstacles. One must determine what would be a satisfactory life for that person and then how it can be achieved. The analysis of failure shows to what extent the patient has not been able to use opportunities or to what extent failure was caused by insufficient capacities or ambition. The analysis of success is just as important and will reveal the positive aspect of these same features. One must know to what extent the patient leads a life which is healthy for his make-up and whether there is a balance of work and recreation according to his individual needs, sufficient time for rest, and ability to take care of the instinctive needs.

It is the physician's task to determine what assets are available and how they can be utilized and to what extent shortcomings are modifiable. It is frequently possible to develop the positive aspects of a personality trend and to change shortcomings into assets. One tries to make personality features which are liabilities ineffective by making the patient aware of them and teaching him to counter-balance them through the utilization of certain assets. It is also important that one determine whether the patient will be able to recognize the underlying difficulties and, if so, whether he will be able to do something about them, or whether one must be satisfied with only a partial adjustment. The physician must be careful not to promise himself, and certainly never a patient, a thorough adjustment, claiming that he will be able to get at the root of things and find the cause for the maladjustment. Correct prognosis and successful treatment depend greatly on our ability to size up a personality correctly.

DEVELOPMENT OF PERSONALITY

A person, from birth, is constantly reacting to, and shaped by, anatomic-physiologic and environmental factors. In reviewing the development of personality, it is understood that physical growth must be considered during any of the phases under discussion as well as living conditions, including economic, social, and cultural factors. Members of the family, persons in one's social group, in school, and at work play a varying role. Their possible significance should not be overlooked and can become clear only with an understanding of the dynamic factors which were important in the individual's life. The developing personality is most pliable and easily affected by persons in the environment. It is therefore of great but not exclusive importance to analyze infancy and childhood by whatever means possible. Identifications in early life form the essential structure in personality development. Repressed and remembered life experiences are not important as such, but how they affected the individual at the time of their occurrence and what their meaning is to the person at the time of the investigation are important.

The setting into which a child is born must be evaluated including the process of delivery and the state of the mother's health, the child's physical condition, whether the child was planned and wanted or rejected, or whether insecurity and friction existed in the family. The role that the child will play among the siblings is determined by difference in age and by the possible threat to the position of these older children in the family.

The infancy period (until about two years) is essentially a dependency period with fast motor and sensory development. Persons in the environment are fully in charge of nutrition, of urging motor activities, and of directing the development of toilet habits. It is obvious that any excessive suppression of the expression of the child's personality by those in the environment, as well as undue stress on body functions (food intake and elimination) and emotional factors which disturb the child's security must have an undesirable influence. Parental influences can be helpful or retarding. The undesirable results are disturbances in appetite, too early or retarded control of elimination, late walking and talking. Physical illness may lead to a regression to an earlier stage of behavior.

Childhood (3 to 12) brings in the problem of adjustment to a wider group with its competition and interferences. In education, the relationship of physical and psychologic growth should be of basic importance. Intellectual development follows an uneven progress. Socialization will be easiest in one's own age group, presenting difficulties if one is pushed into an older or a younger group. Changes of environment may present the need for difficult readjustments or prevent sound progress in the development of self-confidence. Ill health, inadequate nutrition, and poor housing affect children in many different ways and each situation must be studied individually.

Sexual development, in its broad as well as narrower sense, is important, as has now been proved through the study of healthy children in nursery schools and maladjusted children suffering from minor or marked psychopathologic reactions. In the first year oral factors play the major role, e.g., feeding, which therefore should become an opportunity to satisfy the need for love and develop a feeling of security. In the second and third years, bowel and bladder training become important. There is evidence to show that in some children forced excessive cleanliness and suppressed healthy aggression bear a relationship to the earliest beginning of phobias and compulsions. In this period, but more so in the period between 4 and 6, sexual curiosity and the need for information become apparent. In average children, a period of sexual latency, which lasts from 6 to puberty, follows.

In the early phase of childhood (3 to 6) physical illnesses, especially when they are prolonged or lead to crippling conditions, may affect the personality development. The still insecure child is aversely affected by obvious dissension of the parents, and their rejection or overprotection of him. The birth of a younger sibling may create an involved psychologic situation in which the youngest child suddenly becomes an older one. Jealousy and anxieties may be expressed in many behavioristic and physiologic symptoms. Well-known symptoms which deserve careful thought by the physician are temper tantrums, fears, fearful dreams, thumbsucking, nailbiting, lisping, stuttering, and enuresis. All these psychopathologic reactions should be evaluated carefully in order to understand their significance. They may also occur in the second period of childhood (6 to 12) when gastrointestinal disorders (vomiting, constipation, anorexia) are frequent. In this phase, difficulty in social adjustment and minor types of delinquency bring the child to the physician who should then study the degree to which standards have developed.

Adolescence is the period of emancipation with its complexities of sexual and social development. Interest in one's own body appearance and fitness becomes great and insecurities, expressed by overconcern to minor ailments or athletic compensation, are obvious. With the education of the public, menstruation is now considered an inconvenience by girls who are prepared for it and not as a disgusting or frightening experience. Masturbation, which is common especially in boys, may become an anxiety-producing situation. Transient homosexual factors may be disturbing until a full heterosexual orientation has been obtained. Anal-erotic, sadistic, and narcissistic tendencies of early childhood may be reactivated. The desire for affection is now combined with the possibility of offering love and physical satisfaction. The feeling of isolation in the earlier years of adolescence, sensitiveness with regard to the actions of others, egocentric imaginations with desires for success, and discouraging feelings of inadequacy lead to difficulties in group adjustment. Gradually the adolescent becomes part of the group, first of his own age group and then of society in general. Revolt to authority and rejection is seen in his attitude to his parents and others and may lead to delinquency. Around 14 to 16, a constructive attitude begins to solidify. Philosophic and religious concepts may become clarified, changing naïve beliefs to critical acceptance. The tendency to identify oneself with others diminishes and is replaced by increasing individualization. Thinking becomes more abstract and discriminative. These factors are utilized in education.

Maturity should be reached around 19 or 20. Various strivings are harmonized with self-reliance and self-control. There is a need to adjust contradictory strivings, leading to consistency and unity in experience and action. In forming judgments reality is taken into consideration, and the possible is distinguished from the impossible in one's hopes and daydreams.

In mature adult life, minor changes in the personality may take place, but the main tendency is for personality features to become more pronounced but not to change fundamentally. These changes are frequently related to adjustment of interests and strivings by the experiences of life, especially work, marriage, and social relations. (Sexual adjustment is discussed in Chapter XVII and reactions to childbirth and menopause in Chapter XIX.)

One should "consider the person in his relationship to the group, to his changing body, and to his mode of living in ever-changing times and environment. A person may become suddenly aware of aging by noticing changes in his body or in his environment. The death of contemporary friends, meetings with former friends after long intervals, or unexpected difficulties in securing positions force upon him the recognition of his own aging. Gradual changes in himself, obvious to persons in his environment but not to the individual, cause others to form attitudes and decisions which he notices and which worry or bewilder him.

"The important psychological changes include decreased learning ability, which precludes the ready shift to a different type of work or to a new mode of living. Decreased span of attention results in increased fatigability.

"With age, responsibilities increase and may greatly color one's outlook on life. Insecurity develops when confidence in one's body or in one's earning power or social desirability is shaken. This insecurity leads to a need for self-protection, a readiness to defend what one has achieved, caution, and frequently indecision. These reactions are recognized in many of our social attitudes, such as the seniority rule of many working groups. When we consider this psychological development, it is not surprising to find so often irritability, anger, anxiety, and resentment as emotions which interfere in social adjustment and have an undesirable physiological influence. Another expression of aging is the difference in emotional attitudes towards the past and future — a longing for the safety of the past and anxiety regarding the insecurity of the future. There may be a tendency to remember the lost opportunities of youth and the failure to do justice to what one has gained from an active life. The desire to obtain what has been missed may lead to ill-considered adventures. The attitude toward death gradually becomes a philosophical one. Death becomes accepted but anxiety arises in connection with the responsibilities involved. Loneliness may become an important factor in the life of the unmarried person and in that of many mothers whose children have grown out of the home. A narrowing of interests and a tendency to more aversions and to intolerance make a social reorientation difficult. The need for increased recreation may often not be recognized by the active man and woman whose lives are filled with duties and responsibilities."*

Extensive experience, persistence in pursuing goals and a need to keep working "balance the decreasing ability for learning, attention, and imagination. Self-reliance and self-control cause him to be careful and exacting, so that he makes fewer mistakes due to haste and impulsiveness. Greater emotional stability not only produces better work, but may permit a better social adjustment of previously unstable and even psychopathic personalities. Stability of action is also improved by the tendency to take fewer risks and chances. The decline of sexual restlessness may be welcomed by many, especially if married life has been terminated or if the partner has aged sexually. In a wholesome society the conservatism of aging should be blended with the desire for change characteristic of youth. A tendency to turn from the outer to one's inner world results in contemplation, deeper religious appreciation, and philosophical thinking. Although the capacity for enthusiasm seems to decrease, a higher sense of duty and obligation results in stronger social consciousness, permitting participation in the activities of the community. The realities of life are more highly appreciated and necessary adjustments are correspondingly evaluated."*

CONSIDERATIONS IN MENTAL HYGIENE

This discussion is based on the general knowledge of problems of personality in daily life, as gained from personal experience and

* Diethelm, O.: The Aging Person. Psychological and Psychopathological Aspects of Aging. *North Carolina Medical Journal*, 5, 1944.

from literature. In addition, during ten years of teaching the first year class at Cornell University Medical College, the previously mentioned personality outline was used as a basis for obtaining a dynamic understanding of human behavior. From the written reports of 876 students and about 350 interviews, the most frequently recurring difficulties were singled out. The average age of the students was 21 and they came from all parts of the country but with a vast preponderance from the Eastern states and from urban living conditions. The greatest difficulty in writing the personality study was found with regard to recognition and understanding of emotions (about 40 per cent), next, the attitude to sexual desires (about 15 per cent), to standards (12 per cent), and to ability to deal with oneself (10 per cent). The conclusion seems warranted that in the younger generation of our culture the discussion of a person's sexual life does not present the difficulties which one might assume from literature. On the other hand, in the field of emotions, which medicine has recognized as being of great importance in physical illnesses and in physiologic influences, one is confronted with unexpected obstacles of recognition and subjective description.

One frequent complaint in students of varying ages and in adult life is difficulty in concentration which may be related to a lack of interest, to emotional interferences, to finding the problem too difficult to learn, and to fatigue. Learning may suffer because of inability to single out the essential, and anxious overemphasis on knowledge. In hazy thinkers, neglect in considering the situation as a whole and lack of systematization need correction.

Emotional reactions may be hidden and subjectively and objectively difficult to recognize. For example, anxiety may be expressed in fretfulness or aggressiveness, depressed feelings, tension, irritability, fatigue, somatic symptoms, and muscle pains. Frequent help is asked for moodiness in which it is difficult to recognize the role of unimportant situations, including fatigue. It is helpful to advise modification in the routine of living which will permit persons to disregard the unhappy mood by stressing suitable interests, reading matter, social contacts, and recreation. It is often difficult to recognize delayed emotional reactions, especially anxiety and resentment, and therefore the relationship to precipitating emotions. Some undesirable reactions on week-ends are often related to delayed reactions or to an inability to disregard one's worries on days of relative inactivity. Undesirable persistence in pursuing goals is frequently related to the person's unwillingness to accept the inevitable, or to a need to dwell on painful experiences because of underlying guilt. In worrying, the need to dramatize situations may deserve correction. In anxious anticipation, which usually becomes a set tendency, the analysis of the cause, followed by a persistent attempt at control of these undesirable thoughts, may gradually lead to a modification.

Resentment is a complex reaction in which a thoughtful analysis can be helpful. As a rule, to limit the analysis to a few resentful reactions will be desirable. Otherwise, resentment will be kept alive. To tell a person that he is resentful will increase the emotion. The need for tolerance and willingness to forget must be understood. Resentment includes the dynamic factor of projection, which may lead to suspiciousness and, in pathologic exaggerations, to paranoid features. A desire for retaliation may be used as an excuse for satisfying otherwise unacceptable desires and be followed by guilt and resentment to oneself. Resentment implies an underlying feeling of being resented or rejected by others, adding the factor of unhappiness which may overshadow the emotion of resentment.

In all emotions, it is important to establish their specific type, their intensity, and their duration. Then only will a person be able to use his emotional reactions to full advantage, i.e., to consider them indicative of underlying personality reactions which deserve immediate attention. The role of emotions on physiologic functions must be evaluated if one wishes to maintain good health. Suppression of certain emotions is essential for desirable interpersonal relations. On the other hand, suppression, and at the same time keeping the emotions alive by dwelling on them, is unhealthy. Studies of childhood have shown the importance of combining the privilege of displaying emotions with a persistent and patient education of control and suppression.

It is essential that one learn to live in the present with due attention to the future and without undue dwelling on the past. One must be able to throw off disappointments and unhappy experiences and to develop standards which prevent unforgiving attitudes to oneself and persistent guilt and self-blame. Discouragement to failure should be analyzed in the light of the factors which led to non-success, and constructive reassurance can be found in factors which have at other times, or along other lines, given success.

Difficulty in displaying emotion, which may be as great a handicap socially as too-ready display, may be due to an inability or unwillingness to show it. This inability and unwillingness may be related to an excessive egocentric orientation, to fear of revealing oneself, to uneasiness, or even to distrust in group relations. The ability to feel with others without suffering with them is an essential factor in a healthy patient-physician relationship. Insufficient sympathy is found in persons who are too self-centered and incapable of sharing interests with others, and who often suffer from their inability to respond readily with emotion. One's type of humor reveals many of the emotional reactions to oneself and to others and may demand a considerable analysis before a desirable change occurs.

One's ability to transform into action present interests and strivings is closely linked to emotions and standards. The problem of procrastination offers an example of the inhibiting influence of anxiety because one's high goals present too great a barrier. Procrastination may also be caused by the unwillingness to expose oneself to criticism of others. Aversion to a task, or lack of interest in it, distraction by intensive curiosity or by many other interests, or lack of drive related to emotional or physical factors may be important. In laziness this lack of initiative deserves careful scrutiny. Hastiness, which is the expression of anxiety, may be considered by the person as a sign of quickness in decision, and impulsiveness as an indication of healthy spontaneity. Such self-deception should be brought to the individual's attention. Stubbornness is not an expression of strength, but of weakness, a lack of security in giving up or modifying one's position. "Will power" represents the ability to persist in pursuing a goal and depends on the emotional setting, social influences, the clarity of the goals, and their value to the individual.

One's sense of duty to oneself, to one's family, and to society frequently deserves investigation in order to permit a person to take care of his own needs and those of others. The formation of ideals, their stability and lability, depends on early identification with important persons in one's life. It is essential that one prevent or change a rigidity of ideals, and have a sound tolerance. Racial, religious, and social prejudices are frequently not related to one's standards but to insecurities, and express defense reactions. They reveal self-deceptions and excuses to oneself.

It is obvious that a physician must concern himself with the person's attitude to his body. Overconcern, often hidden behind athletic activities and satisfaction in high achievement, may refer to one's appearance or to various bodily functions. The development of faulty standards and insecurities may have started in infancy and relate to the influence of various persons in one's early life. Anxiety in connection with illnesses, or in physiologic expression of anxiety to one's problems, may cause a general body overconcern. Damage to body surface, e.g., scars, or the development of malformations, may be unbearable to narcissistic individuals.

The average person knows little about his need for sleep. He should know whether early retiring or sleeping late will give him the greatest benefit. Incomprehensible differences in sleep patterns of marital partners may lead to unreasonable social and living demands on each other. Fatigue is combatted by various means, depending on whether it be due to exertion which is helped by increased rest, or to emotional factors. For the latter, modification of the situations involved and physical exercise are indicated. Weekends and vacations should be opportunities for recuperation.

Normal and pathologic sexual functions and their means of satisfaction are discussed in Chapter XVII. The questions which are commonly asked of a physician by persons of varying ages and cultural background refer to general sexual information or more specifically to disturbing sexual dreams, ejaculation, the frequency of intercourse, masturbation, and varying degrees of homosexual desires or activities.

Cravings for alcohol and tobacco, as well as for coffee and food, demand a willingness on the physician's part to study the problem objectively and be fully aware of his own bias. In Chapters II and XVIII these cravings are discussed. Increased or decreased food intake is usually related to disturbing emotions when a physical explanation cannot be found. Anxiety, tension, and resentment, and to a far less degree depressive moods, affect the desire for food.

Such observations are frequent in infancy, childhood, and adolescence. Less marked fluctuations in appetite, and therefore frequently overlooked by the individual, occur in adults.

Material security depends on a person's needs and his attitudes. Undue anxiety to debt, to old age, and to assuming new responsibilities with marriage or children necessitates a study of the whole personality if one wishes to understand these involved reactions and offer correct help. Desire for wealth may have its source in the desire for luxury, for power, or social standing and must be studied accordingly.

A certain amount of interest in oneself and willingness to face oneself is desirable. However, a persistent tendency to self-analysis is usually destructive. Most people take health and success for granted and turn to analysis only when confronted with ill health and lack of success. The analysis of situations and factors which permit good health and success offers constructive aspects. Destructive self-analysis undermines self-confidence and leads to increasing self-centeredness. Its correction cannot be achieved in a short time and demands persistent willingness for re-education. Self-reliance cannot be recognized readily from the behavior of persons because aggressiveness, arrogance, stubbornness, or excessive emotional control may hide insecurities and their emotional accompaniments. Apparently even self-reliant people may fail when their personal security is destroyed whether this be the loss of wealth or of health, of husband, parents, or children. A seeming lack of self-reliance is often seen in women and children who grow up in a protected environment and appear submissive and dependent on others. They are able to rise to opportunities and needs, if confronted by special interests, by an appeal to their sense of duty, or by financial struggles. The ability to assume and to carry responsibility varies greatly. In some who enjoy it, it leads to overburdening. Others who feel inadequate shirk responsibility. Feelings of inadequacy may be justified by actual intellectual, emotional, or experiential deficit. More frequently these feelings are related to undue conscientiousness or anticipation of possible involvements, or an unwillingness to feel bound, e.g., marriage, children, or job obligations. In these individuals the concept of freedom and the ability for self-denial must be studied.

Social needs and adjustment to the group vary considerably without ever justifying the evaluation of being pathologic. In lonely persons who have a need to belong to a group, the general emotional setting and insufficient self-confidence which prevent healthy spontaneity and sharing with others must be considered. Being too concerned about the impression one makes on others, for whatever dynamic factors, leads to anxiety and interferes with one's spontaneous expressions. Insufficient emancipation and rigid standards lead to exaggerated devotions and loyalties, interfering with one's healthy need of self-preservation.

The problems which are expressed in lability and immaturity of the personality belong essentially in the field of pathology (especially psychoneurosis and psychopathic personality). However, there is too great a readiness to make such diagnoses and to dismiss the patient as an undesirable therapeutic problem or advise intensive psychotherapy. A sufficient study of the factors involved might show possibilities for modification of personality features and life situations.

BIBLIOGRAPHY

1. LOEB, L.: *The Biological Basis of Individuality.* Charles C Thomas • Publisher, Springfield, 1945.
2. CARMICHAEL, L.: (ed.) *Manual of Child Psychology.* John Wiley and Sons, New York, 1946.
3. ENGLISH, O. S., and PEARSON, G. H.: *Emotional Problems of Living.* W. W. Norton and Company, New York, 1945. (A psychoanalytic formulation of the development of personality.)
4. FRY, C. C., and ROSTOW, E. G.: *Mental Health in College.* The Commonwealth Fund, New York, 1942.
5. PLANT, J. S.: *Personality and the Cultural Pattern.* The Commonwealth Fund, New York, 1937.
6. COWDRY, E. V. (ed.): *Problems of Aging; Biological and Medical Aspects.* The Williams & Wilkins Company, Baltimore, 1939.
7. DIETHELM, O.: The Aging Person. Psychological and Psychopathological Aspects of Aging. *North Carolina Medical Journal,* 5, 1944.

Chapter II

TREATMENT IN GENERAL

PSYCHIATRIC treatment starts with the first examination. Mistakes made during the examination, such as provocative questions, can aggravate a patient's condition, make treatment impossible by the physician who makes them, or increase the difficulties for another physician. It is impossible to see a patient merely for diagnostic purposes. The patient wants, and has the right to expect, an answer to the problems which he should discuss with the physician.

Most patients will be referred to the psychiatrist by other physicians, but every practitioner should know how to deal with emergency cases. This is of the same importance as first aid treatment in physical illnesses. Every practitioner must be able to treat the large number of psychiatric disorders which he meets in his practice and which he should not or cannot refer to a psychiatric specialist.

It is wise in all circumstances to obtain the complaints as fully as possible from the patient and the relatives or friends accompanying him. These complaints are the problems for which help is requested. At the end of the examination, i.e., after the facts have been established, the physician will be in a position to formulate the problem more inclusively and, distinguishing the important factors from the mere incidental, propose the treatment. The physicians who seek the psychiatrist's advice should always formulate the problems clearly with their own observations and findings, as well as the possibilities for treatment which they have mentioned to the patient and relatives.

The indications for the therapeutic approach depend on a clinical diagnosis which includes the recognition of the illness, the personality setting, and life situations. If this is impossible to determine at the first consultation, one should not hesitate to point out to the patient the need for further discussion or observation. Basing his advice on his examination, the physician must decide whether he is sufficiently qualified to treat the patient, whether the patient can be treated while continuing his work or whether he can be treated at home while staying away from work, or whether he should be sent to a hospital and to what kind. The prognostic evaluation permits the physician to outline the expense which will be involved. It allows the patient and the relatives to take care of necessary changes in their occupational and business relations and in family and social arrangements. Whatever is proposed must be formulated clearly and patiently in words suitable to the persons who seek our advice and not in technical terms which are confusing or may have a meaning for the patient which we did not intend to imply.

A psychiatric discussion is a novel and frequently perplexing experience for the patient and for relatives. A person's reserve and distrust of others frequently makes confiding difficult. We physicians must always realize that it is essential first to establish in the patient a confidence that will enable him to trust us and to mention life experiences and desires which he has heretofore considered very private and has not mentioned even to his intimates. We expect him to discuss them freely with us who are strangers, trusting our code of medical ethics. This makes it necessary, therefore, that a psychiatrist discuss his cases with no one. Many factors cannot be mentioned by him in his report to the family physician, but this need not prevent a scientific formulation, which should be in terms of actual facts instead of mere diagnostic terms. It is always wise to ask the patient how much he wishes us to mention in our report and what he wishes to have kept entirely confidential. Few difficulties will arise if this is carried out with tact. Many times we are able to make the patient see the need for discussing certain problems later on with his family physician so that further guidance is possible. The same considerations are even more important in the formulation to relatives. In difficult situations where the danger of misrepresentation of the facts by relatives or patient exists, a three-cornered discussion is helpful. The physician presents his formulation to both patient and relatives together, clears up misunderstanding, and establishes cooperation for treatment and adjustment.

The formulation to the nurse contains only the facts which are necessary for her to understand the patient. More important for her than diagnostic terms is an understanding of the patient's personality, his likes and dislikes, his idiosyncrasies, his interests, and the essential psychopathologic facts. She should be equipped to take care of any situation which may occur during the twenty-four hours and to help the patient to lead a properly adjusted life. It is natural that a patient will get attached to his nurse and may confide in her certain problems which he has withheld from the physician. The nurse must discuss these with the treating physician, and every patient should be made aware of this necessity and understand it. The nurse can act only as a helper and should not attempt to treat the patient independently. It is impossible to carry out a parallel treatment by nurse and physician, although this may often seem desirable to the inexperienced person. The same attitude applies to relatives and friends. All information and observation should be pooled, and used by the physician in his treatment. This attitude is essentially the same as that in the other fields of medicine. It is stressed here especially because the patient, nurses, and relatives frequently feel that the human problems with which the psychiatrist has to deal are intelligible to themselves and adjustable by them. This is only apparently correct. The physician is the only one in the position to recognize the significance of these problems and to treat them according to the need at the time of the illness and according to his whole plan of treatment. This, on the other hand, does not mean an undue curtailment of the treatment by the nurse. One must also realize that a nurse will get tired and that 24-hour duty is therefore undesirable in most cases. It is desirable for the physician to stimulate the nurse's interest and show her the help which she is able to offer and the changes which have occurred in the patient's illness. This is especially important in protracted and chronic illnesses. In order to prevent the feeling of monotony and undesirable allegiance between nurse and patient, a change of nurses is often wise.

In formulating his treatment a psychiatrist must distinguish between what is important and what is incidental. This does not mean that incidental features can be neglected. The patient needs to understand why little attention is paid to symptoms which disturb him. It is frequently necessary to attend to especially annoying complaints or to symptoms which interfere greatly with the therapeutic adjustment at the time. The claim that we should not carry out any symptomatic treatment and only pay attention to what seems fundamental is an extreme point of view which presents an important, but not an exclusive, therapeutic principle. It is our therapeutic task to modify whatever is possible or to enable the patient to endure what cannot be changed.

One should always consider first what is physically accessible, but again with a distinction of what is important and what is incidental. Only a few problems can be attacked fundamentally at a purely physical level. Not all personality functions and dysfunctions have a physiologic or an anatomic basis. Chemical and endocrinologic treatment play the same role as in internal medicine and a discussion of them is therefore omitted; but one must always be clear about their significance and their influence on the whole personality setting. Otherwise, physician and patient will become distracted and neglect a direct approach to the personality. Evaluating the striking results which are occasionally obtained by physical approach, e.g., surgical intervention, it is necessary that one consider the indirect factors which brought the change about, especially suggestive and socializing influences.

The physician should first formulate the problem, singling out the factors involved and determining whether they are modifiable, considering the whole setting of the personality. It is essential that he obtain as clear a time allocation as possible, realizing, however, that this is only possible to a limited extent and that re-formulation will constantly be necessary with increasing understanding of the personality and its development. Illustrations from his history, pointing out the coincidence of certain life situations and personality reactions, enable the patient to see possible interrelations and allow an analysis of certain striking reactions, even in the first consultation. The physician does not try to solve the problems, but tries to show possibilities for investigation and explanation. He therefore puts his formulation best in the form of a question and leaves the solution open if necessary. Every diagnostic examination must end with such a therapeutic discussion. The physician therefore needs to be in command of all the facts. In a diagnostic center, the psychiatrist should be called in after all the physical investigations have been completed.

I personally feel the need for taking notes during my discussions. This prevents my overlooking interrelations and puts the facts

clearly before me for the final therapeutic discussion. It allows me
to make use of the patient's own words. I adhere to the same rule
during treatment. Problems which cannot be settled completely at
the time of discussion will not disappear unsolved. A work sheet
which offers a record of what has been obtained and what investigations have to be postponed can be kept. This forms the basis for
planned treatment. By formulating this to the patient, I have always
been able to obtain his consent to my taking notes. In consultation
practice a patient is willing to recognize that future consultations
may become necessary during his lifetime and that a record taken
now will then prove to be of great assistance to him. In suspicious
patients I have promised that I shall be willing to destroy a record
of certain intimate details if the patient so wishes it at the end of
treatment. Thus far none of my patients has ever requested this.
I prefer to take my notes openly and not to dictate afterwards. This
procedure puts everything above board and allows me to refer to
my notes and prevents falsifications which will always occur when
one depends entirely on one's memory.

A brief example may illustrate the need for combining diagnostic discussion with therapeutic synthesis:

Case 1:

A 31 year old woman was referred to the Johns Hopkins Diagnostic
Clinic because of manifold physical complaints. All the examinations
were practically negative. In the psychiatric consultation the following
understanding of the case was reached:

Shortly after the patient had started to work as a stenographer at 21
she developed a constant soreness on the top of her head and chronic
constipation. In the last two years these symptoms had increased and
the pain in her head was especially marked when she felt tired in the
evening and after excitement. In the past six months the patient had
suffered from several anxiety attacks, usually occurring at night and on
the two days before menstruation. Her sleep had become disturbed
through marked anxiety dreams. The patient was an excitable, quick-
tempered, moody person who enjoyed social activities and athletics but
curtailed them considerably during the winter. When having sufficient
outlets she always felt better. A year after her marriage, i.e., eight years
ago, the patient's parents moved into her home. She reacted with
marked resentment because of the increased financial burden, which
forced her to keep on working, and because her sick parents demanded
much attention. Both parents died two years ago. The patient now felt

that she had not been kind enough to them. Because of severe financial losses she had to keep on working instead of taking care of her household and enjoying life. Her husband, who was not very sociable, was less than ever in a mood to go out with her. Their sexual life had never been well regulated. The patient was passionate and had not been able to adjust to a less passionate husband and especially to his dimininished sexual desires during the last year of business worries. She indulged frequently in sexual fancies (dealing with her husband). Withdrawal, which had been practiced during their whole married life, disturbed her pleasure greatly, frequently preventing an orgasm or sufficient relaxation.

The patient was able to see the correlation of life situations and bodily symptoms. She remembered how her work during the first few years had been a strain because of her great conscientiousness, exactness, and a constant tendency to anticipate difficulties. All these personality traits had made it impossible for her to enjoy married life and housework and to adjust to increasing disappointments.

The need for guarding against these traits and for developing compensatory outlets was discussed. Her church activities offered opportunities for social outlets and for reviving her interest in music. Work as a secretary proved unnecessary when the patient accepted the advice to live on a carefully planned budget. She was able to do her housework, which she enjoyed, and to find time for physical recreation in the form of long walks, skating in winter time, and swimming in summer time. She gained an understanding of the fundamental rules of sex hygiene; i.e., willingness to adjust her desires to her partner's with due attention to situational factors, control of her sexual imaginations, and physical exercise. Birth control by means of a pessary and preventive jelly was urged instead of coitus interruptus.

The family physician explained to the husband, whom I did not see, the social needs of the patient and discussed their sexual life with him thoroughly. I have heard since that the patient is doing well in a life which has been readjusted according to the discussed plans. She has few complaints and seems to take their recurrence more as an indication that there might be disturbing personality problems than as an expression of actual physical illness.

These hypochondriacal reactions form a large group of psychiatric diagnostic practice. By a formulation in terms of the life situation and personality factors, many patients will be benefited greatly and find possibilities for some kind of adjustment.

There is no essential difference in the approach to the problems of the various types and degrees of personality disorders. In certain psychopathologic disorders one may not be able to outline the treatment as fully as in others, but a satisfactory factual formulation is always possible and will help us to gain the cooperation of the patient and family. It is important that we explain routine treatment in detail and clear up misunderstandings and apprehensions. The succeeding steps of treatment, changes, and modifications must be re-formulated from time to time. During this period the physician should consider the patient's ability to grasp his formulation and be guided by possible intellectual deficits, depressive or delirious thinking difficulties, or scattering. We should choose brief sentences and words which are familiar to the patient.

Psychiatric treatment consists of analysis of a patient's reactions and of the dynamic factors involved, physical and psychobiologic, and of an attempt at adjustment in accordance with the individual's needs and possibilities, with due attention to family and group relationships. It cannot be pure analysis. The physician should offer his own formulation, which is more inclusive than the patient's, and explanations which take care of the patient's needs and allow further investigations. He cannot merely pay attention to what seems fundamental in the light of our present scientific understanding. Minor situations and reactions deserve full attention. In every illness we can distinguish phases with special problems and needs. In some illnesses characteristic phases occur daily and should be utilized therapeutically. In his therapeutic procedure the physician should therefore evaluate a reaction in its setting in some special phase of the illness as well as in the setting of the illness as a whole, i.e., the personality and its whole development, with attention to past and future, reality and imaginations, desires and hopes.

In the first and every subsequent contact with the patient we should consider that he comes with definite complaints, his specific attitude and expectations, and a limitation of understanding. It is the physician's task to take care of all these factors. In obtaining the history from the patient and in the direct examination we want to get an understanding of the development of the illness and of the causes, of the modifiability of difficulties, and of the available resources. This includes obtaining an idea of the extent to which the patient can take a helpful point of view and where he falls short. One should, however, be cautious when one is trying to elicit facts which allow one to obtain an understanding of the dynamic factors and be willing to postpone this if it might lead the patient to go beyond the material which he can face safely. One should not put the patient in a position in which he is forced to admit certain facts or may feel it necessary to deny facts against his better knowledge. This would produce conflicts of conscience and guilt or resentment which would impede the progress of treatment or even make the patient worse.

The physician is at great advantage if he knows a great deal about the dynamic factors and problems involved. He can utilize this knowledge in planning his treatment. On the other hand, he must be able to take care of the patient and carry out an active and constructive treatment even if his understanding of the case is limited and must remain so for the time being, or possibly forever. The satisfying of scientific curiosity must give way to therapeutic needs. There is the danger of trying to obtain perfect results as far as an understanding of the case and so-called normal behavior goes. The patient's knowledge is not a measure of therapeutic success. One frequently will find that it may be more helpful for the patient if he is not made aware of certain factors and possibilities.

Every physician should be clearly aware of what he is doing for his patient. A brief formulation of certain procedures which are in common use is therefore necessary. "Reassurance" is used a great deal. By this one means re-establishing confidence, comfort, and ease in the patient. It should be achieved by presenting facts and not by mere words. The patient's own statements about progress should be utilized. It will usually be necessary to re-formulate them so that the facts mentioned appear in their proper significance and in their correlation to the total situation and not as isolated facts. The tone of the physician's voice inspires the most confidence if it is offered in equanimity and quiet assurance. Sometimes one may wish to be more emphatic; according to the patient and the situation, one may prefer to be brief or go more into detail. Mere repetition ought to be avoided. Re-formulation is necessary if a patient is unable to understand or receive the desired comfort from a statement of facts. Using the patient's statement, one should not omit parts of it but explain why and how the emphasis needs to be shifted. Presenting his own observations and those of persons in the environment, the physician wishes to draw the patient's attention to them. This procedure will lead to a broader attitude to the illness and restore or increase in the patient the need to take into consideration the opinion of others, especially that of the physician. Arguments ought to be avoided. Confidence based on acceptance of the illness as a medical problem in the handling of which the physician is competent is a great help in producing reassurance and offers possibilities for suggestive therapy. Every patient will derive considerable satisfaction from the discussions in addition to the therapeutic value which he gets out of them. The knowledge that the physician approves of his discussions and actions establishes more ease and confidence.

Suggestive influences always enter. The therapeutic situation in itself, the physician's personality, nurses, and environment exert their influence. Direct and indirect suggestive factors with their helpful and interfering possibilities have to be considered carefully. The therapeutic use of suggestion is discussed in detail in Chapter III.

Re-education is an important therapeutic measure. It is a medical procedure which influences the patient's habits of thinking, acting, and emotional control (for detailed discussion see Chapter X). It includes the establishing of a healthy life routine with a balance of work and recreation (see p. 43). It is our goal to achieve re-education primarily through the patient's increasing understanding of himself, but this alone is frequently insufficient and constructive suggestions must be offered. This leads to self-restraint and self-reliance, with adjustment to life situations and the necessity for fitting into the group.

Psychiatric treatment should not make use of discipline with its strict rules and demands for obedience. It does not request submission. Treatment depends upon cooperation and although it is necessary to utilize rules of conduct, they must be plastic and adjustable to the individual needs of the patient. Rules upon which one has decided and to which the patient has agreed are adhered to on the basis of a mutual understanding of their necessity. Difficulties in adhering to them should be analyzed with the patient and formulated in such a way that the patient can comprehend their origin. If one can see the necessity, one must be willing to draw conclusions and adjust the rules. Submission should not be gained and threats should be altogether avoided. One does not wish to foster submissive tendencies because the goal is self-reliance with a willingness and need to use self-restraint. This does not lead to abolition of the individual's strivings and efforts, but to moderation, regulation, and adaptation.

Thus far, therapeutic considerations which may apply to any patient have been presented. The remainder of the chapter refers largely to psychiatric patients and includes treatment in psychiatric hospitals.

Only a careful study of the patient's personality allows a plastic and carefully adjustable routine. Re-education and the formation of better habits cannot be separated from routine. There are many cases in which, because of his illness or ingrained features of his personality, the patient's cooperation is not possible. For this situation the law gives us a means in the legal commitment, whereby the physician is privileged to detain and treat a patient. This should not be used in a high-handed manner. The same therapeutic rules apply to a committed patient as to a voluntary patient — the treatment is still based on cooperation. It is always possible to establish cooperation along certain lines, although it may be a tedious and slow procedure. Rules and handling based on the use of force are successful in some cases and bring about cooperation. Nevertheless, force is not desirable because it is a haphazard and therefore unscientific treatment.

Commitment should be simplified as much as possible and should take into consideration the patient's and the relatives' sensitiveness. The fear of abusing this infringement on an individual's freedom has led frequently to deplorable commitment laws, such as public court procedure to determine insanity. In any well-governed state, it should be possible to depend on the physician's judgment and integrity. It should be sufficient to have one or two licensed physicians state that their careful examination and the facts obtained necessitate the patient's hospitalization against his will. Judicious and strict supervision of hospitals which are privileged to accept and detain such patients must be carried out by a state health department. After the admission of a patient to such a hospital the legal responsibility lies with the superintendent. The fear of legal dangers in making out commitment papers, which prevents many physicians from resorting to this necessary means of treatment, is not justified if the physician knows psychiatry and the indications which necessitate commitment (see page 45). It is the duty of every practitioner to inform himself about the commitment procedure in his state and the available private and state psychiatric institutions. Medical societies should be interested in the development of modern commitment laws and should see that the hospitals in their state offer modern psychiatric treatment. Psychotherapeutic effort should always be made to have a patient enter a psychiatric hospital voluntarily. If, later, need for commitment should arise, thorough consideration should be given to the desirability of transfer to another hospital where the patient will be kept under commitment.

Non-restraint and cooperation are of fundamental importance in psychiatric treatment. But here again we must be willing to accept certain limitations. Cooperation may not be possible at certain periods. Nevertheless, it is the ultimate goal. If it cannot be obtained wholeheartedly and in every respect, it should always be possible to some extent and at least with regard to the most important problems. Restraint cannot always be omitted. We cannot permit a patient, for instance, to mutilate himself or to give in to a persistent suicidal need. However, such cases, in which temporary restraint is necessary, are not frequent. Physical restraint because of danger to others can be omitted in a well-managed hospital. (The possibilities and needs for restraint are discussed in Chapter VIII.) It would help a great deal to put patients and relatives at ease if each hospital were required to keep a record of all restraint used and to publish it in the yearly report.

Punishment and reward should not play a role in treatment. It is natural that the patient will take the curtailment of privileges as a punishment. The physician's formulation should enable the patient to see that this is an erroneous interpretation and that the advised modifications are therapeutic aids and necessities. Although in certain cases these may constitute a form of punishment which the patient applies to himself, I would hesitate to offer such an explanation and avoid bringing in the concept of guilt except when the facts obviously present such a dynamic factor themselves. Reward must be reviewed from the same point of view. It is interesting to note that physicians who believe in punishment and reward argue also for the need of discipline and stress re-education to the neglect of a dynamic-analytic approach. The individual will then suffer. These tendencies are therefore mostly found in physicians who want to, or have to, take care of a great number of patients. This is an explanation but not an excuse. Even if a few physicians must take care of a vast hospital population, individualized treatment in a modified form is still possible. Various large hospitals are carrying out such treatment successfully.

Paying attention to the needs of the various phases as well as of the illness as a whole, makes it possible to offer well-planned and individual reassurance which is not mere promise, but is based on, and supported by, facts. In the reassurance the patient is afforded the benefit of medical knowledge and experience. It is best to avoid concrete examples in which personal features of other patients are given. Reassurance should leave open possibilities of unexpected changes and one should only take care of the patient's doubts if it can be done honestly. Both physician and patient should keep the ultimate goal of treatment in mind, but what constitutes the physician's final goal cannot always be presented fully to the patient.

Every physician must heed the patient's religious attitude and needs. However, this will always remain a side issue in the treatment. A physician does not have the right to attempt to change a patient's religious and philosophic conceptions and his political attitude. The physician's own convictions cannot enter into the treatment, and he will always have cause for regret at one time or another if he tries to make use of his own personal tendencies.

The rules for routine are the same during periods of illness and health. The four fundamental factors which should be balanced according to the individual and his present needs are work and recreation, rest and physical requirements. Such occupational therapy is important in the treatment of every illness (for detailed discussion see Chapter X). Everyone should know how these factors are best balanced in his daily life and this should be discussed at the end of any consultation. Work includes healthy mental and physical occupation. For an understanding of the individual's capacity and needs, one has to investigate his whole personality. Recreation embraces not only sports and hobbies but also intellectual and aesthetic enjoyment. Religious activities should find their place.

The need for sleep and rest varies individually. Eating is not merely a physiologic function. Many patients eat in a hurry and irregularly and forget the need for pleasant eating accommodations. It is always more desirable to eat in congenial company than by oneself. During an illness these factors must be modified according to the type and phase with which we deal.

Treatment consists primarily of a co-ordination of facts and participants. The patient is inclined to take his own problems as too important and to use them as a casual explanation for all his life difficulties. The physician must try to reconstruct the difficulty presented by the patient, its origin, and bring in wholesome corrective associations. His formulation is couched in the sort of language used by the patient and the family. He must always be in a position to have all the facts available. In the information the physician offers to nurses it is necessary to stress the patient's needs and personality resources, the activities, actual and potential, that might be carried out in daily life, with due attention to the problems of socialization. His instructions allow the nurse to realize what is important to discuss with the patient and to what he is sensitive. He utilizes the healthy factors of forgetting and losing oneself in group activity. He must take care of the patient's inclination to accept his illness as blameworthy and affecting his self-respect. Every interview should leave the patient with something constructive which should include a vision of what we wish to attain, a correct attitude, and an understanding of the entire procedure which the patient can grasp at that time. The physician should be prepared to end conversations into which he is drawn unexpectedly with a constructive statement which will take care of the situation until the next interview.

The physician should formulate his decision for further consultations or hospital treatment at the end of the first consultation. Ambulatory treatment without disturbing the patient's occupation and duties is most desirable. Often it is necessary to modify the daily routine considerably. Advice for vacation or travel is only justified in the period of convalescence. Distraction through amusements must be guided by the principle of recreation. Treatment by consultation can be adequate in any reaction type, although it will be predominantly used in psychoneuroses and minor personality disturbances. The need for suitable hospitalization arises out of the need to protect the patient or other people or because the facilities of a hospital will offer the best therapeutic possibilities.

The patient may be dangerous to himself because of suicidal urges, the neglect of vital physical needs, financial extravagance, ethical involvements, and the inclination to expose himself to various kinds of risks. He may be a menace to others because he might inflict physical or material harm, but it is also necessary to consider hospitalization when the patient is an undue strain on his environment. The neutral hospital environment removes friction and other obstacles to improvement. Some patients endanger society in general because of their lack of co-operation in the treatment of any infectious diseases from which they may be suffering. Hospitalization is frequently required in order to allow supervision and the limitation of such freedom as the patient is not in a condition to utilize. The use of commitment becomes indispensable in such cases. It is the physician's task to protect the patient from suicide during his illness. A psychiatric hospital therefore needs secured windows and locked doors. The latter restriction is practically absent for patients who do not need it, through the privilege of more or less limited parole. Some hospitals have special wards without guarded windows and doors, while in others all wards are alike in this respect. In the management of a hospital, the psychologic influence of all these precautions upon the patients has to be considered.

The problems of special privileges and parole must be considered carefully, as these are valuable aids in treatment. The utilization of privileges and parole permits patient and physician to recognize to what extent the former can be exposed to life outside of the hospital when discharge and ambulatory treatment become advisable.

Hospitalization is also desirable to create possibilities for socialization and re-education. The routine is designed to accomplish this and helps the patient to recognize that his illness may be an explanation of, but not an excuse for, behavior difficulties, and that even while sick it is necessary for him to use self-control.

The physician's formulation to the patient of the reasons for his hospitalization will help to overcome prejudice against admission to psychiatric hospitals. Correct treatment in a general hospital is usually not possible, or only possible with a modification of therapy within the limits set by the inevitable handicaps. Nursing homes are at best only a substitute. It is our task to overcome prejudice against closed institutions, especially against state hospitals, by thorough education of the public and by meeting the community's need for well-equipped public hospitals. No patient should be advised to enter a private hospital if this means a considerable financial hardship. Patient and relatives must be made to realize that a therapeutic difficulty arises if the patient in consequence has to return to a serious financial situation. The money should rather be saved for the important period of convalescence.

Hospital treatment can be guided by one of two principles: Either a physician is in charge of a ward and all its patients, losing the patients when they are transferred to another ward; or else a new patient is assigned to one of the physicians who will take care of the patient during the whole hospital stay, regardless of ward allocation. It seems to me that this distinction involves fundamental principles of treatment. In the first type of approach, the principle of the adjustment of the individual to the group is of primary importance and the personal influence of the physician secondary, whereas in the other approach the personal influence of the physician is considered to be of primary importance.

When the treatment is carried out by a physician who is in charge of a whole group, much stress is laid on the individual patient's adjustment to the group. The principles which are discussed under group therapy (Chapter V) play an important role. It is accepted that it is the patient's inability to adjust to others that has necessitated his admission. One has to keep in mind, for example, that psychoneurotic patients requiring admission to a psychiatric clinic are unable to get along outside of the hospital. As long as such patients are able to perform the duties of their daily life, ambulatory treatment is usually desirable unless environmental difficulties demand treatment in more neutral surroundings. As a rule, voluntary admission, on the patient's own responsibility, is a fundamental principle. In this treatment a great deal of the burden of treatment is therefore shared by the patient. He is expected to perform his duties and learns to understand himself better through observing his own reactions during the twenty-four hours. A healthy ward atmosphere stimulates mutual cooperation among the patients and a favorable attitude toward hospital routine and treatment. The patient knows that inability to live up to the requirements of the group necessitates transfer to a ward where less is demanded of him. It is important that the admitting officer consider carefully the ward to which the patient should be assigned in the first place. Transfer from ward to ward should be entirely for therapeutic reasons. It is rarely necessary in order to obtain a change of physicians. Having one physician in charge of a ward has the great advantage of uniformity. His group forms a unit and he can regulate and adjust the routine so that he gets the best possible working basis for his more individual therapy. Research work which he, or some other workers, may wish to carry out will be less disturbing to the patient and less likely to be interfered with. A distinct disadvantage is that physicians may have to be changed if one wishes to make use of the most suitable group, according to the patient's changing psychopathologic picture. On the wards for disturbed patients, management is without doubt facilitated by having one physician in charge. He knows how he can use the opportunities (attendants, tubs, etc.) which the hospital offers without interfering with the treatment of other patients. The patient can be guided toward developing allegiance to a ward-spirit rather than a specific transference. A great advantage is that the physician is intimately acquainted with the patient's life on the floor and in making his decisions is less dependent upon the nurse's reports than is the case when several physicians have patients on the same ward. Moreover, his knowledge of the patient obviously includes a knowledge of the total situation, including family relationships and responsibilities and is not restricted merely to personal transference material.

In assigning patients to individual physicians one has the advantage of selecting the most suitable physician, while the latter has the satisfaction of studying and guiding the patient through all the various phases of his illness. The treatment will naturally be a more personal one, and in consequence group life and adjustment may often suffer. Habit training is without doubt easier when one physician treats the whole group.

In the Payne Whitney Psychiatric Clinic (The New York Hospital) both principles of hospital treatment are utilized. The physician follows the individual case through his whole hospital stay. The unity of group life and its activities are preserved and cultivated therapeutically by having one of the more experienced physicians in charge of two floors. He carries the supervision and planning of the group life in addition to the treatment of his individual cases. On the floor for disturbed patients, one physician is in charge of the whole group, but the previous physician will follow for five days a patient who has been transferred. This procedure is beneficial for the general adjustment to such a floor and permits continuation of treatment if the stay on this floor lasts only a few days. In my experience this combined type of arrangement makes optimal use of the hospital facilities.

In such treatment excessive dependence of the patient upon the physician is avoided. The patient is led to develop a feeling of being able to manage himself in daily situations and is therefore sooner prepared to return to life outside the hospital. He learns to understand that individual freedom is relative and to accept his responsibilities to the group, and more and more also to the group to which he belongs outside of the hospital.

An exclusive relationship between one physician and one patient is not possible in a large psychiatric hospital. The chief as well as the supervising and consulting physicians who must take the legal and ethical responsibility have the right and duty to be informed of the intimate details of treatment. It is, however, essential that the patient feel assured that his communications be considered highly confidential. When it is necessary to combine teaching with treatment, it becomes important for the physician in charge of the case to use his judgment in his manner of presenting the case. The case presentation can nevertheless be scientifically adequate.

In most cases private rooms are desirable for personal comfort, but they are not essential therapeutically. Government hospitals with open wards are therapeutically as well equipped as the private hospitals with separate rooms, which naturally increase the expense considerably. Close observation in suicidal cases and the treatment of autistic patients are facilitated on open wards. Therefore many private hospitals combine private rooms with open wards.

It is best to group patients according to the degree of behavior disturbance and not according to diagnostic and prognostic factors. This allows us to deal with group adjustment therapeutically and to establish group cooperation. It removes the stigma of hopelessness from chronic cases.

Isolation in the sense of locking a patient in a room is not in use any longer, but separation is often necessary. This should never be carried out without full supervision. Even in excited patients separation should be used only for relatively short periods. Many times the apparent need for constant separation from the group is merely an expression of the physician's or nurses' inability to deal with the problem.

The introduction of scientific hydrotherapy and of various somatic procedures (Chapter VII) has made the treatment of excitements much easier. Their success depends much on the nurses' and attendants' understanding of the patient and on the physician's ability to individualize treatment. The present tendency to consider continuous baths superfluous is unjustified. Each hospital should have rooms with two or three tubs and, in addition, single tub rooms. Then only will one be able to care for patients who need separate treatment because they become too easily excited or disturb others, as well as patients who can achieve rest with others in the room. The more elaborate hydrotherapy departments with various apparatus and heat treatment are of little importance except for their general stimulating metabolic influence. Electrotherapy is without scientific justification and therefore no longer in use.

Therapeutic activity should be guided by a sound medical judgment. The physician needs to know how to treat the physical and mental aspects of the illness. A brief period of careful physical observation is desirable. In most hospitals patients are kept in bed for at least twenty-four hours. This has also a helpful psychologic influence by impressing the patient with the fact that due attention is being paid to physical factors. Prolonged bed treatment, however, has been abandoned except where definite physical indications exist. Rarely will it be necessitated by a condition of undernourishment. It has been proved that patients regain their loss of weight under a careful routine and individual psychotherapy faster than by milk diet and rest cure. Agitation also will be relieved by planned activity. Excited patients usually refuse to stay in bed. It is inadvisable to struggle with such patients. The use of hydrotherapy, sedatives, and psychotherapy is of prime importance (see Chapters V and VIII).

A healthy, normal diet is offered to the average patient. Through intermediate nourishment and the addition of cream to the diet we help correct undernourishment. When there are specific physical complications the diet must be adjusted accordingly. Atonic patients may need a special diet and modified activity, often combined with massage. In all these cases it is essential to realize that the dietary adjustment may be merely incidental.

Feeding problems need to be studied carefully. By hastily resorting to tube feeding, the patient's tendencies to react with withdrawal into himself or pathologic submission or aversion to the physician will be increased (see Chapters IX and X). One should try to encourage a patient as long as possible to feed himself and if unsuccessful, resort to spoon-feeding as the next step. Only after these persuasive methods have failed and the general physical condition demands it, should one start tube-feeding (see Chapter X, p. 250). Even during the period of tube-feeding, physician and nurses should make tireless efforts to induce the patient to accept spoon-feeding again. Rectal feeding is of little value from the standpoint of nutrition. In some patients, especially latent homosexuals, rectal feeding as well as other rectal manipulation (temperature, enema) are contraindicated.

Fluctuations in weight are important indications. Gain may be the earliest manifestation of improvement in a depression; loss may warn us that the patient needs modification of his routine or that his appearance is deceiving and may conceal an increase in the depth of his depression. One should therefore keep a weight chart on every patient, recording his weight once a week. A daily pulse and temperature chart are also needed. Oral or axillary temperature is sufficiently exact in most cases. In personality disorders a slight temperature increase caused by constipation is frequent. Whether it also occurs under emotional influence is still disputed. More telling is the pulse rate, which is usually more or less persistently high in anxiety states. A decrease goes hand in hand with general improvement. Sudden increases in pulse rate should always induce the physician to look for an explanation in the situational setting (e.g., the influence of a discussion with the patient, visitors, letters). Acute minor sleep difficulties should be viewed from a similar point of view. Constipation is one of the important physiologic complications, especially in depressions, under which heading it is discussed fully. The frequency of bowel movements should be carefully watched. Considerable attention should be paid to general hygiene and especially to skin and oral hygiene.

Drugs which induce sleep or help to control excitement and agitation are necessary, but should be used sparsely. The physician who uses individualized psychotherapy, hydrotherapy, occupational therapy, and a well-planned routine will have relatively little need for them. He will guard against the tendency to substitute chemical for physical restraint and try to avoid both as much as possible. Placebos have no place in well-planned, active psychiatric treatment. A complete discussion of the most important drugs is offered in the chapters on excitement and depression. The physician should not only be thoroughly acquainted with the drugs he may wish to use — how they work, the dangers involved, the optimal dosage — but he should be no less careful to study the patient's reaction to the drug and to modify the treatment accordingly. As a rule, it is wiser to use large doses than to repeat.

Through changes in our therapeutic conceptions, we have been led to insist that all patients receive sufficient fresh air. In some excitements this may not be possible without transferring the patient to a suitable institution, e.g., a state hospital, where outdoor activities can be organized without disturbance to others. Bed patients and stuporous patients should receive special attention in this respect.

In modern psychiatric hospitals alcoholic beverages are omitted completely. In consultation practice their use should be restricted, as the influence of alcohol often conceals the very factors which we are most anxious to bring into the foreground. I personally advise omitting it for at least three weeks in every patient. This gives us an opportunity of understanding those factors which cause the patient to take alcoholic drinks and to determine what course should be followed in therapy. Smoking should also be restricted. Temporary complete abstinence from tobacco will also show certain underlying urges. This is best seen in sexual difficulties. Because of the removal of the anaphrodisiac nicotine, sexual desires occasionally appear frankly or are concealed in general restlessness and dreams. When coffee and tea are taken in excess, the patient should understand his need for stimulants and his potentialities for control. A physician's personal prejudices should not interfere with these conclusions; otherwise, he cannot treat all his patients correctly.

Sexual abstinence is most desirable. It allows the patient to recognize the actual amount of sexual passion which he possesses, by what it is stimulated and to what extent, and what means of control are available. The cooperative patient is usually willing to undergo sexual abstinence for several weeks. The physician must realize that sexual relationship is never therapeutically necessary. By resorting to such unjustifiable advice a physician shows his own limitations.

Patients usually do not need to stay in the hospital until they are entirely well. Discharge is one of the important therapeutic steps. In most cases, one advises a direct return to work and regular life with desirable modifications, instead of a vacation, which is frequently proposed by patient or relatives.

In many cases an adjustment of the patient who has not recovered, or cannot completely recover, must be attempted. This can often be achieved by means of occupation for which the patient is adapted. Many hospitals establish contact with employers and families where patients can be placed suitably. This whole trend toward utilizing outside adjustment needs to be still further developed. Such adjustment will not only bring the patient closer to a normal life but will save much money for relatives and communities. The treatment of personality disorders places a tremendous burden on the public and, if we wish to be able to take care of this increasing expense, it is essential that we psychiatrists direct our treatment accordingly.

A relatively small number of children require treatment in a psychiatric hospital (see Chapter V). The same general principles as for any other psychiatric hospital apply to a children's unit. This unit, for example, must be large enough to allow the grouping of the patients according to their psychopathologic disorders and their behavior. Best therapeutic results would be obtained for most of the children if, according to their psychopathologic needs, they could be studied and treated in well-organized psychiatric units in pediatric hospitals, in nursery schools, and in suitable schools and homes.

Only the general rules of hospital treatment have been presented in this chapter. Many problems, although they are also related to treatment, have been omitted. I am referring to the organization of large hospitals into sub-departments, to the size of psychiatric hospitals and their various buildings, and to the proportion of patients to physicians and nurses. Local problems must be considered in the planning of a hospital which should fulfill an obligation to the community, the local practitioner, and his patients. Therapeutic considerations must remain the decisive factor. It is always desirable that the administration of such hospitals be entirely in the hands of psychiatrists. All the details of routine and management are so closely related to treatment that satisfactory decisions cannot be made by a lay person. The psychiatrist is the soul of such a hospital. High standards of living and pleasant interior and exterior decorating should make it hospitable enough for a stay of any length of time, but the desire to return to the world outside the hospital should be fostered. One should expect the utmost from a patient according to his psychopathologic condition but this can be achieved only if he is urged to live up to high standards of dressing, eating, work, and general behavior.

Psychiatric treatment is important in any general hospital. Best results are obtained if the internists and surgeons have enough psychiatric knowledge to recognize and treat personality disorders. Psychiatric consultants may advise them or carry out the treatment if the skill of a specialist is required. Transfer to a psychiatric hospital should be based on definite therapeutic indications. Small psychiatric units in a general hospital can rarely fulfill all the basic requirements which have been discussed in this chapter.

It is essential that not only the nurses but all the persons who have dealings with patients be selected from a therapeutic point of view. In nurses, knowledge alone is insufficient. On the other hand, the postulate that psychiatric nurses only need sympathy and common-sense, with merely a rudimentary theoretical knowledge, is too extreme. All these factors must be combined. It is desirable that more attention be paid to the training of male nurses. We often need them in our treatment. This point has been overstressed abroad, where they still hesitate to have female nurses attending male patients. Nurses should have an understanding of the psychopathologic aspects of their patients and be made constantly aware of the intricacies of the everchanging nurse-patient relationship. The psychiatrist should be in full control of nursing. Group nursing is therapeutically superior to the assignment of special nurses to individual patients except on definite therapeutic indications. In the selection of a nurse one must be guarded by the individual needs of the patient.

Social workers permit an important extension of psychiatric treatment. Their functions are no longer primarily the alleviation of the economic needs of the poor. They fulfill the much broader role of advising suitable work situations, educational facilities, recreational, and living accommodations. Their important contribution in the treatment of children is discussed in the pertinent literature following Chapter V.

Psychotherapy is used in much the same way whether treatment is ambulatory or in a hospital. For a detailed discussion on psychotherapy the reader is referred to the various chapters on this topic and to case discussions. I would like, however, to point to the error of having too narrow a concept of psychotherapy, considering only well worked out procedures worthy of this name. Psychotherapy includes all kinds and ways of utilizing psychologic means to achieve beneficial psychobiologic changes. Simple explanations and formulations based on the facts obtained as well as more far-reaching analysis, suggestion and hypnosis, and re-education belong to it. It is wrong to stress good intelligence as an essential requirement. By adjusting the procedure to the patient, a physician should be able to help the feebleminded and the intelligent as well as the cooperative, and the confused, or negativistic patient. It is essential that one know the goal of the interview and how to end it constructively. In a state hospital where one physician is in charge of a large number of patients, interviews will necessarily be less frequent, but opportunities can be utilized for personality adjustment which a smaller hospital cannot offer. In a large group, for example, there is the possibility of activities which are closer to everyday life than the limited occupational and social opportunities in a small hospital.

Mental hygiene, i.e., the maintenance of the health of the personality and the prevention of personality disorders, has received great attention in the last thirty years. Every psychiatrist must know the fundamental principles of mental hygiene. Efforts have been primarily directed to the formative stage of personality development, i.e., children and adolescents. The mature adult, however, also has need of a better physical and mental hygiene and much constructive work can be done in this field. Every physician is confronted with the problems of alcoholic abuse and narcotic addiction, venereal disease, and sexual hygiene. These are important topics in mental hygiene. The physician should be equipped to assist in the choice of suitable vocations and to give advice on the problems of marriage and of having children. Strict rules cannot be offered. Studies in heredity have not yet proceeded far, partly because too much attention has been paid to the question of the inheritance of disease entities instead of reaction tendencies, and partly because of the complexity of the human personality. It is wise not to give dogmatic and final decisions but to consider the whole family setting. Marriage and procreation should not be proposed as therapeutic measures. In recommending either, we must always consider the influence both upon the patient and upon the well person. In patients who are not sufficiently recovered, or in whom there is reasonable danger of serious recurrences, or where hereditary dangers are known to exist, the physician should advise against marriage. If marriage takes place in spite of his advice, he should urge birth control or the sterilization of the patient. If pregnancy occurs, the possibility of abortion with sterilization has to be considered. Abortion may be indicated by the danger of increase in an already existing illness or of recurrence of a previous serious illness. In the first case we must also consider the nature of the illness and the possibility of a later healthy pregnancy. This is the exception, and in addition to abortion, sterilization should always be considered seriously. On the other hand, in considering the child, abortion can only be urged when sufficient proof of dangerous inheritance exists.

Eugenic procedures have not yet been sufficiently studied to be used therapeutically. The physician must concern himself with individual adjustment.

Sterilization should not be advocated too freely and should be discussed thoroughly with the patient. It may often have to be proposed to the man instead of the woman. One should keep in mind that a marriage may terminate and a remarriage with a healthier partner may offer the possibility of healthy childbearing.

BIBLIOGRAPHY

1. JANET, P.: *Psychological Healing.* 2 Vols. The Macmillan Company, New York, 1925. (Historical review and discussion of various methods.)
2. NOYES, A. P.: Psychotherapy in State Hospitals. *American Journal of Psychiatry,* 91, 1935.
3. BRYAN, W. A.: *Administrative Psychiatry.* W. W. Norton and Co., New York, 1936.
4. McLESTER, J. S.: *Nutrition and Diet in Health and Disease.* W. B. Saunders Company, Philadelphia, 1940.
5. MEYER, A.: Organization of Community Facilities for Prevention, Care and Treatment in Hospitals for Mental Disorders. *First International Congress on Mental Hygiene,* 1930.
6. CRUTCHER, H. B.: *Foster Home Care for Mental Patients.* The Commonwealth Fund, New York, 1944, (Includes a detailed bibliography of the topic.)
7. SMILLIE, W. G.: *Preventive Medicine and Public Health.* The Macmillan Company, New York, 1946. (The chapter on mental hygiene presents a good orientation.)
8. CRUTCHER, R.: Child Psychiatry. A History of Its Development. *Psychiatry: Journal of the Biology and Pathology of Interpersonal Relations,* 6, 1943.
9. ZILBOORG, G., and HENRY, G. W.: *A History of Medical Psychology.* W. W. Norton and Co., New York, 1941. (This book offers a broad historical background for the student of treatment in psychiatry.)

Chapter III

SUGGESTION AND HYPNOSIS

IN ANY FORM of treatment the physician's personal influence necessarily plays an important role. This influence may take the form of direct instruction or authoritative advice, or it may operate in a less obvious manner through the indirect effect of suggestion. It would not be judicious at this stage to attempt an inclusive definition of suggestion. This would inevitably lead to an elaborate and unprofitable discussion of theoretical material. Instead, I prefer to present the outstanding factors in suggestion and their significance with regard to treatment.

Suggestions are exerted by one individual upon another. Through words or actions, there is produced in the patient a result which not only corresponds to the stimuli offered but goes far beyond an adequate response. The patient is in a state of expectancy, and his attention is considerably narrowed. His critical ability is diminished and he is willing to submit to the influence of the physician. This does not mean that he is aware of any of these factors. Often a patient seems to doubt the physician's ability, or is convinced that he has a highly critical attitude. Some authors state therefore that suggestion takes the patient by surprise. It is an indirect influence on the personality in which emotional factors play a considerable role. We know from the ordinary experiences of daily life that we are easily influenced by the emotions of others and that certain emotions can be suggested to us. Through the suggestions the patient is led to believe that the results indicated will occur, and as a result they actually do take place. One is in this way able to produce emotional changes, to influence the patient's strivings, thoughts and actions, and to cause far-reaching physiologic reactions.

There is for each individual a tendency to accept and submit to suggestion, and this phenomenon is termed, "suggestibility." It varies greatly and cannot be easily determined for a given individual. We must also realize that every person has not only a positive suggestibility, i.e., a susceptibility to suggestion, but also a corresponding negative suggestibility, i.e., an impulse not to follow suggestion, or to do the opposite of that which is suggested. This inherent connection of positive and negative suggestibility explains the fact that so many patients whom we know to be suggestible are refractory to our suggestions. This is seen especially in children and old people. They are open to suggestions which appeal to specific interests, but impregnably resistive to all others. The same is observed in feebleminded persons and in those who have a tendency to hysterical reactions.

Suggestion and beliefs are somewhat similar phenomena but suggestion has a more far-reaching psychobiologic influence. Suggestion can affect our moods readily, eliminate our critical ability, and dissociate ideas and tendencies. It exerts a marked influence on the heart and vasomotor system, on the intestines, and on the functions of glands. The vegetative nervous system and those organs influenced by it are accessible to suggestion.

It is impossible to outline the limitations of suggestion as it affects the whole integrated personality with all its interrelations. Suggestion plays a role in every treatment, even though it is frequently negligible from a practical point of view. It is quite evident that many physicians who believe in the specificity of their chemical, endocrinological, or surgical treatment overlook the suggestive influence of the treatment and of their own belief in its efficacy.

Suggestive influence can be exerted in such a form that the patient is not aware of it. We then speak of indirect suggestive methods. The assurance that a certain medicine will help constitutes an indirect suggestive approach which plays an important role in any treatment of physical ailments and is utilized to a varying degree by the physician. In this way a physician may influence the whole psychobiologic personality in the treatment of any physical illness. Indirect suggestions are therefore a valuable aid.

In certain treatments, especially in physio- and electrotherapy, the suggestive influence plays an important, and frequently the main, role. The physician should keep this in mind so that he does not become fascinated by a successful method and overlook the more essential suggestive factors in his treatment.

There is a marked tendency to use indirect suggestion in a purposely hidden form. Medicines are offered in functional disorders with the explanation that they perform a change or cure. The physician himself knows that his medicine cannot produce the desired effect, but that it may be accomplished through the suggestions included in his explanations. Internists and surgeons and especially the general practitioner use this method frequently. It is not necessary to offer examples. Every physician knows that functional gastrointestinal and cardiovascular disorders, abdominal pains, menstrual complaints, headaches, and pains in various joints are treated in this way.

Indirect suggestions which are offered in this hidden form should be avoided. They have no place in modern psychotherapy. Instead of misleading the patient, the physician should offer a frank formulation of his findings and encourage the patient to discuss his problems. It is therefore essential that every physician understand personality problems and be able to treat them. The results in psychiatric out-patient departments prove that such adjustments are possible even in feebleminded persons. It is true that indirect suggestion plays a considerable role in this treatment. It is not, however, used in a purposely misleading form but is inherent in the physician's personality, the adjustment to home and work, and the helpful influence of relatives and employers to whom the patient's difficulties have been explained. For such treatment in an out-patient department, well-trained social workers are indispensable assistants.

The physician's office, his nurses and aides, and the hospital environment also influence the patient. It is therefore possible to secure results earlier in a patient in a well-managed hospital. The ward and group spirit affect the patient either in a salutary or in an adverse way. Many psychiatrists, who unknowingly work almost entirely through indirect suggestion, believe that their convincing or authoritative explanations have made the patient understand the dynamic factors of his illness and that the symptoms in consequence disappear. Others do the same by shouting at the patient or by appealing to the emotions of fear or shame.

In any kind of suggestive therapy one should consider the patient, the physician, and the means used. The patient does not need to offer active assistance so much as a passive readiness and a positive suggestibility. The physician should know whether his personality is able to exert strong suggestion. Certain suggestive methods will appeal to him more than others. The choice of the method and the content of the suggestions which one wishes to use depends on the nature of the patient's illness, his personality, and the interests and personality of the physician.

All psychobiologic functions can be modified through suggestion. Suggestion can be used as the main therapeutic factor, or may be merely an aid in another psychotherapeutic procedure. The main indication for suggestive treatment is the presence of symptoms which are not based on a marked personality involvement and which frequently persist after the main factors have become clear to the patient. The best examples are offered in many of the war neuroses, in fright symptoms after explosions or accidents, and in hysterical reactions in poorly organized individuals. To this latter group belong psychopathic and immature personalities, children, and feeble-minded persons, who often react easily with hysterical motor symptoms or various pains to minor difficulties in life. Furthermore, suggestion is of valuable help in many hypochondriacal complaints, especially various pains, cardiovascular and gastrointestinal complaints, difficulty in bowel movements and urination, and sleep disturbances. Suggestion encourages a depressed patient and diminishes his anxiety and fear.

Direct suggestion never has as far-reaching effects as hypnotic suggestion but many of the above-mentioned symptoms yield to well-planned suggestions, especially if this treatment is combined with some kind of re-education. The appeal to the patient's will and advice as to how he may strengthen his will-power represents a direct suggestive approach. This method, which has been proposed especially by neurologists for the treatment of tics and stuttering, will be discussed in Chapter XVI.

A psychiatrist should know what all the current fashionable medical ideas are and understand with which psychobiologic factors they work. All these methods take some of the principles of the many procedures which we use, consciously and unconsciously, every day in psychiatry and elaborate them to an extreme, to the exclusion of everything else. We will be able to gain the patient's confidence and cooperation if we can re-interpret this to him in terms of the dynamic therapeutic factors involved. We physicians will then be able to utilize some of the features of that mode of treatment in which the patient has faith. If this is not possible because of the patient's personality, we can adjust our approach to the patient's belief.

Everyone is susceptible to suggestions which are produced in himself. This tendency is termed, "auto-suggestion." It has always played a certain role in psychotherapy. The patient substitutes faith in the outcome for effort. Coué tried to develop this helpful tendency exclusively, but he overlooked the fact that the physician's personality and belief in his method were of primary importance and that his treatment was therefore primarily suggestive. The same factors explain the results which are obtained by Christian Science. Together with muscle relaxation, suggestion and auto-suggestion have been utilized by psychiatrists.

Of even greater influence than individual suggestion is suggestion by the mass on the individual. Mass suggestion is used freely in various religious healings. In recent years it has been utilized in group psychotherapy.

Hypnosis occupies a special place in treatment by suggestion. This method utilizes the sleep mechanism. Hypnosis has been well known in all ages, but scientifically it was first worked out by Bernheim and Liébault, who were able to prove that suggestion and not mystical tendencies, as Mesmer had argued, is the dynamic factor in hypnosis. As a result of their studies, the method of hypnosis has been simplified. Verbal suggestions are now used almost exclusively. Modern textbooks neglect to give a clear presentation of the technique. I consider it essential for every psychiatrist to master the technique and for every general practitioner to understand the working factors. There are still many prejudices against the medical use of hypnosis, but it definitely has its place in medicine as a form of therapy. Through its use one can also demonstrate the factors of dissociation; and it offers a greater possibility for the understanding of suggestion.

In hypnosis, the patient's attention is drawn to the physician's procedure and away from the stimuli of the surroundings and from stimuli arising within himself. Therefore his field of consciousness becomes gradually narrowed, and in a certain stage there does not exist anything else for him but the hypnotizing physician. The patient is then entirely relaxed and has lost the volitional control of his body. This is accompanied by increasing drowsiness leading to a sleep-like state. The physician utilizes these tendencies by suggesting sleep. Whether the final sleep, which can be very deep, is the same as spontaneous sleep is as difficult to determine as whether sleep in narcosis is the same as normal sleep.

Awakened from a deep hypnotic sleep, the patient may have amnesia for most of the events which have occurred. A total amnesia is usually not obtained without a corresponding suggestion to that effect during the hypnosis, and even then the patient frequently begins to remember some details after a few hours.

It is impossible to determine the onset of the hypnotic stage. It is a fluent process and there are no definite known limits between the waking state and the slight hypnosis. For practical purposes different stages of hypnosis have been distinguished. This has been misleading, as it fostered the belief that certain signs indicated the same depth in everyone and that a so-called deep hypnosis was necessary for therapeutic suggestions. Experience has proved that the same sign, e.g., catelepsy or amnesia, may be produced easily in some and only with great difficulty in others, and that this has nothing to do with therapeutic suggestibility. It is often possible to affect symptoms in some patients in slight hypnosis whereas a deep hypnosis must be achieved in others.

An important characteristic of hypnosis is the post-hypnotic suggestion. Such suggestions, given during the hypnosis, still hold after the hypnosis has been terminated or may function at a suggested time after the hypnosis. A person who has received a strong hypnotic suggestion to carry out a certain act when he is awake will, at the appointed time, have a feeling that he wants to carry it out as if it were his own impulse. Posthypnotic suggestions are of great therapeutic importance. They allow the physician to influence symptoms permanently or over a certain limited period. He is thus able to regulate the patient's sleep, its onset, as well as its duration. We must, moreover, realize that all changes produced in hypnosis have a tendency to persist afterwards. A person educated to rest in hypnosis will therefore utilize this tendency whenever he gets ready to sleep. The posthypnotic suggestion will then be an additional factor in producing sleep in such a prepared person.

The hypnotic technique is based on an imitation of sleep, utilizing an impressive description of relaxation. Verbal suggestions are now used primarily. Previous to the studies of Liébault and Bernheim, hypnotic suggestions were frequently given in more or less elaborate mystical procedures. Charcot and his school used fright hypnosis which was based on the hypothesis that through fright a patient develops the special hysterical reaction which is called hypnosis. This misconception and technique led to poor therapeutic results and brought hypnotism into disrepute, which has not yet disappeared. (Animal 'hypnosis" is primarily based on fright. It would therefore be best if this term were generally substituted by "cataplexia.") Braid used fixation — the patient had to look at a sparkling silver ball very closely until he was tired and fell asleep; Faria asked the patient to look in his eyes, believing that fascination produced the sleep. Mesmer stroked the patient's skin lightly. He believed that these so-called "passes" allowed a magnetic fluid to go from him to the patient. In all these methods, the suggestive influence is the only dynamic factor. In scientific hypnosis, one should therefore avoid methods which appeal to the sense of the mystical, and use frank suggestion instead.

Almost everybody can be hypnotized, but the result depends very much on the circumstances. If a patient goes to a man who is famous for this kind of treatment, one may be sure that he is already under a marked suggestive influence before the physician even starts. What is called "will-power" has not much to do with the possibility of being hypnotized, because people with "will-power" may be very suggestible. The physician should be aware of the possibility of certain disturbing factors. A person who is under the influence of strong emotions is less suggestible. It is therefore wise to discuss acute worries before any hypnosis is started. Fear of the treatment has to be dispersed by an explanation, suitable to the patient, which presents hypnosis as a special kind of suggestive treatment in which a sleep-like state is produced with the passive cooperation of the patient.

In offering suggestions the physician utilizes the knowledge of those sensations which accompany normal sleep. When difficulties are encountered, it is helpful to inform onself more closely about individual sleep habits and observations. A patient should lie comfortably on his back. Anything which interferes with free breathing should be removed. Collars and belts may have to be opened, or a patient may have to be advised to come in more comfortable clothes the next time. The room should be quiet and bright lights eliminated, although I have rarely found it necessary to darken a room. Any interruptions such as telephone calls must be prevented. It is essential that the physician himself feel at ease; otherwise, his suggestions will not carry well. In the hypnotic relationship a patient easily senses the physician's mood disturbances and is affected negatively. Haste and restlessness inhibit hypnosis. The physician must be sure of his technique. Uncertainty or hesitancy in offering suggestions, the mere stumbling over a word, will prevent suggestions from working. I always urge therefore that a physician learn the technique from somebody who is experienced, if this is possible, and that he know the exact wording of the suggestions which he intends to give and how to proceed from one step to the next. In order to establish sufficient self-confidence, I assign a new physician a patient who can be readily hypnotized. Hypnotizing the patient in this physician's presence, I also give the post-hypnotic suggestion that the hypnosis by the other physician will be immediate and deep. A physician should not attempt to hypnotize a patient before he knows the technique well and has confidence in his own ability.

In order to fix the patient's attention and to get his eyes easily tired, I hold a coin about a foot from the patient's eyes, at a height which will not make looking at it a strain. I explain to the patient the reason for this fixation. Usually I put my other hand on the patient's forehead. At the same time I start with the suggestions, advising the patient to breathe deeply and quietly, not to try to help but to take a passive attitude, merely listening to my voice and not paying attention to noises. The next suggestion is that he begins to feel relaxed and notices a heaviness in his arms and legs. He feels drowsy. The coin therefore becomes blurred. (As a result of the immobility of his eyes and the lack of moving of the lacrimal fluid, vision actually does become blurred.) His forehead feels warm (due to the warmth from my hand). This warmth is agreeable and is noticeable in his whole body. His eyelids become heavier and heavier and gradually fall (much attention is paid to closing of the eyes as this is part of normal sleep). Tingling sensations are noticed in the arms. Again the patient's attention is directed to actual sensations, utilizing and enforcing them through suggestion. Spontaneous closing of the eyes, which develops through a gradual lowering of the eyelids, occurs in one to two minutes. If this does not happen after two minutes, the patient should be asked to close them voluntarily and then one proceeds with the suggestions. Voluntary closing is not desirable, but does not mean that hypnosis will not be successful. In this early stage of hypnosis the patient is frequently still able to open his eyes and to resist the influence of the hypnosis, but for more volitional acts he needs more will-power. He feels tired; his muscles are relaxed; his thoughts wander aimlessly, and suppressed and repressed thoughts come more easily into awareness.

The next suggestions attempt to increase the patient's attitude of passivity. I point out to the patient that his arms are actually heavy, and lifting his arm, let it fall down heavily. I state that he is not aware of the noises any longer; that his quiet respiration and his relaxed face indicate that sleep has started, and that in his sleep he is under an increasing influence of my suggestions. A few passes over the arms increase the suggestion that I am exerting a definite influence over his motility. This can then be easily proved to him by catalepsy or by his inability to open his eyes against my order. The demonstration of these facts is therapeutically desirable only in that it is proof to the patient of the truth of our suggestions. In most cases I do not even attempt to show catalepsy if the general relaxation indicates a sufficient hypnosis. It is important not to attempt to show catalepsy too early. A failure disturbs the physician's and the patient's confidence in the strength of the suggestion.

In deep hypnosis, amnesia may occur spontaneously, but it usually must be suggested. Amnesia is therapeutically important only if the physician has stirred up in a hypnotic discussion material which he feels would disturb the patient afterwards. It is one's aim to prevent such an occurrence. In deep hypnosis, fancies and forgotten experiences come easily to the foreground, and the patient is able to discuss problems about which he cannot or does not want to talk in the awakened state. Deep hypnosis is desirable for therapeutic suggestions, but it is not a requirement, and no undue delay should be caused by the inability to produce catalepsy or amnesia. Both phenomena may occur easily, or only after prolonged treatment, and are not always indicators of therapeutic suggestibility.

Each hypnosis should be terminated carefully. It should never be done abruptly, but, on the other hand, one should avoid unnecessarily elaborate suggestions. I merely tell the patient at the end of the hypnosis that he will wake up after I have counted (slowly) to three, and that he will feel relaxed and at ease, with no after-symptoms in the form of fatigue, dizziness, or headache. When he has been awakened, I advise him to rest a few minutes before getting up. Many suggestible persons otherwise experience the above-mentioned harmless but annoying after-symptoms.

It is essential that all suggestions be given in a quiet, somewhat monotonous, and impressively assuring voice. The sentences should be short and clear so that the patient can grasp their meaning easily. In offering suggestions one should consider the patient's personality and cultural background. For example, a physician whom I hypnotized successfully several times was disturbed by the suggestion that his pulse was slower, because he was not able to check up on this statement. Knowledge of hypnosis by the patient is not desirable, but when present, is not necessarily a handicap. Each physician has to find his own mode of offering suggestions. Some prefer a clear and rather loud voice, others a low or even whispering one. On the whole, commands and authoritative words have been given up in favor of carefully phrased and persuasive suggestions.

In resistive patients, special modifications are necessary. One may have to offer a great variety of suggestions, utilizing one's knowledge of normal but usually unobserved sensations and physiologic changes, such as slight paresthesias in the motionless arms and hands or the absence of blinking to touching the conjunctiva sclerae. In many patients a "fractioned" hypnosis will overcome the difficulty: one produces a slight relaxation, with closed eyes, and asks the patient afterwards to describe the changes he has noticed. In the immediately following hypnosis the physician utilizes this knowledge in his suggestions. Through four or more brief (about two minutes), successive, and increasingly deep hypnoses, a sufficiently deep hypnosis can frequently be reached in less than half an hour. It is also wise to give at the end of a hypnosis the post-hypnotic suggestion that a deeper stage will be reached easily the next time.

Some patients in early hypnosis exhibit a sneering grin. This happens frequently when they try to overcome the suggestive forces but are unable to do so. It is therefore a sign of already established hypnosis. Less frequent is compulsive laughing. When a patient blinks his eyes constantly or is unable to lie still, one should proceed with mere verbal suggestions, and, in addition, must resort to sudden commands producing immobility or catalepsy. In most of these cases it will be found best to look for a more suitable psychotherapeutic method.

In the beginning hypnosis should be repeated daily, the duration always relatively short (ten to fifteen minutes), except when exploration is attempted. After one or two weeks it is desirable to begin restricting the procedure to alternate days and then, by gradually increasing the interval, lead eventually to complete cessation of hypnosis. A physician should not expect sudden, spectacular results. It is preferable to train difficult patients gradually to the hypnotic suggestions. There are naturally many exceptions, e.g., the need for rapid removal of dangerous hysterical symptoms or acute sleep difficulties. It cannot be emphasized too strongly that verbal suggestions are the only desirable means of inducing hypnosis. Physicians who claim that the use of special apparatus is necessary or advisable show that their personality is not suited for this treatment.

Most physicians are not aware of the more recent development of therapeutic hypnotic technique. They still believe that it is only necessary to give suggestions for a symptom to disappear and not recur. This purely symptomatic treatment is insufficient. In order to give well-planned suggestion, the whole reaction and personality setting must be understood. We want to make use of the psychobiologic functions and tendencies which play a role in the normal personality and therefore go beyond mere symptomatic cure. Instead of giving commands, one should try to lead the patient through individually adjusted descriptions to experiencing sensations and emotions, increase his self-confidence and self-reliance, loosen and change habits of thinking and actions, and make him attain a perspective toward his illness. It is therefore wrong to use hypnosis to the exclusion of analysis. Exclusive, protracted hypnosis leads to failure because after a time the suggestions lose their effect.

In hysterical paralysis one does not only confine oneself to suggesting a strengthening of the muscles through relaxation and rest and a better blood supply, and to asking the patient to carry out certain exercises, but one also investigates the underlying factors and gives suggestive advice accordingly. In a young woman with a contracture of the right foot which occurred after a sexual assault, the main problem was to desensitize her to sexual pleasure, which she had experienced during the assault, and to change her attitude of resentment to one of constructive acceptance. Similar factors played a role in the hysterical vomiting of one of my patients which I was able to stop easily through hypnosis. Good results with hypnosis have often been obtained in the primarily psychogenic vomiting of pregnancy.

In gastrointestinal disturbances hypnosis is frequently used to eliminate highly disturbing symptoms, followed afterwards by analysis and adjustment. In chronic constipation, urinary disturbances, and bronchial asthma, in which we frequently find important contributory or precipitating psychogenic and emotional factors, hypnosis helps greatly in re-education. The same is true in tics and stuttering.

Hypnosis may help considerably in menstrual difficulties, frigidity, and sexual impotence. In the treatment of frigidity, the production of an attitude of acceptance of, and submission to, sexual relations is the goal. In addition, one increases the patient's spontaneous awareness of pleasurable physical sensations and of the pleasure experienced by the partner. In impotency, after the underlying factors have been carefully investigated, hypnosis not only helps to increase self-confidence and to overcome anticipation of failure, but stimulates sexual desire and increases actual potency. We should also utilize the patient's preoccupations and day-dreams. Dreams of satisfactory intercourse, even with discharge, can be suggested and used as a proof of completed treatment. Hypnosis is especially valuable in cases in which we know that analysis, with awareness of the underlying factors, would lead to results that would be more destructive than constructive from the point of view of the personality. In one of our patients, impotency was caused by a justified suspicion of his wife's unfaithfulness during a brief interval. The family life was otherwise happy, but a clear understanding of all the factors would have led to divorce, as the patient would not have been able to forget the episode.

When sleep difficulties are the only complaint, a successful re-education is possible through hypnosis. The patient first learns that he can get drowsy. Then confidence in his ability to sleep is established, and this overcomes his fear of a sleepless night so that he remains relaxed and will fall asleep. This confidence is of great importance in cases with difficulty in falling asleep, and in those with early awakening and inability to resume sleep. Light sleep which is disturbed by any noise can be increased in depth through direct suggestion and by educating the patient to pay less attention to disturbances. A good example of the value of a knowledge of hypnosis in general practice is illustrated by the case of a young woman who was unable to adjust herself to her husband's suicide. Her family physician was able through hypnosis to suggest sleep after three sleepless nights.

After a prostatectomy a 60 year old man developed persistent hiccough diminished after two days, allowing retention of food, The fear that he would be unable to overcome it increased rapidly. After a few days he was in a serious general condition. Hypnosis was administered twice daily and, with the decrease of his fear and an increasing belief in his satisfactory abdominal condition, the hiccough diminished after two days, allowing retention of food, and ceased entirely a few days later. Suggestive and hypnotic therapy is valuable also in postoperative prolonged inability to urinate.

Many isolated pains, especially headaches, often yield to hypnosis in a short time. This result, however, cannot be obtained when it occurs in a setting of well-established habits of self-observation and hypochondriacal invalidism. It is, moreover, possible to use suggestion and even hypnosis in the re-education of hypochondriasis. It increases confidence in one's own body, establishes courage to go on in a normal life, and corrects anticipation and anxiety. The patient is urged to let himself go, not trying to elaborate on thoughts or sensations. Special attention should be paid to the time before falling asleep and to preparing the patient for specific situations which produce or increase anxiety. In trying to produce relaxation, the physician will always combine re-education with suggestion. The physical means of producing relaxation are not sufficient in themselves. Hypnosis is rarely indicated for these conditions.

If we wish to use hypnosis, it must be based on an understanding of which suggestive influences on the psychobiologically integrated personality are especially powerful. We know, for instance, that we can affect motility easily and we therefore use hypnosis for cramps and various functional disturbances of motility. The influence on sensibility is utilized in the correction of hysterical paresthesia and anesthesia and localized genital irritations. Various types of hysterical skin disorders, such as urticaria, vesicular and eczema-like disturbances, respond well to suggestion. One is able to influence vasomotor and secretory functions, but this is of little therapeutic value except for re-education in connection with analysis. Hypnosis is helpful in functional disorders of the bladder, large intestines, and rectum (urine retention, painful hysterical spasm of the bladder, incontinency, and occasionally in enuresis, hysterical constipation and mucous colitis). As a result of the strong influence of emotions, we can produce affective changes to one's experiences, i.e., desensitization, and thus the ability to forget. Hysterical blindness and mutism are cured by general suggestion. Of no therapeutic value is the physician's ability to suggest and influence illusions and hallucinations, changes in orientation with regard to time and space and to one's own personality, except, according to some authors, when there is a need to terminate an hysterical delirium or fugue.

Dysmenorrhea is often best attacked with hypnosis, whereas amenorrhea, which frequently responds, is preferably treated by other psychotherapeutic methods. We also rarely need to resort to hypnosis in the treatment of functional cardiac disorders. Of mere scientific interest are changes produced by hypnosis on blood calcium and blood sugar, bile secretion, and kidney functions.

Few physicians use hypnosis in the treatment of alcohol and drug addiction, although some striking results have been obtained through changing the patient's emotional attitude, e.g., causing a disgust reaction to the actual imbibing of alcohol, and effecting relaxation and adjustment of the personality.

Hypnotic clearing up of hysterical amnesia has been abandoned for the more direct psychotherapeutic approaches because they offer the patient an understanding of the working factors. In attempting to have a complete, dissociated scene re-experienced, we do not obtain an accurate re-experience. Part of the forgotten material is substituted by displacement and condensation, as in dreams. The reproduction of a forgotten scene in hypnosis is accomplished piece by piece, and gaps may be concealed by distorted material. What is reproduced is always presented in condensed form. Physicians who still retain cathartic methods now combine them with analysis in the hypnosis. To this they may even add the method of free association under hypnotic influence. There is no need to suggest amnesia because this treatment leads to understanding and not mere suppression of the reproduced life-experiences. This modern cathartic-analytic procedure may be desirable in patients who are unable to discuss their problems and in whom a waking analysis can proceed only very slowly. For practical reasons the time-consuming factors must be evaluated in every treatment.

It is not only the suggestive factors that are therapeutically important in hypnosis. The healing influence of sleep itself is also valuable. Some physicians have therefore urged prolonged hypnoses (two hours, several times a week for months) on the assumption that similar benefit may be obtained from hypnotic sleep.

Obsessions and phobias are not affected by hypnosis, although these symptoms, especially in children, are said to be much relieved by suggestion and re-education. Hypnosis is rarely used any longer to produce anesthesia or sleep in connection with general narcosis or in the attempt to diminish pain in childbirth.

It is unimportant to distinguish between pre-, intra- and post-hypnotic influences. It is more important that we utilize them carefully. The suggestive preparation of the patient is frequently overlooked.

The combination of hypnotics or sedatives with hypnosis is seldom therapeutically necessary. The chemical influence is used to decrease the patient's resistance and to cause in him a more passive and suggestible attitude.

There are few contraindications. It is most important that we select monosymptomatic cases and avoid this treatment in patients who have a tendency to successive symptomatic variations. Otherwise, after having cured one symptom, the patient will react with something new. Prolonged treatment must be avoided in erotic patients and those who develop a dependence on the treatment. In all these patients skin passes or any mechanical manipulations which increase the skin eroticism have to be excluded. No accompanying organic illness, not even organic cardiac lesions, is a contraindication if the patient is treated with care (dispelling fear), and if one is satisfied with slight hypnosis. Relaxation and direct suggestion are helpful. The attempt to change a depressive mood or to eliminate hallucinations by hypnosis has long been given up. On the other hand, suggestions are highly important. The beneficial influence of the hospital atmosphere is largely on a suggestive basis. Contraindicated are patients with a tendency to paranoic and paranoid reactions. The delusions frequently crystallize on the physician. Hypnosis in children was used more frequently in years past; it has now been replaced by brief analysis and social adjustment, but I still might advise it in distressing tics and stuttering. Children after the age of five are usually hypnotized without difficulty and no damage is done to the further development of the personality if verbal suggestion and explanation of the procedure are used. Because of the loss of plasticity of the personality, people over fifty are usually resistant to hypnosis, but a trial is frequently desirable. I know, for example, of a 52 year old chronic alcoholic who was cured by a physician in three hypnotic treatments. The occasional occurrence in hypnosis of spontaneous hallucinations or convulsive attacks is no contraindication if the patient remains in suggestive rapport with the physician. These symptoms, however, are rare if one selects cases carefully. The development of full-fledged delirious reactions demands a change of treatment. Persons who show some tendencies to somnambulistic twilight states should not be hypnotized, as their auto-suggestibility will lead to spontaneous use of the hypnotic experience.

Much has been written about the dangers of hypnosis. They do not exist in medical treatment, if one carefully considers indications and contraindications and uses verbal suggestions exclusively. Hypnosis in the hands of lay people is dangerous, as is any other medical procedure. The possibility of suggesting crime in hypnosis is very slight and no greater than through skillful direct suggestion.

Practically all cases of accusation against hypnotizing physicians have proved groundless. Many accusations of sexual misdemeanor have been made by hysterical patients and patients with delusions. It is, therefore, important that no physician hypnotize a patient of the opposite sex without a chaperone.

Hypnosis does not appeal to every physician. Many have given it up because of its monotony. In modern hypnotic treatment, in which the suggestions are not purely symptomatic and general but formed in accordance with the patient's personality and illness, and changed according to the whole development, much depends on the physician's constructive imagination. Hypnosis is now an individualizing and active treatment.

BIBLIOGRAPHY

1. FOREL, A. H.: *Hypnotism or Suggestion and Psychotherapy.* Translated from the 5th German edition, Rebman, New York, 1906. (This book is interesting because it contains many examples which illustrate the far-reaching results of hypnotic suggestions.)
2. HULL, C. L.: *Hypnosis and Suggestibility, an Experimental Approach.* D. Appleton-Century Company, New York, 1933.
3. ERICKSON, M. H., and KUBIE, L. S.: The Successful Treatment of a Case of Acute Hysterical Depression by a Return under Hypnosis to a Critical Phase of Childhood. *Psychoanalytic Quarterly,* 10, 1941. (An illustration of the psychodynamic understanding and use of hypnosis.)

Chapter IV

PSYCHOANALYTIC PROCEDURE

IN PRESENTING psychoanalytic treatment, I shall limit the subject as much as possible to the therapeutic procedure and discuss theoretical aspects only as far as seems necessary for a correct understanding. The practical application of some of these theories becomes evident in various chapters. On the other hand, I shall devote more space to dream analysis than modern psychoanalytic treatment demands because of its importance in psychotherapy in general. The "free association method," resistance, transference, and countertransference are discussed at some length. Every physician should understand these concepts. A psychiatrist should be able to recognize and deal with these phenomena whenever he is confronted with them in his treatment whether or not he can accept psychoanalytic theories and interpretations. After an introductory discussion, I shall present Freud's analytic procedures and additional suggestions of his pupils. This chapter offers merely a summary. The reader should keep in mind that the actual method should be learned by a thorough analysis of the student himself under the skillful guidance of a qualified psychoanalytic teacher. Well-planned programs are presented by various psychoanalytic training centers. Training in psychoanalytic treatment has advanced considerably in this country in the last fifteen years and has become available to an increasing number of psychiatrists.

In recent years emphasis has been placed on analysis of the patient's defenses. In addition, the technical procedure has become more elastic. Modifications, which are signs of healthy growth, are included in this chapter if they adhere to the fundamental rules of psychoanalysis. For practical reasons, the psychoanalytic procedure of the Washington School and the psychoanalytic contribution to brief psychotherapy and to the treatment of children are presented in Chapter V, and specific therapeutic aspects are referred to in various chapters. The interspersed quotations are taken from Freud's publications which are mentioned in the bibliography of this chapter.

A brief historical survey is necessary to make the reader aware of the great changes which this method has undergone in the fifty years of its existence. The existing literature is bewildering to the physician who is not psychoanalytically trained because much that has been claimed at previous stages of psychoanalysis has later been greatly modified. Treatment has changed according to new observations and theories.

Psychoanalytic theory and treatment originated in the observation of Breuer and Freud that repressed life experiences play a role in hysterical phenomena. They found that patients lost their hysterical symptoms when treated with hypnosis, in which they were able to talk freely about forgotten experiences and re-experience them, together with the emotions which had accompanied the original experience. However, the symptoms disappeared only when the causal experience had been reproduced in all its details and the patient had described it fully, expressing his emotions freely. Remembering and abreaction with the help of hypnosis was the goal. This treatment, called psychocatharsis, was discarded by Freud because of its technical difficulties when he found that by means of free association he was able to get at the underlying forgotten experiences without hypnosis and suggestion. The task now was to offer interpretations and thus get around resistance. Attention was still directed at gaining an understanding of the formation of symptoms. The uncovering of "complexes" instead of symptoms became the goal.

Abreaction was substituted by the effort which the patient had to put forth to overcome the critic against his free associations. Finally, the present method, in which one does not try to single out certain situations as more worthy of analysis than others, was reached. The physician reveals the various resistances to the patient. When the patient has succeeded in overcoming them, he is able to tell of the forgotten situations and their interrelations. The goal remains the same, i.e., to fill in the gaps of memory, or, to express it dynamically, to overcome the resistance of the repressive forces. Specific complex-situations are no longer singled out, but are studied whenever they occur. Dream analysis is considered important whenever dreams occur in the procedure of free association. Whereas previously dreams had been utilized as special points of attack, the analyst does not concentrate on dreams although he welcomes the opportunity to analyze them. Symbols are interpreted less freely and their individual setting and meaning carefully taken into consideration. The transference situation has become of utmost importance and a special transference technique has evolved. The analysis of more specific strivings and developmental situations has developed into the study of the whole personality.

In using the free association technique, the physician plays a passive role, listening to the patient, but not interfering or offering active help. The patient is told to be passive, trying not to observe himself or to find ideas which he wants to reproduce, but to voice any associations without attempting to decide whether or not they are worth while. He is requested to say whatever comes to his mind, even though he may think that certain ideas are not important, do not belong to the topic under consideration, are mere nonsense, or are too objectionable to be mentioned.

The physician's passivity does not mean inactivity. He does not actively interfere but guides the patient and offers interpretations to the patient, who may accept, reject, or ignore them without special attention. The patient proceeds with his associations accordingly. The physician offers interpretation only with careful selection of the therapeutic moment. In this way the patient proceeds, telling actual events of the present and past, fancies and elaborations, attitudes to specific events, persons, and in general, without trying to find connections. Sometimes these relationships become spontaneously clear to the patient. More frequently, the physician has to point them out through a question or by offering his interpretation. These interpretations should be taken as tentative, and future associations will show the patient whether or not they are correct and to what degree. This procedure is obviously quite different from a discussion by the patient, although it may be compared to it. Relationships, explanations, and solutions which seem clear at one time may be modified or rejected later. In well-organized patients this procedure leads to a constructive end.

In the classical method, the patient lies relaxed on a couch, the physician sitting behind the patient where he can observe but cannot be seen. This prevents the patient from looking constantly for the physician's response. The associations are not really free, how-

PSYCHOANALYTIC PROCEDURE 77

ever, because the entire analytic situation exerts its influence. Resistance prevents the patient from arriving at the repressed material. It can be recognized in the patient's inability to produce associations, in restlessness, and in his facial expression (blushing, tears, anger). It may also happen that a patient reproduces too many associations in order to conceal more important ones. An outstanding sign of resistance is that nothing essentially new is brought forth. Resistance indicates repressed material which can only be reproduced with much difficulty and which has usually exerted an important influence on the patient. All these mechanisms are unconscious. It is important that the analyst think over the last few therapeutic sessions in order to find out whether he has not overlooked something which might explain the resistance or whether he might not have initiated it. Resistances should not be pointed out to the patient, but each occurrence should be investigated. This procedure subjects the patient to as little force as possible, keeps the contact with reality, and provides that no factor in the neurosis is overlooked and that the physician does not inject his own anticipations.

"It may seem surprising that this method of free association, carried out subject to the observation of the fundamental rule of psychoanalysis, should have achieved what was expected of it, namely, the bringing into consciousness of the repressed material which was held back by resistances. We must, however, bear in mind that free association is not really free. The patient remains under the influence of the analytic situation even though he is not directing his mental activities on to a particular subject. We shall be justified in assuming that nothing will occur to him that has not some reference to that situation. His resistance against reproducing the repressed material will now be expressed in two ways. Firstly, it will be shown by critical objections; and it was to deal with these that the fundamental rule of psychoanalysis was invented. But if the patient observes that rule and so overcomes his reticences, the resistance will find another means of expression. It will so arrange it that the repressed material itself will never occur to the patient but only something which approximates to it an allusive way; and the greater the resistance, the more remote will be the substitutive association which the patient has to report from the actual idea that the analyst is in search of. The analyst, who listens composedly but without any constrained effort to the stream of associations and who, from his experience, has a general notion of what to expect, can make use of the material brought to light by the patient according to two possibilities. If the resistance is slight he will be able from the patient's allusions to infer the unconscious material itself; or if the resistance is stronger he will be able to recognize its character from the associations, as they seem to become more remote from the subject, and will explain it to the patient.

"Uncovering the resistance, however, is the first step towards overcoming it. Thus the work of analysis involves an art of interpretation, the successful handling of which may require tact and practice but which is not hard to acquire. But it is not only in the saving of labor that the method of free association has an advantage over the earlier method. It exposes the patient to the least possible amount of compulsion; it never allows of contact being lost with the actual, current situation; it guarantees to a great extent that no factor in the structure of the neurosis will be overlooked and that nothing will be introduced into it by the expectations of the analyst. It is left to the patient in all essentials to determine the course of the analysis and the arrangement of the material; any systematic handling of particular symptoms or complexes thus becomes impossible. In complete contrast to what happened with hypnotism and with the urging method, interrelated material makes its appearance at different times and at different points in the treatment."*

An understanding of dreams is obtained through the technique of free association. The patient is asked to tell what comes into his mind with regard to certain parts of the dreams, using either the chronological order of the dream or allowing the patient to select the most outstanding parts. The patient proceeds with free associations, which are again under the influence of this specific analytic situation.

Freud found that we must distinguish between the manifest and the latent material of the dreams. By manifest content he means the dream as one experiences it, continuous or disconnected, apparently sensible or nonsensical, clear or vague, with or without clear emotions, and often using material taken from experiences of the

---

* Freud, S.: *Autobiography,* pp. 77-80.

last twenty-four hours. This manifest material, which on the whole is of little importance, he also investigated. The real content of the dream is the latent content, i.e., the hidden material which we get through free association. The dream's function is preventive — to keep disturbances away. It also tries to satisfy the desire to sleep and at the same time to gratify underlying strivings of the personality. The stimuli may be sensations in the body (hunger, thirst, pain, sex). There is a marked difference in the ability to obtain satisfaction of these stimuli in dreams. Psychic stimuli which might disturb the sleep are kept away through the satisfaction obtained in hallucinatory projections in the dream. Dream experiences are always distorted. Even in dreams the personality seems unable to accept all strivings and desires openly. Various tendencies may be unacceptable from an ethical, aesthetic, or social point of view. The elements of the dream are therefore translated or distorted into other elements, which Freud calls symbolic, and these are symbols of the unconscious dream-thoughts. Many of the symbols which we find in dream life are also found in daily life. Others cannot be found in modern language but only in the more symbolic language of primitive peoples and times.

Freud states that the distortion of the dream is caused by the "dream work," which converts the latent dream into the manifest dream. Through his method of interpretation, the physician's aim is to do the opposite, i.e., to reach the latent content from the manifest dream. In the actual analysis of the dream, the physician must sometimes offer symbolic interpretations to the patient, but he should do so as little as possible and should always try to select the most suitable moment. A "censor" between the latent and manifest material of the dream does not allow the underlying strivings to enter the dream fully. This censor works out the compromise of the repressed desires. In the analysis the censor shows itself as resistance. Parts of dreams are frequently temporarily forgotten. Experience shows that these dream elements are usually of utmost importance and their recollection and analysis is often the shortest way to an understanding of the whole dream. A striking feature in the dream work is the tendency to condensation, i.e., to the fusion of two or more different thoughts, persons, events, or desires into one. Words which have a double meaning are therefore often used. Another feature is the mechanism of displacement. This means that the latent element is replaced by something that does not seem to have much to do with it, or frequently the old order of the element is changed. Freud calls these features archaic features because the same symbolic language preceded our present word language and is characteristic of the earliest stages of our intellectual development. The study of the working of dreams will therefore give us an understanding of our own intellectual development and will take us back to our earliest childhood and the earliest stages of our race. Through the interpretation of our dreams we can see that there is no void of memory during the first two years of childhood, but that all these memories have been forgotten or repressed. Of minor importance, and in contrast to the censorship which achieves a distortion of the dream, is the tendency toward secondary elaboration, which often fills in gaps in the dream and gives the appearance of something logical.

Dreams are wish fulfillments, or at least attempts at such. In many dreams, anxiety or punishment is the outstanding feature. Some dreams are the gratification of purely sexual desires; others of hunger, thirst, desire for liberty, and egotistical or revengeful tendencies. The dream is a translation of desires and strivings into a more primitive form. Some dreams express the present state of the person in symbolic form; others show a tendency to make a readjustment and to give a solution of certain problems with which the dreamer is at that time especially occupied. Where two succeeding dreams are experienced, the second dream frequently explains the meaning of the first dream or contains the wish fulfillment. It is important to realize that the meaning of the symbol depends on the personality setting. Through free association, the patient will therefore have to arrive at an understanding as to whether or not the interpretations offered are correct.

Because of the censorship, thoughts and desires are allowed to enter from the unconscious in a concealed form only — i.e., in pictures and symbols. Two tendencies which we find in dreams play a role in daily life. The first one is repression. This is the process through which instinctive desires or their ideational presentation are rejected and kept out of consciousness. It is the result of a psychic conflict, a struggle between two desires. This leads to an external and internal privation. Through external privation real gratification becomes impossible. Internal privation tries to destroy even imaginary gratification and tries to make the whole problem non-existent. In the analysis the censorship appears as resistance. The second tendency which Freud pointed out is the process of regression, which has purely to do with sex. Fixation of sexual desires may take place at any stage of development of the sexual life, and libidinous strivings have a tendency to return to the point of fixation. These mechanisms are also seen in the dream.

Freud found that these same mechanisms which we find in dream symbolism are at work in neurotic reactions. The neurotic symptoms are symbols like the symbols in the dream. He also saw that the same mechanism works in our daily life. Phenomena which are well known but not considered important, such as slips of the tongue, mistakes in reading and listening, forgetting, losing things, and errors frequently deserve to be analyzed. These actions are termed symptomatic acts. There is often a motive behind these mistakes and after the motive has disappeared the mistake will not occur again. This does not mean that all these mistakes have a meaning, but many of them do. An error is sometimes the result of two tendencies which interfere with each other. There is an impulse to say or do something, but a counter-impulse, which is hostile to the intention, causes the mistake. We also forget names and experiences in order to keep disagreeable things out of our memory.

In order to understand the present procedure, Freud's fundamental concepts should be briefly formulated. "The theories of resistance and of repression, of the unconscious, of the aetiological significance of sexual life and of the importance of infantile experiences — these form the principle constituents of the theoretical structure of psycho-analysis."* He feels that psychologic factors which have a pathologic influence are always unconscious. The symptom is a substitute for important desires and experiences which have become unconscious. Experiences of earliest childhood which we may remember here and there and which do not seem to have a special meaning are frequently a disguise for important unconscious experiences. It is essential that we uncover the unconscious relations and motives.

* Freud, S.: *Autobiography*, p. 76.

The unconscious consists of forces and drives which cannot become conscious at will. The proof of the existence of an unconscious is obtained through the analysis of dreams, phantasies, mistakes, and neurotic symptoms. The material which forms the unconscious has once been conscious but not being acceptable to the personality, was therefore repressed. Environmental influences in childhood and, later, in addition, the development of the personality cause this process of repression. Repressed activities still maintain a great deal of energy and try to force their way into consciousness. They never succeed directly but appear in changed form. The emotions which are linked to the unconscious forces may be attached to quite unrelated drives and activities (displacement). They may change their direction, or be greatly modified, or appear as symptoms. Material of which we are not aware, but which can enter our consciousness at will, forms the preconscious. This is not repressed material, and is therefore not subjected to the distortive influence of the censor. It can be recalled directly. The unconscious is characterized by its content and methods of working. In the content we find repetitions of desires; i.e., effects, which frequently find a pathologic outlet physically. In every neurosis therefore we find part of the unconscious instinctive life and all the repressed desires and emotions. The object of these repressed desires is also represented in the unconscious. The characteristic features of the working of the unconscious are the ease of displacement and condensation and the tendency to identification and to projection. Further characteristics are the existence of the possibility of contraindications side by side, the leaving out of the associative links, the absence of the concept of time and space, symbolic language, and the substitution of external reality by internal reality.

Freud has paid special attention to analysis of the forces which rule the unconscious. They are formed by the drive for preservation of the self and by sexual instincts. It is important that in reading psychoanalytic discussion, Freud's concepts of sexuality be kept in mind. Sexuality is not merely related to the genital organs but is formulated as a broader function of the body which strives for pleasure. It enters only secondarily into procreation. He further includes under "sexual" all the affectionate and friendly emotions and strivings for which one usually uses the word "love." He postulates therefore that sexual drives do not begin with puberty, but with infancy. Infantile sexuality is the outstanding formative factor in the development of the personality and its analysis is of utmost therapeutic importance.

In the child, sexual instincts first turn to the self as object, later to outside objects. In the first two or three years of life, which form the pre-genital phase, two main phases can be distinguished — the oral phase, in which the mouth is the erotogenic zone; and the anal-sadistic phase, in which the anus and organs of excretion are erotogenic zones. In the latter phase, and also to some extent in the oral phase, aggressive tendencies, which are the forerunners of sadistic tendencies, develop. Between the third and sixth years, all these sexual strivings are united and centered in the genital zone. At this stage of development the heterosexual tendency is fully established. In the pre-genital, and in the early part of the genital, phase, the self is the object of libidinous desires. This tendency is termed, "narcissism." Conflicts with the outer world develop especially at this time, when the child selects as a definite sexual object the parent of the opposite sex. Toward the parent of the same sex the child develops hatred. This triangular situation is called the Oedipus situation. It forms the nucleus of every neurosis, and I shall therefore refer to this, as well as to other features of the sexual development, in the discussion of the treatment of various neurotic reactions. A boy makes the mother his love object and wishes to take the father's place. The relationship of the girl is similar — an affectionate dependence on the father and a need to get rid of the mother, who is superfluous and in the way. When other children arrive, the Oedipus situation expands itself into a family complex. Hate may develop towards the new and undesired arrival and resentment towards the mother, who allows the child to be pushed into the background. With growing up, important changes may occur. A boy may choose his sister as a substitute for his faithless mother. Among several brothers, jealousy and rivalry may develop around a sister. A little girl may take an older brother as substitute for the father or a younger sister as substitute for the child which she has desired in vain from her father.

At the age of about six there follows a period of latency, in which the child uses his energy in the formation of the personality, but the whole genital development is stirred up violently and repeated in an abbreviated form during puberty. In boys, fear of castration closely follows the Oedipus situation. In girls, this is expressed by envy of the male genitalia (referring to the small size of the clitoris). This reaction precedes the Oedipus situation in girls.

In childhood, and therefore in analyzing patients, phantasies play an important role. There are certain phantasies which are present in every child; namely, phantasies about birth, notions of procreation, of assault by adults, and phantasies arising from observations of sexual acts in human beings and animals.

Tendencies which affect the individual development of the sexual life may occur in every phase and may be on an accidental or a constitutional basis. If sexual instincts receive satisfaction at a certain stage of development, the instincts have an urge to repeat themselves, and this then leads to fixation. These points of fixation always exercise an attraction to the sexual instincts and later in life, when actual satisfaction is not possible, the instinctive desires may return to these points of fixation. It is possible that the same individual may have such points in various phases of his sexual development. Regression will then come to a standstill partly at the point of fixation in the latest phase, and will partly proceed to points in earlier phases. One speaks of sublimation when infantile sexual desires are no longer related directly to sex but have been transformed into strivings and activities which relate to ethical, aesthetic, and social aims. The factor of sublimation plays a formative role in the development of the personality and is expressed in many of the interests and strivings of adult life.

Freud offered a theory of the structure of the personality, distinguishing three parts: the ego, the super-ego, and the id. This theoretical subject will be presented briefly. The ego is the personality as it appears to others. Its task is to act and adjust to reality. Part of the ego develops a critical and constantly observing attitude to the ego; in other words, it makes the rest of the ego the object of observation. This part is called the super-ego. In addition to this self-observation, the super-ego comprises the conscience and the ideals of the personality. The development of conscience is a reaction to the Oedipus situation. The formation of ideals is based on early admiration of the parents or of others in authority. Identification with the beloved object, e.g., the mother, and with the feared object, e.g., the father, is the important dynamic factor. This cannot be taken too literally. A cruel mother, for instance, can become an object of fear in a boy and play a corresponding role. Love, related to ideals, and hate, related to persons one fears and connected with anal-sadistic tendencies, are present in the super-ego. Feelings of moral guilt express the conflict between the ego and the super-ego. The id is formed by the instinctive life and receives all the repressed material. The id and the unconscious, however, are not identical, as part of the ego and super-ego are also unconscious. Repressed aggressions, which arise from the conflict between the super-ego and the id, are important in the analysis of many neurotic patients and psychopathic personalities.

Resistance is an unconscious function of the ego and super-ego. Not only the recovery of lost memories, but also the analysis of resistance is important therapeutically. The ego must defend itself against the outer world, the id, and the attitude of the super-ego. Resistance is the force which opposes all these influences and leads to repression as a defense mechanism. Resistance also causes identification and projection, displacement, transformation into the opposite, and transformation of activity into passivity. The ego has a tendency to develop special personality features as a reaction to particular difficulties (the most important characteristics are described under anal-erotic and oral-erotic personalities).

Anxiety has become one of the central problems in psychoanalytic thinking. Although it is present in every neurosis, it is frequently absorbed into the symptoms. With suppression of the symptoms, anxiety will therefore appear. This should be utilized analytically. Anxiety develops in the personality as a reaction to a disturbance in the instinctive life, to dangers in the outer world, and threats from the conscience. It signals danger to the person. Whenever anxiety appears in the treatment, it indicates that repressed forces are coming close to the surface and are threatening the patient. The result may be increased defenses or a working through. It is also possible that the analyst may have created too much anxiety by giving a premature interpretation. Psychoanalytic investigations seem to show that anxiety is of instinctive nature. Its biologic prototype is seen in birth-anxiety. This later develops into psychologic anxiety, which is the basis for later anxiety and is closely related to infantile sexuality, especially the castration complex.

Special attention is paid to the relation between patient and physician. An intensive emotional relationship of the patient to the person of the analyst, for which no explanation can be found in the real circumstances, develops in many analyses without the help of the physician. The patient projects upon the physician the emotions which he has experienced with regard to other people in his life. Marked emotional factors, which vary according to the material elicited, enter into this relationship. Freud calls it transference. It is a re-enactment of old relationships with those people who have been important in the child's development. The most important of these relationships are those with the parents. On the whole, the patient develops an attitude of affection and dependence (positive transference). In some cases a hostile attitude may become dominant and persistent (negative transference). Less frequently the patient's affection may take a sublimated form. During the treatment, one observes the opening phase of the transference situation, which develops into a full-fledged transference (transference neurosis) in which the whole infantile experience with all its attitudes and taboos is repeated. It is important that a dissolution of the transference be achieved at the end of the analysis. The physician must constantly scrutinize his own attitude and investigate the unconscious factors of his counter-transference. Counter-transference which is not analyzed may impede the analysis.

Freud classified the neuroses into "actual" neuroses and psychoneuroses. To "actual" neuroses belong neurasthenia, anxiety neurosis, and hypochondriasis. He feels that these disturbances are due to the inadequacy of the somatic gratification of sex. Personality factors enter, but the psychogenic material in these neuroses is of secondary importance. Freud therefore did not consider pure "actual" neuroses suitable for his treatment. In recent years, however, a less sharp distinction is drawn in the therapeutic procedure between "actual" and psychoneuroses. It is especially felt that the adjustment of psychogenic material in anxiety neuroses is important. The psychoneuroses include hysteria (conversion hysteria), phobias (anxiety hysteria), and compulsive neuroses. Symptoms of an "actual" neurosis frequently precede a psychoneurosis, or symptoms of an "actual" neurosis may arise in the setting of a psychoneurosis.

The psychoneuroses are the field for psychoanalytic treatment. They permit the development of a transference neurosis whereas schizophrenic and paranoic illnesses, being of a narcissistic type, do not yield to the development of a manageable transference. However, in recent years an increasing number of authors have obtained good results in schizophrenic illnesses.

In the beginning, Freud believed that an infantile sexual trauma caused the neurosis. The treatment was conceived to reveal these repressed experiences. This concept has been given up in its original form. Freud soon pointed out that there is a predisposition resulting from the libido fixation plus the accidental traumatic experience. The libido fixation is caused by the sexual constitution, i.e., the ancestral experience, and the patient's infantile experience. More recently some of his followers have reformulated this theory according to present conceptions. The traumatic situation develops when the person (ego) is not able to deal with indistinctive dangers. The trauma is the amount of libido which the individual cannot master at a given time. However, there are children who are subjected to trauma to such an extent that they cannot avoid developing a neurosis. Studying the infantile trauma, one should look for the possibility of external infantile experiences and internal trauma. The internal trauma depends upon constitutional factors, i.e., fixation, or, in other words, disturbance in the libido development. Predisposing constitutional tendencies are considered but are less utilized in treatment than the analysis of the factors for their development into the present personality traits. The main therapeutic issue is to make the patient understand why he was not able to deal with his desires, which were repressed. This leads to a classification of the role of his standards (super-ego) and unconscious forces and drives (id). The neurotic conflict is the struggle between the personality (ego) and repressed desires. The frustrated desires find their expression in neurotic symptoms. The reappearance of repressed phantasies is the first sign of unsuccessful repression.

Instead of trying actively to overcome the difficulties of reality, the neurotic patient escapes from them into the illness. The symptom formation is different in the various types of psychoneuroses. In conversion hysteria we deal primarily with repression and the displacement of the genital libido to a non-sexual organ. Displacement and condensation are used by the unconscious. The hysterical symptom has absorbed the anxiety which was caused by the danger of a situation. In phobias, the object of the instinctive desires is repressed, but the desires themselves have been only partly repressed. The patient therefore must struggle against these partly repressed desires and experiences anxiety, which is displaced by the substitutive symbol. Phobias are of genital origin, but show a definite sadistic tendency. In obsessive-compulsive neuroses, we deal not only with a refusal of the instinctive desires and their repression, but with a more important regression to the earlier points of fixation and a reaction to the anal-sadistic tendencies. This leads to a change of the personality and the development of an intolerant character. The desires are unsuccessfully repressed, and therefore appear in obsessions and compulsions. In perversions, the object of the desire has been repressed, but the desire itself remains conscious and the patient becomes enslaved.

I shall not go further into a discussion of the various psychoneuroses, as I will refer to the pertinent psychoanalytic conceptions in the chapters on hysteria, phobias, obsessive-compulsive neuroses, and sexual maladjustments.

Based on these concepts, psychoanalytic treatment is interested in the underlying motives and factors (primary disease process) and not in symptoms (secondary process). The goal is not sexual freedom, but the freedom of the instinctive life in its broadest sense. The patient learns to understand what his desires are (the understanding of the id); what the attitude of the personality is to them (attitude of the super-ego); to what extent it is desirable to modify this attitude, and how he can and wants to deal with his desires (attitude of the ego). This leads to an adjustment to reality. Energies which have been penned up in the struggle with the instinctive strivings are freed for other uses. The insufficient harmony of the personality is changed to a synthesis of the personality with continuity and uniformity. By means of the transference relationship, the conflict between the patient and physician is substituted for the inner conflict. The patient is not only in a love relationship to the physician, and therefore able to overcome his resistance, but he also feels protected and therefore has the courage to find the repressed material. This leads to a retrograde analysis of the development of his personality, making conscious the conflicts which caused specific developments based on the factors of fixation and repression. The patient learns to view the repressed material as unreal and to lose his anxiety with regard to it. He also learns to accept painful experiences. The need for causality is highly utilized in the treatment and it is the physician's goal constantly to instill doubt as to the correctness of the patient's formulation.

If a case is found suitable for psychoanalytic treatment, the physician should offer a few explanations before the actual treatment starts. The patient is advised not to expect recovery in a definite period of time, and guesses as to duration are declined. If an estimate is urgent, a rough indication may be promised after a few weeks' analysis. It is advisable that a whole hour be given to the treatment, daily, or at least several times a week. The patient and the physician should adhere strictly to the time allotted. Exceptions to this rule may be necessary when the patient is going through a crisis. The financial question ought to be settled before treatment begins. Free treatment is inadvisable, not only because it demands too time-consuming a sacrifice from the physician, but also because the financial responsibility is a therapeutic stimulus for the patient. Whenever possible, the patient should pay at least a token fee.

The opening phase covers the period from the beginning of the treatment until a reliable enough transference has been developed so that one can proceed with interpretations. At the start, the patient is made acquainted with the fundamental rule that he shall say whatever comes to his mind. From the moment this has been accepted, a large part of the physician's work until the end of the treatment will consist of an endeavor to circumvent its evasion. Difficulty in producing associations, as well as too easy associations, may be indications of resistances. The amount of affect accompanying them must be observed. During this phase, encouragement and active help may be offered, but on the whole, it is the rule that the physician should never become too far removed from an expectant, passive attitude. Interpretations are offered merely to ease obstacles in the progress of the associations, and are rarely deep. Unconscious drives electively influence the flow of associations and it becomes gradually obvious in which way the pleasure principle tends to operate. Floating positive and negative transferences are expressed frequently. The goal of these phases is to allay anxiety, to allow for preliminary modification of the patient's super-ego, and thereby permit a more or less unhampered development of the transference situation. The preliminary floating transferences merge impercep-tibly with the affects which are caused by the analytic situation and the fundamental rule. This may cause the first crisis in the analysis. Many of these crises can be avoided by the analyst's awareness of the presence of transference from the start and the recognition of the patient's expectations of him. Because his symptoms have dis-appeared or because of a frankly hostile attitude, the patient dis-continues the treatment. The defense forces (resistances) now work more openly than previously.

The resistances which appear during the entire analysis are recog-nized in the general negativistic behavior of the patient, his inability to live up to the free association rules and to accept the physician's interpretations, his dearth of associations and silences, new symp-toms or exacerbations of old ones, and slips of the tongue. The most successful resistances are unobtrusive and the physician may not be aware of them. They can, for example, be recognized in the standstill of the analysis. Resistances may utilize projections, dis-placement, distortion, rationalization, or amnesia. Both positive and negative transference can be used as defense mechanisms. According to their origin, five groups of resistances can be distinguished: (1) repression or defense resistances — to prevent unconscious presenta-tions from becoming conscious in the analysis; (2) transference-resistances — the patient evades recollection through the re-enact-ment or repetition of infantile experiences (see also p. 93); (3) resistances caused by the gain through illness; (4) resist-ances caused by guilt feelings and a need for self-punishment; (5) resistances caused by the inertia of instinctual urges, i.e., of the id. In addition, resistances can be set up by the analyst's counter-transference. It is the task of the analysis to release the dammed-up instinctive desires and find for them a way into consciousness. Re-sistance is the patient's attempt at self-protection and cannot be overcome by direct attack but has to be undermined. It is not only necessary that the patient's repressed material be made conscious, but also that interrelations are recognized. The process of making repressed material conscious leads to a freeing of psychic energy and is therefore more than mere abreaction.

Resistances are not merely uncovered, but the patient is urged to go deeper into his unknown resistances by means of free associations. He "works through" the resistance and overcomes it by going on with free associations despite the resistance. Only thus will patient and physician succeed in finding the underlying repressed strivings. Through this experience, the patient becomes convinced of the existence and strength of resistance. The physician cannot force this result and must wait patiently. He should not offer deep interpretations until a strong transference has developed. It is not the aim to offer solutions but to present ways which are unknown to the patient. If interpretations are offered too early, the patient will stop treatment either because he develops marked resistance or because he obtains relief. One should remember that the desire to get well, which comes from suffering, is the main therapeutic force until a strong transference has developed. Even later, suffering forms the drive for recovery, diminishing with improvement. The patient's intellectual interest, which develops with the progress of treatment, is a far less important therapeutic factor than this desire for recovery. The secondary gains from the illness, which are found in the analysis, work against these forces. A patient may be masochistic, continuing analysis although he is not helped by it. Interpretations show the patient the unknown ways to recovery, and transference allows him to overcome resistance. Transference alone may remove symptoms but this will last only as long as the transference persists. This phenomenon corresponds to that of suggestive therapy. In psychoanalysis, the intensity of the transference is used to overcome resistance. If this has been done, the patient cannot remain ill even when transference is dissolved.

In the transference phase, the ground of the patient's conflict has been shifted to the analytic situation itself. The previous discussions had dealt with external situations and maladaptations of a symptomatic kind. An almost imperceptible change in the atmosphere of the analysis has taken place. The free associations produce more and more material which deals with the present day. The patient becomes preoccupied with the situation in the physician's office and his immediate relations with him. The main therapeutic task is to make this unconscious set of attitudes conscious. Interpretations are now expected by the patient. They should only be given if they explain unconscious factors and not because the patient demands them. Everything which transpires during the analytic situation relates to the transference situation. Numerous fragments of information about the infantile development and modes of thinking are accumulated and many minor reactions noticed. All these facts refer to both the instinctual and conscious development of the personality. In the interpretation of transference manifestations, these two aspects have to be kept separated so that the patient is led back to the unconscious roots of the transference-phantasy from the point of view of both the libido and ego. In addition, interpretations aim to overcome immediate obstacles.

When the patient's thoughts lead him into the realm of the unconscious, he does not necessarily remember his unconscious strivings but may express them in action. It is important that the analyst anticipate and prevent acting out by means of proper interpretations. It is the physician's task to make the patient "fit these emotions into their place in the treatment and in his life-history, subject them to rational consideration, and appraise them at their true physical value. This struggle between physician and patient, between intellect and the forces of instinct, between recognition and the striving for discharge, is fought out almost entirely over the transference manifestations."*

In transference two kinds of libidinous strivings are active — the strivings which are conscious to the person and at his disposal and those which have become arrested and are either unconscious or expressed in fancies. These libidinous strivings turn towards the person of the physician. ". . . the patient will weave the figure of the physician into one of the 'series' already constructed in his mind. If the physician should be specially connected in this way with the father-imago . . . it is quite in accordance with his actual relationship to the patient; but the transference is not bound to this prototype; it can also proceed from the mother- or brother-imago

* Freud, S.: *Collected Papers*, Vol. II, p. 322.

and so on. The peculiarity of the transference to the physician lies in its excess, in both character and degree, over what is rational and justifiable — a peculiarity which becomes comprehensible when we consider that in his situation the transference is effected not merely by the conscious ideas and expectations of the patient, but also by those that are under suppression, or unconscious." *

In contrast to the abreaction of the emotions which accompanied the original experience, the patient projects onto the physician. The analyst becomes to him the figure under discussion. He represents, at various times, various people who have played a role in his life, especially in childhood. These identifications throw light on the nature and development of the ego-ideal. As soon as one identification is analyzed, an earlier one takes its place, leading further backward in the personality development. Emotions of love as well as hate, resentment, and fear are projected onto him. Phantasies or real experiences are re-enacted. Specific situations, such as the Oedipus and castration situations, are re-enacted many times over a prolonged period. The analyst "must guard against ignoring the transference-love, scaring it away or making the patient disgusted with it; and just as resolutely must he withhold any response to it. He must face the transference-love boldly, but treat it like something unreal, as a condition which must be gone through during the treatment and traced back to its unconscious origins, so that it shall assist in bringing to light all that is most hidden in the development of the patient's erotic life, and help her to learn to control it."** An argument against the genuineness of this love is the unmistakable element of resistance and the fact "that it shows not a single new feature connecting it with the present situation, but is entirely composed of repetitions and 'rechauffes' of earlier reactions, including childish ones. One then sets about proving this by detailed analysis of the patient's behavior in love. When the necessary amount of patience is added to these arguments, it is usually possible to overcome the difficult situation and to continue the work, the patient having either moderated her love or transformed it; the aim of the work then becomes the discovery of the infantile object-choice and of the phantasies woven round it."† In the patient's behavior and feelings

* *Ibid.*, pp. 313-314.
** Freud, S.: *Collected Papers*, Vol. II, p. 385.
† *Ibid.*, pp. 386-387.

towards the physician the patient can see his original reactions which had been repressed.

Transference is the mirror of the patient's development. The patient presents infantile demands which cannot be gratified by the analyst, and resistances which must be analyzed may result. If transference becomes erotic, it is a means of avoiding the study of the real infantile desires. The intensity and extent of transference is the result and expression of resistance. One can only gain an understanding of the role of transference in the treatment if one studies its relation to resistance. The physician should not touch upon the transference problem as long as thoughts come freely and until a strong transference has developed. When the patient is unable to proceed, or mentions thoughts which are connected with the situation of the moment, the physician points the resistance out to the patient and states that it most likely has to do with the person of the physician. This serves as an opening for uncovering the transference. One should never urge a patient into transference. It takes from the phenomenon of transference the convincing character of spontaneity and creates for the physician handicaps which are difficult to overcome.

Freud insists that the physician should merely guide the patient and not take any active part. This type of passivity does not mean inactivity. The physician offers interpretations, never dogmatically, however, but merely as possibilities. He does not wish to appear infallible and is willing to admit readily his incorrect interpretation if further material proves this. Interpretations are essential. The physician not only has his experience through which he is equipped to understand unclear reactions better than the patient, but he also has the advantage of the detached onlooker. He can see connections and casual factors while the patient is struggling with repressions and resistance. The patient needs a guiding interpreter to understand the unintelligible language of symbols. Many of them have an individual meaning whereas others are of more or less universal significance. Interpretations offered at a suitable time clarify bewildering situations, help to overcome resistance, and further the production of more unconscious material. Premature interpretations may increase resistance temporarily and delay further analysis. It is important that a physician guard against the dogmatic interpretation of symbols or too readily consider the meaning of symbols universal.

Interpretations will vary according to the progress of the analysis and the patient's understanding of the dynamic factors and their interrelations. The patient ought to take a critical attitude toward the interpretations offered (those dealing with dreams, resistance, symptoms, and symptomatic reactions) and try to lead to a discovery of the underlying strivings and desires. The first interpretations deal with motives that are on the surface; later ones go deeper and often stir up the whole personality. The patient at first may reject these interpretations, but he will accept them as correct when he can see their validity himself. He then develops a feeling of conviction.

Analysis of dreams is important whenever dreams are brought up. The patient is not advised to report dreams as had been practiced previously, and he is not even asked about them. While in practice it is not possible to reach a thorough understanding of each dream element, it is wise to go as far as possible. The underlying wish fulfillment, anxiety, or punishment factor should always be uncovered. The overproduction of dreams may be an expression of resistance. The physician will then have to omit the analysis of some dreams. The insufficient reproduction of dreams may offer an excellent opportunity to get at repressed material.

The physician may frequently be unable to recognize the dynamic factors in the disguised form in which they appear. He then tries to utilize his own introspective knowledge, picturing himself in the same situation in order to find out to what it corresponds in his own experience. This is done quite spontaneously by the physician, who is urged to abstain from making conscious effort to retain the material which the patient offers and to give his "unconscious memory" full play. The physician's unconscious is the receiving organ for the patient's unconscious. Taking notes is considered undesirable because it leads to a selection of material, the significance of which cannot be fully recognized yet, and focuses the physician's attention on special parts instead of letting him accept the entire material in an unprejudiced way.

Difficulties in the analysis arise with the physician as well as the patient. ". . . every analyst's achievement is limited by what his own complexes and resistances permit and consequently we require that he should begin his practice with a self-analysis and should extend and deepen this constantly while making his observations on his patients."* Through his own analysis the physician is equipped to deal with the reactions which are stirred up in himself. It is also the only way in which he can learn to understand psychoanalytic psychology thoroughly, and develop a strong belief in its correctness. This is the essential basis for a treatment in which the utilization of transference and of interpretation are the main tools. The physician should be neither hypersensitized nor immune so that he is able to listen to the patient's pleasant and unpleasant description of himself. He must guard against being guided too much by his own conceptions and aggressions and a desire for mastery. He may be too eager to indicate points of fixation in the patient's development and to offer explanations. There may be a tendency to talk too much or too little. The patient's resistances may cause corresponding reactions in the physician. In dealing with silences, he needs to find the best way of overcoming the difficulty and has to try encouragement, interpretation, or silence according to the individual case and the occasion. His own oral and anal-sadistic tendencies, homo- or heterosexual urges may become stirred up. A physician must recognize whenever counter-transference and resistance develop and know how to deal with them. He should consider the need for self-inspection when he acts in a stereotyped way, or cannot immediately justify his interventions or silences on good analytical grounds, or cannot explain to himself satisfactorily why the patient is still in difficulty.

In the terminal phase, the physician is under obligation to dissolve the patient's transference. Criteria of termination are not limited to symptomatic considerations. Symptoms may disappear earlier in the analysis. On the other hand, some symptoms may persist even with successful treatment, but merely as husks, drained of their affect. The physician has to be guided primarily by the degree of successful analysis of the instinctual urges and of the ego. He should not rest until he is reasonably certain that he has exhausted the infantile sexual theories and linked them up with the most primitive forms of instinctual expression. "The patient must have made the

---

* Freud, S.: *Collected Papers*, Vol. II, p. 289.

regressive identification already referred to of analyst with super-ego; he must have worked it through and he must, abating his demands on analytic protection, be ready to permit a modified super-ego to function in his own mind. When the analyst feels that these conditions have been satisfactorily approximated to, he may, judging the tempo of the patient's mental adaptation, indicate that the time is approaching for the termination of the analysis." (Glover, p. 96.) Confirmatory evidence of the patient's readiness for termination is found in lack of new material, modifications of recurrent dreams or in dreams which reveal the altered attitude of the patient, in having cleared up childhood memories which had been used as screens for important libidinal urges, and in finding through an exhaustive survey of the infantile sexual theory that all points have come up for thorough discussion. One can also notice changes in the patient's social reactions. In the terminal phase, the usual psychoanalytic rules and technique of interpretation are utilized to dissolve the transference. Plans and dispositions relating to future life will come up spontaneously. The analysis of the problem of being healthy and the reasons for it will achieve the dissolution. One can then frequently see that one no longer deals with a transference neurosis, but with the usual patient-physician relationship and that the neurotic, frightening aspects of the Oedipus situation have subsided. The terminal phase should not be hastened. After a long analysis, it may take from three to nine months. To the danger of separation, patients often react with anxiety symptoms and new phantasies and resistances which need working through.

The original indications and contraindications are still the guiding principles, although some authors have enlarged the therapeutic field to include selected schizophrenic, paranoid, and depressive illnesses and the analysis of young children. The patient should be of rather high intelligence and a somewhat stable personality. Psychoanalysis, except with definite modifications, is not a treatment for psychopathic, inferior personalities. Persons who are older than forty-five or fifty years should also be excluded. They would have to produce too much material, so that a complete analysis would take far too long. In addition, such a personality would be too rigid to expect modification. This point, however, has been revised and age is no longer considered a contraindication if the personality involved seems to be plastic enough to hold out hope for reasonable modification. Psychoanalysis is a slow procedure and therefore is not useful for acute, dangerous, hysterical symptoms in which we need hypnosis (see Chapter III). Psychoanalysis should also be used carefully in patients who are overwhelmed by their tendencies toward rumination or self-analysis, as in some compulsive patients. Moreover, physician and patient should realize before he begins that this kind of treatment takes a long time and is expensive.

Some followers of Freud have proposed technical changes. Ferenczi felt justified in proposing an "active therapy" in which he urged the patient to carry out definite tasks in his daily life, e.g., modifications in the relationship to his family and environment and in his personal habits. This procedure was based on Freud's advice that analysis should be carried on in a state of abstinence because privation is a therapeutic force. This does not mean sexual abstinence, but the attempt to deprive the patient of actions which offer neurotic satisfaction. Sexual satisfaction may be included in certain cases. Substitutive gratification must be forbidden. In anxiety hysteria, Freud even urged patients to expose themselves to the critical situations which caused anxiety attacks. All these interferences led to a stirring up of repressed material. This type of interference is most important in obsessive-compulsive neuroses. Ferenczi interfered with the free flow of associations and directed it back to an earlier topic if he felt that the patient was unconsciously avoiding problems. Habitual day-dreams should be forcibly interrupted. He suggested to patients who were little inclined to produce phantasies that they imagine pictures they ought to have in given situations. He usually requested the following phantasies: 1) positive and negative transference phantasies, 2) phantasies of infantile memories, 3) masturbation phantasies. This is followed by a discussion of the phantasies. Such active therapy should only be used in the later stage of the analysis. Discussing these proposals, Glover warns not to resort to them too readily because the analysis does not seem to progress. One is bound to allow the patient time and place in the transference neurosis to work through certain repetitive scenes. Glover urges the analyst to examine his counter-resistance before he resorts to active interference. Analysis must insist on interpretation

of the patient's material along the lines which are considered fundamental (e.g., repression, infantile sexuality culminating in the
Oedipus complex) and on complete detachment on the analyst's
part.

Others feel that passive therapy should be utilized to the utmost,
as little interpretation as possible offered, and warn against forcing
transference. All agree that the physician should not lose himself
in symptoms and topical analysis, but should consider the analysis
of the personality as the goal. Educational factors play only an
indirect role. The physician forms an ego-ideal for the patient and
acts as an unconscious influence. Freud declined to take an active
part in the synthesis of the personality, but was willing to use a
certain amount of active education in psychopathic individuals who
could not utilize without help the material which analysis brought
to light.

On the whole, analysis should be carried out while the patient
leads a normal life and attends to his interests and duties. Many
authors have argued against hospitalization because transference is
more difficult to establish and resistance more difficult to overcome.
Successful psychoanalytic treatment in hospitals has demonstrated
that these difficulties can be surmounted by having another physician make necessary decisions for the patient. The objection that
hospital life is not a suitable substitute for reality should not be
valid in a psychiatric hospital which is guided essentially by therapeutic principles. There are patients for whom a hospital environment is most beneficial, and analysis should then be carried out
there. The time factor is important and many practitioners therefore
cannot follow Freud's advice that each analysis ought to recover the
infantile sex life before the age of five.

The modern technique has developed from abreaction, primarily
through association technique, to a highly involved procedure which
should be adjusted to the individual case. Instead of exclusive attention to the traumatic theory, the modification of the personality
occupies the physician, taking into consideration psychic and outer
reality and phantasies. The Oedipus complex is the nuclear complex
of the neurosis and the significance of its repetition in the analytic
situation (transference) is highly important, but it is also important
to detach and set free the infantile libido from its fixation on the

first object. The emphasis is laid not only on remembering but also on experience and reproduction. Instead of seeking memories for the purpose of reaching the affect (abreaction), affects are provoked for the sake of uncovering the unconscious. It is also important that one analyze the unconscious factors which caused the patient to seek analysis and the conditions and requirements which he associates with the end of the analysis. The whole development of the individual does not need to be repeated in the analysis, but only those phases in which libido fixation occurred.

Ferenczi and Rank pointed out the following faults in analytic technique: the mere listening and the belief that it is a process of "talking out," with neglect of the dynamic factor of experience; the collecting of associations as if they were in themselves the essential thing; a fanaticism of interpretation; analysis of symptoms; analysis of complexes; indulgence in sexual factors; the dwelling on the analysis of all the elements known from the normal sexual development; use of speculative principles; neglect of the present reactions by paying exclusive attention to the past; offering too much, and prematurely, theoretical knowledge; the tendency to excuse difficulties by the patient's narcissism; the adherence to rigid passivity or "wild" activity.

There are many suggestions as to how Freud's technique can be modified, but it is impossible to present them all here. I have tried to give the fundamental principles and have limited myself to a presentation of Freud's method and have not included in this chapter the theories and methods of former pupils of Freud who have developed their own schools. According to Freud, only those physicians who can accept his concept of the unconscious and his ideas of resistance and repression, his evaluation of sexuality and the Oedipus complex have the right to call themselves psychoanalysts.

BIBLIOGRAPHY

1. FREUD, S.: *Introductory Lectures on Psycho-Analysis*. G. Allen and Unwin, London, 1929.
2. FREUD, S.: *New Introductory Lectures on Psycho-Analysis*. W. W. Norton and Co., New York, 1933. (In these two books Freud presents his psychoanalytic teaching. They should be used as the basis for orientation in this field.)

3. FREUD, S.: *The Interpretation of Dreams*. The Macmillan Company, New York, 1922. (The standard work of dream analysis, offering numerous examples.)

4. FREUD, S.: *Autobiography*. W. W. Norton and Co., New York, 1935. (An autobiographic presentation, offering an understanding of the historic setting and development of psychoanalysis.)

5. FREUD, S.: Papers on Technique. *Collected Papers*, Vol. II. The Hogarth Press, London, 1924.

6. GLOVER, E.: The Technique of Psycho-Analysis. Supplement No. 3 to *The International Journal of Psycho-Analysis*, Baillière, Tindall and Cox, London, 1928.

7. GLOVER, E.: *An Investigation of the Technique of Psychoanalysis*. The Williams & Wilkins Company, Baltimore, 1940.

8. LORAND, S.: *Technique of Psychoanalytic Therapy*. International Universities Press, New York, 1946.

9. FERENCZI, S., and RANK, O.: *The Development of Psycho-Analysis*. Nervous and Mental Disease Publishing Company, New York, 1925.

10. FERENCZI, S.: *Further Contributions to the Theory and Technique of Psycho-Analysis*. The Hogarth Press, London, 1926.

Chapter V

VARIOUS PSYCHOTHERAPEUTIC PROCEDURES

THE TREATMENT of personality disorders by psychobiologic methods has been developed systematically along many lines. The multitude of theories and approaches is bewildering. This is primarily due to the fact that physicians develop specific features of their treatment exclusively because these have been most successful. Most of these methods therefore exert only a temporary, and often merely a local, influence and die with their authors. In this chapter I shall try to give an objective orientation by selecting a few of the most important presentations of those treatments which present different features of fundamental importance.

Three fundamental directions can be distinguished in psychotherapy: suggestion, analysis, and re-education. In the various methods one or the other, alone or in combination, is used. Except for the brief discussion on catharsis, suggestive methods will not be discussed here since this has been done in Chapter III. The analytic approach deserves considerable space for the presentation of various deviations from Freud's psychoanalytic treatment. Re-education receives special consideration as a supplement to the general rules offered in the second chapter.

An analytic treatment with considerable stress on re-education has been outlined by *Alfred Adler*. His theoretical foundation is presented in his *Individual Psychology*. Greatly influenced by Freud, Adler accepted much of the psychoanalytic procedure but modified it on the basis of a theory of "organ inferiority" and its compensations. Rejecting Freud's causal point of view, he proposed the hypothesis that the expectancy of a final goal is of outstanding dynamic importance in the development of the individual personality. In place of Freud's libido theory, he emphasized the striving for self-assertion and superiority. The attitude and adjustment to the group are considered of high importance.

In the first five years of life a goal is set for the need and drive of the personality development. This goal determines the direction of the functions of the personality, offering a promise of security, power, and perfection. In addition, this portentous goal awakens various gratifying feelings of anticipation. A feeling of inferiority is, for instance, diminished by the hope for success. To understand a person means to understand his goal. "Inferiority of organs" leads to biologic and psychologic compensation and frequently to over-compensation. The social and economic conditions in the person-ality development are important. The child's position in the family must be carefully analyzed as well as his attitude to the role of masculinity. Neurotic symptoms arise from inner insecurity, ego-centric orientation, and so great an ambition that it cannot succeed in the conflict with reality. The patient, a discouraged, ambitious person, unwilling to admit defeat, saves his self-esteem by neurotic self-deception.

Treatment consists of an effort to bring all these factors into awareness, as well as re-education which leads to encouragement. The patient is led to try himself out in practical life and to learn from the analysis of arising difficulties how to deal with himself. Tendencies to self-deception are constantly pointed out. The physi-cian should establish a companion-like relationship which will form the first real social relationship in the patient's life. By the con-scious evolution of a feeling for the commonweal and the conscious destruction of the will-to-power, a re-enforced sense of reality, a feeling of responsibility, and a substitution for latent hatred by a feeling of mutual good will develop. With this treatment many authors claim good results in the various types of psychopathic per-sonalities and in the education of difficult children.

In many ways a synthesis of Freud and Adler, but developed along independent lines and always with great emphasis on the per-sonality, is the treatment on which *Jung* based his *Analytical Psy-chology*. He points out four stages in the development of analytical therapy: (1) confession, which utilizes catharsis and attempts to release repressed affects; (2) explanation, in which transference enlightens the patient concerning the factors of unconscious fixation by means of interpretation and a retrograde explanation (Freud); (3) education, based on the principle of finality and the need for power (Adler); (4) transformation of the whole personality lead-ing to self-education (Jung). According to the latter, the personality

as it appears to us is a compromise between the individual and society. Analysis should lead to an understanding of one's self, to
a liberation from the great influence of unconscious pictures, and the
correction of the mask which our personality has constructed as a
concession to the outer world. A thorough analysis is not always
necessary; a brief discussion may often be sufficient. Treatment is
the product of a mutual influence in which the patient's whole
nature as well as that of the physician participates. The physician
should be willing to accept the fact that he also changes during the
treatment. It is therefore essential that he know himself from his
own analysis and that he analyze himself carefully during the treatment of every patient. The physician's transformation, i.e., the self-
education of the educator, is a significant factor in the cure. The
results of psychotherapy depend on the physician's and patient's
personalities.

Considering socially disintegrative forces the dynamic factors in
the individual disturbance, *Burrow* states that unrecognized destructive features of the normal social background are expressed in
neurotic manifestations. He urges the study of the disintegrative
tendencies of the collective socially accepted behavior. The ordinary
everyday reactions of all normal people reveal a deviation of which
the neurotic's socially destructive disposition is but a special instance. In the transference situation the repetition of early social
habits in the patient and in the group is emphasized as well as the
reappearance of poorly assimilated infantile fixations. Any statement, question, or emotional response appearing during the discussion is utilized for an analysis of the motives or of the subjectively
assumed role giving rise to it. In this way the patient becomes aware
of the conflicting tendencies he is expressing.

Rank, a pupil of Freud, considers the analysis of will power the
central therapeutic problem. The psychoanalytic situation is a duel
of the will in which the physician plays the role of counter-will.
He does not attempt to break the patient's will but offers him possibilities for the strengthening of his will. The goal of the analysis is
the transformation of the negative expression of will in the neurosis
into a positive and, if possible, creative will. A constructive therapy
should not attempt to change the individual personality but to develop it so that it can accept itself as it is. In order to provoke ex-

pressions of will which appear in the analysis as the various forms of resistance, Rank fixes a date for the termination of the treatment. The ambivalent attitude of the patient, who desires at the same time the end and the continuation of the treatment, can be recognized as a struggle within himself because of conflict of will. This represents the fundamental conflict of the patient's whole life. The symbols of father and mother represent the two principles of force and love, and the guilt feeling results from the individual's struggle against the will of these two. In the therapeutic links in the love situation, guilt develops as a reaction to wanting to enforce one's own will, and in the third stage it is the reaction to the wish to give oneself through love. From this point of view, transference and resistance must be considered.

Horney deviates considerably from Freud's concepts. She stresses that the character structure is the nucleus of neuroses which needs to be understood. The characteristics are "compulsory strivings, conflicting trends, ... impairment in the relation to self and others, marked discrepancy between potentialities and actual attainments."* It is erroneous to try to "arrive at a direct understanding of the symptomatic picture without first having a grasp of the particular character structure"** and to "relate the patient's actual peculiarities directly to certain childhood experiences and to establish a quick causal connection. . ."† The main effort should be directed at discovering the ways which basic anxiety forces the personality to use in coping with life and how it affects the personality. Instead of investigating the origin and development of neurotic trends (Freud), one should study the actual functions and their consequences. This procedure leads to lessening of anxiety and improved relations to oneself and others. Active interference in a patient's genetic analysis will cause him to study the consequences of particular trends on his character and his life instead of causation. Laying the main emphasis on the study of the actual character structure should not lead to neglect of childhood experiences. To mobilize the patient's constructive forces is just as important as to uncover neurotic forces. Activity on the part of the physician is advised. The analyst should conduct the

---

* Reprinted from *New Ways in Psychoanalysis* by Karen Horney, M.D., by permission of W. W. Norton & Company, Inc. Copyright 1939 by the publishers.
** *Ibid.*
† *Ibid.*

analysis deliberately, urge the patient to arrive at decisions if this seems indicated and to recognize moral values. In many cases an active and direct study of the actual problems will be sufficient and make a systematic analysis unnecessary.

The *Washington School of Psychiatry* accepts the influence of past events, including early childhood, but looks for the dynamics in psychotherapy in the present status of the patient and in his relationship with his physician. The physician assumes an active role. But even when he behaves merely as an observer he is participating and the patient, who senses these reactions, will react to them. Progress will be made when persistent strivings toward success and contentment appear in the patient-physician relationship. The physician must supply foresight to the patient and prevent impulsive acts. The patient must learn to understand his actions and his relationship with others. The degree of awareness of one's interpersonal relations indicates whether or not a person has obtained satisfactory mental health.

One form of treatment which is much used by general practitioners, especially in minor disturbances, although they are usually not aware of its author, is the "persuasion" of *Dubois*. In this method, the physician tries to clarify the development of the symptoms and their relation to situational and personality difficulties. He also explains to the patient the interrelations of these factors and how the difficulties and symptoms can be overcome. He points out how past emotional disturbances were reactions to certain difficulties, how such tendencies have been developed, and how habits of behavior have been formed. The connection between emotional disturbances and physical manifestations is presented, especially influences on cardiovascular, respiratory, and gastrointestinal functions, and on the skin. Examples are utilized freely for illustration. The importance of anticipation, fear, and self-observation is emphasized; thus, anticipation and fear precipitate symptoms which are increased by self-observation. They increase harmless sensations of which we are usually not aware. Difficulties in concentration, fatigue, and various sensations are caused by emotional excitability, instability, and irritability. A vicious cycle is established and has to be broken. Through chance, or because of emotional factors, various symptoms develop and are then increased by fear and self-observation, leading to an increase in symptoms, and this, in turn, to more fear and self-observation. In such a way, unhealthy habits are formed and finally the neurotic picture results.

The patient must learn to understand through the physician's explanations that he has overevaluated his illness and now needs to diminish the importance of his complaints, that he has had a wrong conception of his illness, and that he must correct the faulty intellectual and emotional attitudes that are increasing his symptoms. Different explanations are offered according to the patient's personality and his intellectual capacity. After the patient, as a result of these explanations, has developed an understanding and is willing to accept the physician's formulation, he must be encouraged to draw practical conclusions. He must be willing to accept his difficulties and to correct his habits.

Dubois believed that his treatment appealed entirely to the patient's intellect, making him master of himself through the education of will and reason. The problems which the patient does not understand are those of liberty, will (choosing, resisting, and yielding), and responsibility. The physician is the educator whose task it is to give the patient a more realistic attitude. He emphasizes the need to impress the patient with one's conviction of the cure and to develop this conviction in the patient. In this there is naturally a strong element of suggestion. Explanations offered authoritatively are also suggestions and therefore carry far toward influencing symptoms. Dubois' treatment is the basis for Déjérine's therapeutic approach.

Persuasion is valuable in combination with re-education in the treatment of minor complaints, especially in hypochondriasis and anxiety symptoms. It is essential that correct time allocations be made possible. In cases of long duration the use of A. Meyer's life chart is especially valuable. In abbreviated form this procedure is used in the formulation offered at the end of a diagnostic consultation.

Many methods have been advised to establish relaxation, some working primarily from the psychologic, others from the physiologic, level. Massage and gymnastics belong to the latter group. Emotional catharsis as a psychologic means for producing relaxation was outlined by Frank. Similar procedures have been outlined recently by other authors. The patient is advised to lie on a couch and to let himself reach a slightly drowsy state by assuming complete passivity. Looking straight ahead, his eyes usually soon get tired. When closing his eyes, still looking straight ahead, first dots, and then scenes, or symbolic expressions will appear in the visual field. These reproductions, accompanied by strong emotions, appear suddenly and with great strength. Emotions may also appear without being accompanied by images. The patient remains in a passive attitude and does not try to guide or push away the scenes. The persistent absence of pictures is taken as an indication of resistance. Sessions last 15 minutes to an hour. Each session is followed by a brief, constructive discussion of the emotional experiences. This type of treatment is little used although good results have been claimed in patients with persistent tension, sleep difficulties, and gastrointestinal or cardiovascular reactions caused by emotions. In children and adolescents relief from pent-up emotions and an understanding of spite reactions may be obtained, and an inability to discuss problems can be overcome. The therapeutic goal is not only elimination of emotional tension but to obtain through the ensuing discussion an objective attitude by the patient to his emotions and undigested past experiences. This type of treatment is symptomatic and insufficient without an analysis of the personality.

Analytic treatment leads to an understanding of the factors which play a role in the illness and in personality difficulties. Analysis is insufficient in many persons who, in addition, must be taught how they can change well-established habits and make constructive use of the acquired insight. This is also true of other psychotherapeutic approaches, and physicians should therefore always resort to re-education in certain cases, especially in the poorly organized psychopathic personality. Re-education is used in many ways. To deserve the term psychotherapy, it should be based on an understanding of the personality so that the patient's resources are utilized. It is working with the patient, not forcing him into the correction of old, and the development of new, habits. A helpful attitude on the part of the patient, based on as thorough an understanding of his difficulties as is possible under the circumstances, is necessary to produce lasting results.

Planned re-education as an adjunct to dynamic psychotherapeutic methods is valuable. Based on an understanding of personality factors and on the psychopathologic findings, re-education may be directed to achieving a change in the patient's attitude to himself, to the group, to difficulties in his life, faulty habits of thinking, and unhealthy imaginations. The patient must learn to recognize and accept his responsibilities.

The physician should be willing to use whatever method promises best results — analysis, suggestion, or persuasion. An understanding of the patient and his difficulties is of fundamental importance and permits a clear vision of what can and should be achieved. A certain plasticity of the patient is necessary for successful treatment. Symptoms should be taken as an expression of the whole personality. The main problem is to change the patient's attitude. The training and education of the will, which has been exclusively emphasized by some authors, is therefore merely of secondary importance, although it should be stressed especially in certain cases. Training of the whole personality and formation of better habits is achieved in the course of dealing with specific demands and situations. Through success, increasing self-confidence develops, and the patient is then able to deal with more difficult problems. Best results are obtained in fatigue, hypochondriacal reactions, and general poor life adjustment. The stress on re-education is valuable in dealing with psychopathic personalities, with adolescents and difficult children, and with severe psychopathologic disorders of the adult and of the aging period. The most frequent serious mistake in re-educational therapy is over-emphasis on training and work with neglect of psychotherapy.

Analysis of actual situations is most helpful. The resultant understanding is not sufficient if it does not lead to a realization of what the goals should be for the patient's strivings. Accordingly, rules for normal behavior must be offered to the individual. Cooperation of the physician with persons in the environment is necessary in treating children, especially with parents and teachers. To be adequate, the treatment must establish a philosophy of life, persistence in pursuing a goal, control of one's sexual desires, and an ability to deal with the traumas of life. The patient should learn to derive satisfaction from life. Extreme idealism and extreme scepticism such as seen in adolescence, exaggerated realism or materialism —

all these should be corrected. A practical adjustment of these attitudes is necessary as well as the adjustment to school and work and to other people. Escape from one's own difficulties by forgetting in intoxication or pleasure must be avoided. The educational factor of self-denial is highly valuable.

In recent years considerable effort has been directed toward the development of the techniques which will permit a shortened duration of treatment.

Brief psychotherapy may use the technique of shortening the course of treatment, using fewer interviews, or limiting the therapeutic sessions. The technique is not satisfactorily worked out yet nor are the indications for it well defined. There is obviously a grave danger that brief psychotherapy may become superficial. It can be used only by a psychiatrist who knows psychopathology and dynamic psychotherapy.

In shortening the course of psychoanalytic therapy as presented by Alexander and French, the therapeutic success depends on the following factors — the physician's ability to recognize the precipitating difficulty in relation to the patient's personality, the patient's capacity for gaining insight and his ability to utilize this insight to make changes in his life, and the patient's ready confidence in his physician who should be well fitted to help the particular patient. In each case the plan of treatment should be based on the appraisal of the patient's personality and the problems in his life which he has not been able to solve. The physician must decide whether he should use a primarily supportive type of treatment, or an analysis of the underlying dynamic factors, or direct his efforts at changing external conditions.

Supportive therapy aims at supporting the patient's ego without attempting essential changes, e.g., the reduction of the disturbing emotions which affected the patient's self-confidence, of his guilt feelings, and of chronic anxiety. An analysis and manipulation of the personality, or of the environment, or of both, may be indicated. By drawing constantly on one's knowledge of psychodynamics one can plan the procedure and consider possible modifications. Brief psychotherapy is an active treatment in which the physician should interfere with the patient's acting out. Therapy is intense and effective if the patient can be kept close to his actual life problems. As this treatment is based upon emotional support, the establishing of a transference neurosis should be avoided. A good transference relationship, however, is important for therapeutic success. The patient's personality and the conflict which is presented as well as the physician's personality and his particular skill should determine the type of transference relationship which the physician should actively encourage or discourage. The physician's attitude, for example, may encourage or discourage dependence. The skillful use of interpretation (of the patient's actions, attitudes, dreams, and phantasies) permits the physician to foster the type of relationship which seems indicated.

The above-mentioned authors consider emphasis on the traumatic infantile experiences in the etiology of neurosis justified only in severe chronic psychoneuroses and psychoses, but do not consider it valid for the "acute nervous breakdown." The patient's ability to express his aggressiveness to the physician is the outstanding therapeutic factor. By means of the transference relationship, the patient learns to overcome emotional conflicts which were unbearable. A genetic reconstruction of the past is necessary for the physician but not for the patient in whom emotional experience should replace an intellectual genetic understanding. The time in the patient's life when he refused to mature by yielding to the constantly changing requirements of life is considered the beginning of the neurosis. Recalled material which antedates this phase is an expression of resistance and not of deep penetration into the sources of the neurosis.

Brief psychotherapeutic interviews make use of the principles of distributive analysis in which various degrees of transient or permanent patient-physician relationships may develop, from mere rapport to the above-described transference relationships. A psychodynamic analysis, based on the modern genetic-dynamic approach, is important in every patient. General dynamic principles must form the basis of this treatment, and, "whenever possible, should be supported by the dynamic study of the individual patient. The knowledge of dynamic psychopathology permits the physician to recognize unclear factors and deal with them instead of having the patient make an attempt at analysis of all repressed factors. The result is an active guiding of the patient by means of constant evaluation of the changing psychopathology as well as the underlying psychodynamic factors. For general guidance concerning the pace of the treatment, one should be directed by the patient's success in dynamic adjustment, by his symptomatic improvement, and by warning signals which demand a decrease of psychotherapeutic pressure or a new orientation in the therapeutic plan.*

"At the beginning of treatment, discussions of one hour's duration are indicated, even in patients with marked psychopathology, until one has obtained a good understanding of the psychopathology, of the life development, of interpersonal relationships, of present life adjustment, and of obvious difficulties. During this phase a positive patient-physician relationship will become established.**" After these initial interviews, the physician should select the therapeutic goals and focus the therapeutic attack on specific facts and factors. With the progress of treatment, the original plan will become modified. "The subsequent interviews, once a week to once a month, may last from fifteen minutes to an hour. It is possible to shorten the interviews because one has become intimately acquainted with the life pattern, the personalities in it, and the repetitious emotional involvements. The progressive treatment usually leads to a marked dependence on the physician, who should utilize this relationship to make the patient carry an increasing amount of responsibility.

"The goal of treatment should be a new orientation to the problems related to the illness and to interpersonal relations. Increasing self-reliance should go together with better socialization. The modification of rigid standards will permit a better dealing with the problems of reality. A more detached and tolerant attitude to body appearance and somatic functions should be striven for. Planned re-education must be pursued to modify and, if possible, change the patient's undue attention to detail, his indecision, egocentricity, and indulgence in phantasy life."*

This type of treatment may become superficial, because the analysis of the psychodynamic factors may not be far-reaching enough; the emotional reactions and resistances may not be worked through sufficiently; the analysis may be symptomatic; the physician may be guided by impression instead of dynamic understanding; he may lec-

* Brief Psychotherapeutic Interviews in the Treatment of Epilepsy. *American Journal of Psychiatry*, 103, 1947.
** *Ibid.*

ture instead of offering formulations based on the facts obtained, or he may make decisions instead of letting the patient reach them. The treatment will be safe if it is based on sound genetic-dynamic psychopathology and a judicious use of the patient-physician relationship.

Brief psychotherapeutic interviews are desirable in patients who suffer from psychopathologic disorders in which dissociation plays a minor role and in which the main dynamic factors are readily available (recurrent emotional reactions with somatic symptoms). They are also indicated in chronic conditions in which a correction of the psychodynamics is possible to only a limited extent (chronic schizophrenic, paranoic, arteriosclerotic, and chronic psychoneurotic illnesses). Patients in whom continued psychotherapeutic support is part of life adjustment react well to this procedure. To this latter group belong many psychopathic personalities, epileptic disorders, and oligophrenic maladjustments.

Group psychotherapy has been practiced extensively in the armed forces, but the leading principles have not been well established as yet. It is comforting for a patient to know that he shares his symptoms and psychopathologic reactions with others and his anxieties may therefore diminish. Mass suggestion may have a strong healing influence. Catharsis of strong resentment, and to a less extent of other emotions, may be helpful if one does not permit it to become repetitious. Confession in public may be helpful in some individuals and destructive in others. Through planned information by the physician the patients may learn to recognize the relationship of isolated features to the total situations. With recurrent group meetings a positive relationship to the other participants will develop and lead to an integration which may become helpful in daily life. The personal relationship of the physician to the individual patients and to the group as a whole will become strong and many of the well-known features in the patient-physician relationship will be apparent. On the other hand, this dynamic factor is insufficiently understood in group therapy.

The technical procedure varies considerably but it seems to be generally accepted that the group should not be larger than about a dozen participants from similar age groups, with similar psychopathologic conditions and intelligence. It is important that every patient be carefully studied before he is included so that his psychopathologic and personality features are known. Some physicians like to influence patients primarily through lectures in which they apply Dubois' persuasion technique, suggestion, and the general principles of re-education, while others present psychodynamic principles. Dramas may be used by the members of the group for living out emotions and psychodynamic factors, for getting enjoyment from play, and for socialization. Other physicians prefer seminar discussions or combine group psychotherapy with individual discussions. At present group therapy is dependent on the enthusiasm of a few but, with better understanding, it may become a therapeutic tool which can be applied in in- and out-patient treatment of well-selected psychotherapeutic problems.

Child psychotherapy — Psychotherapeutic procedures for children are greatly influenced by the theories of various authors. Two divergent viewpoints will be mentioned because they underlie current dynamic therapeutic procedures. M. Klein is interested in the unconscious phantasies which she believes can be reached through offering the child an interpretation of symbolic expressions of his play and other actions. Her advice is to disregard the unconsciously biased reports of the parents and the actual problems of the child's life. A. Freud bases her therapeutic approach on the understanding of the child's personality. Her method is to keep in touch with the patient's daily life and to use reports offered by parents as a welcome source of information. The treatment consists of the study of the defenses of the ego against instinctual drives. Psycho-dynamic interpretation should be offered when the child is ready for it. The physician must gain the patient's confidence, playing the role of the helpful adult to whom emotions are transferred. This transference relationship (not a transference neurosis) is an essential therapeutic factor. A special problem in gaining the child's confidence is presented by the fact that he frequently may not suffer from his symptoms and is not coming spontaneously for help but is being brought by the parents. The parents' cooperation is of utmost importance. The role of the mother is especially important — the child's illness is hurting her self-pride, and the child's sharing of his secrets with the physician, to the exclusion of the mother, causes jealousy. The mother, even if she is not suffering from a psychoneurosis, therefore deserves constant therapeutic attention. Some psychiatrists prefer to offer this help themselves, whereas others help the mother through specially trained social workers and reserve their therapy for the child exclusively. While all psychiatrists stress the need of advice from the psychologist, some, in addition, like to combine their efforts with psychologically trained educators.

The use of play as a therapeutic means of expression has proved to be most valuable, especially in children from about two to seven, and in more modified form till an age of eleven to twelve. Any play activity as well as any other kind of action during the therapeutic session (drawing; clay modeling; conversation; as well as the telling of stories or actual experiences, day-dreams, and dreams) are used therapeutically. It is essential that the physician, as observer and interpreter, be patient but primarily passive. The degree of therapeutic activity depends on the child, his therapeutic problem at the time, and the physician's therapeutic concepts. Play therapy should be based on a sound understanding of the varying modes of play in various age groups. In nursery school age (two to five) Despert developed the technique of offering dolls, which represent in facial expression and dress a man, a woman, and two children. One of these latter dolls becomes the patient, and the other a sibling. These dolls are chosen because the life of the children of this age group is primarily related to father, mother, and sibling. In older children other toys and other play activities are indicated. It is important that children be free in their play and interfered with only if aggressiveness against the physician or destructiveness go beyond acceptable limits. There are obviously marked differences of opinion with regard to the limits of free expression.

In older children and in the early adolescent groups, the therapeutic methods of psychiatric investigation are adjusted to the child's development. In all children the learning to share experiences with somebody else is important. Through the patient-physician relationship, relief from anxiety and other disturbing emotions can be achieved; security can be established within himself and to his parents; stable standards with social integration can be developed, and a clear perspective obtained.

Well-planned re-education is of great importance in the minor adjustment difficulties in childhood and adolescence, and this is also true with many adults. It therefore has an important place in mental hygiene.

Indirect Methods: Many patients have great difficulty in discussing their problems, or are unable to see that they have problems which deserve full investigation. It is therefore desirable to have available *indirect methods* which reveal underlying strivings or preoccupations. Material which has been obtained in this way serves the physician not only as a guide for his approach but, after due explanation, demonstrates to the patient the need for discussion. The dream analysis of Freud and the analysis of certain mistakes and errors, slips of the tongue, and incidental forgetting belong to the group of such indirect investigation.

One should always note the patient's behavior and gestures during an interview and draw his attention to them if this goes with the plan of treatment. One patient, for example, played with her engagement ring while discussing a previous love affair which she insisted was settled. At a later interview, when reminded of the ring-play, the patient realized that she had not been able to free herself completely from her previous lover, and was uncertain about her present engagement. Another patient in the first interview, when asked about her father's death, reached for a cigarette and then proceeded to discuss this apparently well-adjusted fact of years past with ease. This and two other similar motions on two different occasions were pointed out to her. It led to an understanding of a still persisting hate of her father.

Dreams offer many possibilities of therapeutic attack, but "typical" dreams are not frequent enough to be used in general psychotherapy, especially in treatments which need to be of more or less short duration. The indirect approach through hypnosis is also rarely fitted for such occasions.

An especially helpful method has been worked out by Jung in his *association experiment*. He presents verbally one hundred words to the patient, who is requested to answer with the first thought which comes to him. Delay in answering or unusual associations indicate that a sensitive problem has been touched. At the end, the one hundred words are repeated with the request to give the same answer as the first time (in the repetition the reaction time is not measured). The inability to do this may indicate that the person used a cover answer the first time and is unable to remember it. He answers in the repetition with the thought which occurred to him originally or he again tries to find an evasive answer. The reaction time is then frequently prolonged. When a patient cannot understand the word or repeats it before he gives an answer, he is usually stirred up by the stimulus. Other indicators are answers with more than one word, slips of the tongue, perseveration of words or mood seen in the answers or reaction time to the stimuli which follow.

In using this test one must realize that Jung prepared it especially for German use. A verbatim translation into another language is futile because many of the words with ambiguous meanings, which were purposely interspersed, lose their special significance. Following is a modification which has been in use at our clinic for a number of years and in which substitutions are made for words which cannot be translated correctly. Words of a special stimulating significance should not follow too closely upon one another so that the emotional reaction can settle down and does not blur the reaction of other stimuli. This must be kept in mind if the physician wishes to inject some special words which he feels will evoke a definite reaction in his patient. Words which in most patients have no specific meaning are therefore used freely in the test to allow a certain rest. The association test is valuable because it allows an orientation and offers the possibility of a direct approach. In modern treatment it is no longer considered as "a valuable means to find the pathogenic complex" (Jung). The theory of complexes and of association laws is not the basis for the present therapeutic use of this test. We use it to find sensitive experiences and tendencies.

Case 2:

The following results in a 27 year old unmarried man, who for six weeks had had a series of hysterical convulsions, is an illustration of our procedure. We knew from relatives that financial and family worries played a considerable role, but when he was free from symptoms after a few days in the hospital, the patient felt that there was no need for any specific discussion.

The average reaction time in this patient seems to be between 1 and 1.6. Durations of longer than 1.8 were considered definite delays.

ASSOCIATION TEST

Stimulus Word	Time in Secs.	Reaction	Reproduction
1. Head	1.0	ache	+
2. Green	1.0	dress	color
3. Water	1.0	bucket	drink
4. Sing	1.8	song	+
5. Dead	1.2	man	+
6. Long	1.2	time	+
7. Car	2.9	game (understood "card")	wreck
8. Pay	2.0	money	+
9. Woman	1.8	child	+
10. Friendly	1.0	people	+
11. Cook	2.0	woman	food
12. Ask	2.4	question	+
13. Cold	2.0	weather	+
14. Save	1.8	money	something
15. Dance	2.2	money (Don't know why I said that)	girl
16. Village	2.0	town	+
17. Lake	1.8	water	+
18. Sick	1.6	person	people
19. Pride	2.0	hard	things
20. Table	1.8	top	+
21. Ink	1.4	well	+
22. Angry	1.6	person	people
23. Needle	1.0	point	+
24. Swim	1.8	water	+
25. Savage	2.6	person	people
26. Blue	1.8	weather	color
27. Lamp	2.4	desk	light
28. Sin	(Did not catch it) (Repeat)	I got to think of that. (15 sec.)	waves
29. Bread	2.0	eat	+
30. Suck	2.0	shoe	thought "sock"
31. Tree	1.4	leaves	+
32. Punish	1.4	crime	+
33. Pity	2.4	sorrow	+
34. Yellow	2.0	dog	+
35. Mountain	What was the word? (10 sec.)	top	+

Stimulus Word	Time in Secs.	Reaction	Reproduction
36. Die	2.0	hard	+
37. Salt	9.0	rag	food
38. New	2.0	car	thing
39. Habit	1.2	bad	+
40. Pray	3.0	prayer	+
41. Money	1.8	debts	+
42. Foolish	2.0	ways	+
43. Fairy	2.0	tale	+
44. Despise	2.4	people	+
45. Finger	2.0	nail	tip
46. Expensive	5.4	sickness	things
47. Bird	2.2	wing	fly
48. Fall	2.0	down	+
49. Book	2.2	back	read
50. Unjust	2.8	crooked	ways
51. Frog	2.0	water	+
52. Separate	8.8	milk	people
53. Hunger	2.0	food	eat
54. White	1.8	color	+
55. Child	2.0	boy	ways
56. Rear	2.0	back	+
57. Pencil	1.0	write	tip
58. Sad	1.8	sorrow	+
59. Spirit	2.0	poor	bad
60. Marry	2.0	girl	+
61. House	2.0	live	top
62. Dear	2.0	one	+
63. Glass	1.4	window	+
64. Quarrel	1.4	fight	+
65. Future	2.0	time	+
66. Big	1.4	person	large
67. Service	3.8	children	trouble
68. Paint	1.0	house	color
69. Depart	2.0	leave	+
70. Old	4.2	old man	money
71. Flower	2.0	spring	weather
72. Beat	2.0	whip	one
73. Fast	2.4	speed	+
74. Wild	2.2	waves	+
75. Family	3.8	trouble	people
76. Clean	2.0	water	clothes
77. Low	2.2	mash	+
78. Strange	1.8	people	unusual

Stimulus Word	Time in Secs.	Reaction	Reproduction
79. Luck	1.0	door	+
80. Lie	2.0	falsehood	down
81. Bear	6.0	animal	room
82. Narrow	1.4	way	ways
83. Brother	2.0	sister	boy
84. Fear	2.2	afraid	anger
85. Stork	2.6	baby	+
86. False	2.0	lie	+
87. Anxiety	2.0	worry	+
88. Kiss	1.4	girl	+
89. Bride	2.4	girl	+
90. Purse	1.8	money	+
91. Door	2.0	knob	+
92. Choose	1.4	one	+
93. Bed	1.0	sleep	sleepless (laughs)
94. Contented	2.0	happy	sad
95. Ridicule	2.8	people	worry
96. Sleep	1.6	bed	+
97. Mouth	1.4	talk	+
98. Nice	1.2	people	+
99. Woman	1.0	girl	child
100. Abuse	8.0	people (I don't know what I thought)	people

Based on the principles which have been outlined above, the following grouping was made and used as a guide for discussion:

1—home and family—9, 11, 16, 17, 20, 24, 26, 27, 35, 37, 53, 55, 61, 67, 69, 71, 75, 81
2—financial situation—8, 14, 15, 38, 41, 42, 46, 69, 70, 90
3—ethical problems—39, 40, 50, 67, 74, 77, 80, 82
    (sin)—28, 86
    (pity)—33
4—attitude to himself—19, 24, 33, 84
5—social adjustment—15, 19, 22, 25, 44, 52, 75, 78, 79, 95, 100
6—attitude to the future—60, 65
7—women and sex—9, 11, 15, 60, 85, 89, 93
8—illness—18, 46
9—car accident—7, 38, 73
10—unclear answers—12, 13, 43, 45, 52, 55, 56, 81

1. *Home and family:* The patient was very attached to his mother. After his father's death three years before, he felt it his duty as oldest

son to take the place as head of the family, but was unable to cope with these responsibilities. He was anxious to keep the family homestead and therefore left college, but he proved to be a poor farmer and was unable to do as well as his father, whom he had always disliked and easily criticized.

2. *Financial problem:* Incapable of supporting his family with the farm, he had to borrow money from relatives. In the last year he had worked as a salesman, but with insufficient income. Many times he had spent money thoughtlessly and blamed himself for his inability to establish financial security.

3. *Ethical problems:* Marked conscientiousness and a scrupulous attitude to business dealings made competition with other salesmen difficult and he was unable to accept the somewhat lax attitude of his superiors. Giving in to these demands, he felt that he definitely committed a serious sin. He was in conflict about the need for saving and his desire for a gay and sociable life. This was increased because of his sympathetic attitude to his mother and feeling sorry for her financial distress.

4. *Attitude to self:* An exaggerated pride in himself and his family background and an unwillingness to accept defeat or to modify the demands on himself were strong factors. He had not been able to adjust to failure in college, where he had tried to excel socially and in athletics and had therefore been unable to reach satisfactory scholastic results like some other students. He was never willing to admit his intellectual limitations. In athletics he was only moderately successful because he lacked courage. Being a physical coward was to him an unforgivable fault.

5. *Social adjustment:* Self-conscious and shy, never developing sufficient confidence in himself, he frequently assumed a boisterous and aggressive attitude which made him disliked by others. At the same time he had a marked desire to be liked and appreciated and wanted to be in the limelight. As a salesman he was sensitive about calling on people with the possibility of being rudely repulsed. The social decline of his family made it more unbearable.

6. *Attitude to the future:* His plans did not materialize. There seemed to be no hope to escape giving up the homestead. His mother would remain a burden. There was little hope for advancement in business. We dealt with a man who was often day-dreaming about future solutions without being able to stand the test of the present reality. He anticipated difficulties and tried to picture how he would meet them, thus undermining his confidence, and therefore was even less able to deal with difficulties when they actually arose.

7. *Women and sex:* Being a passionate person, he had indulged since adolescence in promiscuous intercourse but had never been able

to form a lasting attachment. He had a high ideal of womanhood as represented by his mother and a longing for finding such a wife for himself. His financial difficulties forced him to put off plans for marriage and home indefinitely.

8. *Illness:* A hospitalization because of kidney stones seven months before the onset of convulsions had forced him to incur debt. He was also afraid of recurrence of the pains. The present illness worried him because no physician was able to formulate its meaning to him. When ill he demanded much attention and expressions of sympathy.

9. *Car accident:* When intoxicated he had an accident which involved a relatively high expense. He felt considerable guilt about occasional alcoholic excesses, especially because of his mother's attitude to it and because it had caused difficulties in college.

10. *Unclear answers:* These were taken up last because I felt that they might deal with more sensitive or less clear problems. The answers 43 and 56 dealt with homosexuality. Two years before his illness the patient had received money from a Negro for allowing passive fellatio. Shortly before the onset of the present illness, the same Negro approached him again and threatened exposure when refused. The same factor entered into the answer 80, when we therefore see clearly two factors to the same stimulus—honor and homosexuality. The marked reaction to 80 exerted still a delaying influence in finding an answer to 81. In the repetition, the word "bear" was taken as "bare" and related to the distressing home situation. The marked emotional reaction to stimuli referring to homosexuality is also well seen in the delaying influence on the answers 44 and 45. These stimuli brought also to the foreground the social aspect of homosexuality (44), and the actual manipulation (45). Stimulus 52 referred to the necessity of leaving the farm and its impending loss, with all its family and social implications. Reactions 2 and 3 belong also to this topic. They were not put with any of the groups because the first four words should be taken as a neutral introduction to the test and delays or failures of reproduction evaluated only cautiously. Stimulus 55 refers to his childhood, his behavior difficulties and the severe punishments by his father. Word 12 brought to the fore his social difficulties as a salesman, 13 the life on the farm.

Many stimuli have to be grouped under several headings. It is important that we do not consider groupings as something absolute but look for interrelations. The test itself, and even more, the working out of the many possible tendencies, is an illustration of the dynamics of the personality. The final result is therefore a constructive synthesis in which the various strivings and tendencies are adjusted to each other, and as part of the whole integrated personality.

Less content is obtained through the use of Rorschach's experiment with a standardized set of ink blots. Many patients, taken off their guard, give answers which are highly informative. Anatomic content, for example, is rare and when present in more than two answers points to specific body concern. Sexual answers are usually absent. They are mentioned readily when corresponding preoccupations are present, because the patient feels certain that these interpretations are obvious and generally given. Such answers might reveal interest in one's own sexual organs and functions, latent homosexuality, or anal-erotic interests. The longing to travel or to live close to nature (love of flowers, the countryside, animals) appears clearly. Many answers are more or less clear symbols. They can be used by the skilled physician for a guide in his procedure and for a direct analysis, e.g., by free association (see Case 4, Chapter VI).

Rorschach's method is of great importance as a personality test. Many features of various personality aspects appear clearly and the interpreter can arrive at assets and shortcomings in the person's make-up which form the basis for our therapeutic approach and expectations. The only other valuable personality test is the analysis of handwriting following the method of Klages or his pupils. Because of many practical reasons, this method has not received the attention it deserves in psychiatry.

BIBLIOGRAPHY

1. ADLER, A.: *The Practice and Theory of Individual Psychology.* Harcourt, Brace & Company, New York, 1927.

2. JUNG, C. G.: Problems of Modern Psychotherapy. *Schweiz. med. Wochenschrift,* 12, 1931.

3. BURROW, T.: *The Social Basis of Consciousness.* International Library of Psychology, Philosophy and Scientific Method. Harcourt, Brace & Company, New York, 1927.

4. RANK, O.: *Technik der Psychoanalyse.* F. Deuticke, Leipzig, 1929.

5. HORNEY, K.: *New Ways in Psychoanalysis.* W. W. Norton and Co., New York, 1939.

6. SULLIVAN, H .S.: *Conceptions of Modern Psychiatry.* William A. White Psychiatric Foundation, Washington, 1947.

7. DUBOIS, P.: *The Psychic Treatment of Nervous Disorders*, 6th ed. Funk and Wagnalls Co., New York, 1909.
8. FRANK, L.: *Die psychokathartische Behandlung nervöser Störungen*. G. Thieme, Leipzig, 1927.
9. ALEXANDER, F., and FRENCH, T. M.: *Psychoanalytic Therapy*. Ronald Press Co., New York, 1946.
10. DIETHELM, O.: Brief Psychotherapeutic Interviews in the Treatment of Epilepsy. *American Journal of Psychiatry*, 103, 1947.
11. THOMAS, G. W.: Group Psychotherapy; a Review of the Recent Literature. *Psychosomatic Medicine*, 5, 1943.
12. FREUD, A.: *The Ego and the Mechanisms of Defence* . . . Translated from the German by Cecil Baines. The Hogarth Press, London, 1937.
13. *The Psychoanalytic Study of the Child*. International Universities Press, 1, 1945.
14. DESPERT, J .L.: A Method for the Study of Personality Reactions in Preschool Age Children by Means of Analysis of Their Play. *Journal of Psychology*, 9, 1940.
15. LEWIS, N. D. C., and PACELLA, B. L.: *Modern Trends in Child Psychiatry*. International Universities Press, New York, 1945. (Discussions by various authors of divergent viewpoints, including the therapeutic role of social workers and psychologists.)
16. JUNG, C. G.: *Studies in Word-Associations*. William Heinemann, London, 1918.
17. RORSCHACH, H. (OBERHOLZER, E.): The Application of the Interpretation of Form to Psychoanalysis. *Journal of Nervous and Mental Disease*, 60, 1924.

Chapter VI

DISTRIBUTIVE ANALYSIS AND SYNTHESIS

THIS TYPE of treatment uses analysis as a means to achieve a synthesis of the various factors and strivings — a synthesis which will offer the patient security. The physician may assume a more or less active technique in analysis or in synthesis, according to the patient's personality and the psychopathologic picture. This method, the name of which was proposed by A. Meyer, is based on his main therapeutic principles. The material for synthesis is obtained by analysis of all the factors and situations which are of importance in the study of the human personality and, more specifically, in the pathologic reactions which bring a patient to the physician. The analysis is distributed by the physician along the various lines which are indicated by the patient's complaints and symptoms, by the problems which the physician himself can recognize, by the patient's imaginations concerning the present and the past as well as by actual situations, attitude to the future, and outstanding features of his personality. Every analysis should lead to synthesis, and after each consultation the physician and, to a considerable extent, the patient also should be able to formulate what has been obtained from the analysis and how it can be used constructively. The treatment is guided by the need to achieve a wholesome integration of the total personality as well as of various functions. Psychogenic and non-mental (somatic, social) factors are studied from the point of best modifiability. Therapeutic leads may be seen in psychologic, psychopathologic, or physiologic findings. The analysis of the personality may be very intense, bringing to the fore repressed material and leading to a prolonged working-through of resistances in the setting of a strong and active patient-physician relationship. In some cases the physician will assume the directing role, based on his dynamic understanding of the patient's problem. Distributive analysis and synthesis is an elastic and far-reaching psychotherapy, and its principles can be applied to all types and degrees of personality disorders.

The patient's complaints are seriously investigated. They are never minimized but are reduced to their actual value by a careful formulation. This formulation should, of course, take into consideration the patient's capacity for understanding at the time. One should use brief and clear sentences which the patient can grasp without effort. The clinical setting determines whether this formulation is offered in definite terms and perhaps linked with direct suggestions, or in the form of probabilities with the advice to have the physician and patient investigate the problems further. The succeeding analysis may be distributed along the lines of the various complaints. In the term, "complaint," in its broadest sense are included symptoms, difficulties with oneself and with others, and problems for which the physician will offer aid. In some cases the patient is advised to neglect his complaints for the time being and to direct the analytical scrutiny to possible underlying factors.

Psychogenic factors which are manifest or suspected are traced in concrete episodes in which symptoms and abnormal reactions appear. These factors are studied for any common elements, for their origin and conditioning. Characteristic situations are carefully analyzed. The theory that certain factors are always present and are therefore of fundamental importance is tested on actual material; it is not accepted offhand as a basic principle. The setting up of one factor as the common denominator for all reactions is avoided. Analysis of the past, for instance, is of great importance because it offers historical material for an understanding of the original personality make-up and its development. One must constantly keep in mind, however, that the history and interpretation are given by the patient in terms of his present attitude. Whenever possible, one should try to check with the accounts of others. Distortions and misinterpretations will occur and have to be clarified as treatment progresses. The patient must not be considered dishonest, for often obvious experiences cannot be associated in their entirety. Furthermore, an isolated experience cannot be seen correctly by either physician or patient.

Analysis should not be carried out along preconceived lines of dogmatically accepted leading situations and reactions. Plasticity is always necessary in the physician's procedure. Inquiry should be distributed along all possible lines, especially those offering opportunities for action. This does not mean that one should be guided primarily by symptoms but rather by those factors, situations, and symptoms which seem important and workable to the physician. One should be guided by the development under treatment and should not follow a rigid, systematic outline. Opportunities for therapeutic attack arise constantly and should never be overlooked, although one may frequently have reason to postpone an analysis and synthesis until later. Acute problems which demand immediate study and attention may arise. In every case it is important that one investigate all the factors and situations which play a role in the person. Distributive analysis, therefore, includes not only the present personality, but its past as well, and future possibilities.

Every treatment must be ultimately constructive. Mere analysis is frequently destructive if the physician does not take a guiding hand. Through analysis one becomes aware of one's shortcomings and failures, and there is an inherent tendency in every one to study failure more than success. No doubt, because of a certain synthesizing tendency of the human personality, many patients spontaneously make constructive use of what has been obtained through the dissecting procedure. One may expect this in the average, well-organized personality whose problems do not seem insurmountable to him. In less fortunate persons, however, or those in whom the illness does not permit the ready functioning of associative healing tendencies, analysis may easily leave the patient with much material which he cannot use constructively. It is therefore essential that constant attention be paid to synthesis. After every analysis of situations or symptoms, whether this be in one consultation or after several, the patient should be directed to a synthetic review of what has been obtained and the physician should always take an active part in the final synthesis.

In many patients frank re-education is necessary in order to correct long established habits and reactions. This should be combined with analytic-synthetic treatment. In psychopathic personalities and in many other cases in which prolonged treatment is necessary, the personality discussions should be spaced sufficiently to allow the patient to put into practice whatever he has learned from the interviews. Examples of this treatment are Case 28 (hypochondriasis) in Chapter XV, Case 41 (homosexuality) in Chapter XVII,

Case 13 (schizophrenia) in Chapter X, and Case 26 (epilepsy) in Chapter XIV. In psychopathic individuals, and also in many other patients who have difficulty in making associative connections spontaneously, a constructive summary should be expected from the patient at the end of every consultation. If the patient cannot summarize the results of the analysis, the physician should devote sufficient time at the end of the therapeutic interview to reach with the patient such an understanding. It is wise to put the patient under the responsibility of producing something new in each consultation to prevent mere repetition and waste of time. In this way, one not only offers the patient a better understanding of himself but practices active re-education of faulty habits of thinking and of tendencies to evasion, to procrastination, and to a waste of time and effort. The consultation becomes a task for the patient to carry out, and he receives pleasure from having done it satisfactorily. In treatment in which the physician shares with the patient the responsibility for his behavior during the whole contact, direct or indirect re-education must constantly enter. Not only will a patient get well in a shorter time if his whole life is adjusted and supervised during treatment, but it prevents the patient from losing sight of his responsibility to himself and to the group.

Distributive analysis and synthesis is a treatment which can and must be adjusted to the patient's needs and psychopathologic picture. It does not exclude other therapeutic procedures, psychobiologic and physiologic, although as a rule in psychoneurotic and minor personality reactions it is used as the main therapy.

In this treatment a clearly defined diagnostic formulation is necessary. This formulation should include the main reaction type, the phase of the illness, and the personality setting. Many factors which cause great distress during a certain phase may be of secondary importance if one considers the illness as a whole. The physician must decide whether he wishes to attempt to eliminate these symptoms immediately or whether he prefers to neglect them and utilize their disagreeable or painful influence as an incentive to get well. In the latter method, a provocative type of therapy may be carried out.

The complaints, which should be carefully obtained, show whether there are symptoms or factors which should be taken care of immediately and what kind of routine is most desirable. The development of the illness, the life setting, and a preliminary understanding of the personality should always be obtained in the first few consultations, in order that the treatment may be planned. In the distributive-analytic approach it is frequently necessary that the physician keep a work-sheet showing along what lines he should proceed, what has been covered, and what had to be left at loose ends, and when a change in treatment will be necessary. In this treatment the physician cannot be guided by rigid rules and preconceived ideas, and his results will, to a large extent, depend on his own plasticity, knowledge, vision, and imagination.

It is essential for every physician to have a good knowledge of his own personality, not only because it will increase the possibilities of understanding his patients, but also because it will enable him to recognize his own tendencies and potentialities in the relationship between patient and physician. In this way he will be able to avoid many pitfalls, the most common of which is the tendency to become emotionally involved in the patient or his problems or to have his own emotional ease disturbed by preoccupations with problems to which he is sensitive.

Distributive analysis is usually carried out in a direct approach in which physician and patient discuss the problems in the form of an ordinary conversation. By means of questions, the physician directs the patient's attention to definite situations and reactions, in order to obtain an understanding of the factors at work and the management of each factor. It is usually best to begin by analyzing past occurrences. Everyone has a greater tolerance for the past than for the present. It is therefore easier to establish an objective attitude which is the basis for control and synthesis. This direct approach is not a question-answer treatment. The physician submits problems in the form of questions or as facts with the advice to investigate them, and the patient studies them for the factors involved. The patient's own statements are offered freely for critical review. Whenever arguing or rationalization occurs, it is made the topic for a therapeutic discussion. Diffuseness or dearth of ideas may cause a change to another topic but not the inability to talk about a certain topic. If such an inability occurs, the difficulty is submitted to discussion. Many times, however, discussion along other lines may be more fruitful and the topical difficulty overcome more easily after the patient has gained a better understanding of himself.

In the indirect method, one may utilize association tests, Rorschach's ink blot cards (see Chapter V), dreams and symptomatic acts (see Chapter IV), with or without the use of free association. The material which has been obtained in this indirect way is either used as guidance by the physician for singling out problems which deserve special attention, or it is directly pointed out to the patient with the advice to investigate carefully the factors involved. It depends on the patient and his reaction which procedure one should follow. Interpretations are best avoided until the patient has proceeded far enough in the understanding of the problem to be able to accept them as possibilities which he has to consider. On the whole, therapeutic interpretations are far less indicated than literature leads one to believe. The Rorschach experiment has the advantage of eliciting the preoccupations of the patient in a form which he can readily accept and the material obtained can therefore be made the basis of discussion. Free associations may be used somewhat differently from Freud's original procedure. On the other hand, it may be wise to adhere strictly to his rules in cases where a long-term treatment is planned. In the average case, however, better results are obtained when the physician interrupts the free flow of thoughts whenever it seems best to him, guiding the patient's attention in another direction by a brief question or remark, or by a formulation which includes dynamic factors in addition to those which the patient has accepted. At other times, the physician may recognize an opportunity which the patient overlooks. With the active use of free association, one adheres to the general principles of distributive analysis and synthesis.

A brief analysis will sometimes be sufficient to achieve personality synthesis and greater attention will have to be paid to a practical life adjustment. It may be necessary to create a situational arrangement which will, as far as possible, do justice to the needs and opportunities of the patient. We should, however, offer opportunities for expansion and try to find those which really fit the case. For example, in an attempt at socialization, we should avoid forcing recreation and constant group contact on a patient.

In this treatment the physician plays an active role, guiding the analysis along the lines of inquiry which seem most profitable and terminating it when it seems wisest. At times, termination may be necessary because the patient enters a realm of his personality where constructive understanding is impossible for him. A good example is latent homosexuality. Similar difficulties are frequently encountered in ethical and religious problems. Also, the physician may terminate the analysis of one problem because it may seem at that time premature or may take too long. The goal may be reached more rapidly after the patient has obtained insight along other lines through the investigation of other life situations which the physician feels must be subjected to scrutiny.

The ultimate goal of the treatment is to establish in the patient a feeling of security based on self-dependence, combined, however, with the ability and willingness to be an integrated part of the group in which he lives and of society in its broadest sense. Constant attempts at restoring or increasing self-reliance will allow the physician to proceed on more or less safe ground and will not lead to disastrous results if the treatment has to be stopped for financial reasons before the goal has been reached. It is not necessary for all the symptoms to disappear, but the patient should be able to consider them as incidental, or as an indication of a disturbance within himself which should be investigated. To this group belong the many reactions which involve the vegetative nervous system and which occur in a more or less specific form in every individual who is under strain. Some constitutionally disposed persons react readily with emotional changes. Tendencies to hypochondriasis and anticipation, compulsions and obsessions, tics and stuttering, and undesirable sexual strivings, rarely disappear completely under treatment. One should not expect to achieve "perfect" results but should keep in mind the fact that no one is without some of these tendencies, and the "normal" person can deal with them constructively.

Frequently, one is not able to reach this goal and the patient may need guidance for years, or even during the rest of his life. A more or less permanent relationship of physician and patient is, however, based on cooperation and collaboration and is not cultivated as a dependence upon the physician.

The contrast with other methods, especially the analytic treatment of Freud, is obvious. I shall emphasize only a few important points. While the relationship between physician and patient receives much attention, it is not used as a basis for the analysis but only in order to reach a better understanding. One cannot avoid the help-seeking attitude of the patient, but this is not encouraged and from the beginning one tries to dissolve dependence upon the physician. The actual fostering and utilization of transference in the sense of psychoanalytic transference neurosis is considered undesirable in most cases, especially in the definitely sexual realm. Case 41 in Chapter XVII (homosexuality) illustrates the way in which one can handle such situations constructively. However, the physician works with a transference relationship in the psychoanalytic sense. Counter-transference is not stressed in the psychoanalytic way but the interesting and valuable observations of the Freudian school are considered important indications of disturbing possibilities. Physicians are therefore advised to undergo a thorough study of their own personalities which allows them to gain the necessary understanding of themselves. Free associations are utilized, but not exclusively, and always under the active guidance of the physician. Active synthesis and even advice is considered necessary; spontaneous synthesis is usually not sufficient. In the largest group of patients interest is directed more to actual situations and symptoms than the detection of unconscious attitudes and mechanisms. The factors of repression and also regression and resistance are accepted, but they are not looked upon as the dominating principles in personality disorders. One should not analyze problems in order to find these dynamic factors but be willing and able to recognize them when they actually appear. One should distinguish between the healthy repression of experiences to which the patient has made an adjustment, and the unhealthy repression which serves as an avoidance of understanding and adjustment. Infantile sexuality also is viewed from such a standpoint. The goal of analysis is less to have the patient relive early experiences than to have him understand the present meaning of these experiences and his present attitude to them. It is emphasized that many of the patient's experiences may be conscious, but for various reasons he hesitates to associate and to utilize them. The therapeutic goal is thus a complete integration instead of mere desensitization. This goal, however, cannot always be reached and desensitization is important in cases where experiences cannot be changed. Desensitization based on a genetic-dynamic understanding, is also used to overcome certain undesirable tendencies, such as oversensitiveness to one's inadequacy. Resistance is analyzed carefully whenever it occurs, but may be studied and handled on the basis of the whole personality setting as well as through the uncovering of unconscious motivation. The contributions of the psychoanalytic school to all these factors should be recognized. However, they are not used as guiding principles but as possibilities which the physician should keep in mind and be able to recognize. The occurrence of situations which indicate resistance or repression is considered an opportunity for therapeutic help which is offered immediately when those factors appear or is delayed until later, according to what seems more advisable. Sexual difficulties and the expression of, or even tendencies to, sexual perversions are evaluated in the whole setting. Their presence does not necessarily prove their fundamental dynamic importance. They may form a leading issue or merely be incidental. Their thorough analysis may be indicated, or, in some cases, a less aggressive treatment may be more constructive.

The problems of self-reliance, self-assertion, and the need for independence receive much attention but are not made the main issue (see Chapter V). Restrictions are advised not as a disciplinary measure but to permit the person to recognize his needs and his reaction to the interference with the gratification of his desires. Sexual abstinence, for example, will show the degree of actual sexual desire and how the person can deal with it. Instead of conflicts, one may think in terms of achievement and non-achievement, or of success and failure, and look for the components which can be utilized by the patient.

Re-education is adjusted to the individual's need. The discipline of the treatment is a cultivation of the ability to follow as well as to lead. Advice is offered in the form of questions, which should be left sufficiently broad so that they do not contain an answer for the patient. In encouraging the development of a philosophy of life, one should not furnish the patient with an outline, but urge sufficient plasticity to allow adjustment to experiences that cannot be foreseen. It is his ability to use opportunities that one wishes to develop. The treatment should never lead to an attitude of futility. Most patients who undergo intensive analytic investigations reach a feeling of futility at one time or another. It is the physician's task to look for such reactions and, when they occur, change to a constructive discussion of assets and possibilities. It is important that one recognize feelings of futility early and treat them, because such moods may cause suicidal impulses or frank depressions. Of considerable practical importance also is the fact that many patients discontinue treatment if the mood of futility persists, and they are then worse off than before the treatment. A physician who plans long-term analytic treatment has to be willing to change his procedure according to problems which arise.

The physician shares with the patient the responsibility for the latter's behavior during treatment. An exclusive relationship without contact with relatives or friends is considered undesirable and many times dangerous. Although one must agree to absolute privacy, one should stress frankly to the patient the desirability of objective data. This does not interfere with the attempt to create situations in which the patient can find illuminating data in his own experiences without dictation from the outside.

Suggestion and hypnosis, catharsis, and the various psychotherapeutic approaches previously discussed can be used as aids where they seem desirable.

The following case illustrates the direct method of distributive analysis and synthesis:

Case 3:

A 25 year old clerk entered the psychiatric clinic in October, 1927, with the complaint of spasms of the left side of his face and left shoulder, and a feeling of constriction in his neck when wearing a collar. In 1923, after a long train journey to visit his fiancée's relatives, he had an attack of unconsciousness during which his face was drawn to the left and he felt "something coming up in his neck." Then spasms of the jaw, attacks of dizziness, and a tight feeling around his abdomen started. The patient stated that he had always been in good health. Having left school at 15, he took up work as a clerk in a steel corporation, and gradually advanced in position and salary. His family surroundings had been unhappy. His father and mother did not get along well because of his father's drinking sprees, in which he spent all his money and mistreated his wife. The patient was devoted to both of his parents and had been dependent on their judgment all his life. He had always been a shy person, his feelings easily hurt, but he was well liked, cheerful, and a good worker. He married in 1925. All these facts were obtained from the patient in the first consultation. He was advised to enter the hospital because organization of outside routine and treatment was not possible, as he lived in a small town far from Baltimore.

On admission, the patient, a tall and asthenic individual, was in good general health. His teeth were in poor condition and he had two diffuse masses in the subcutaneous tissue of his neck. He was pleasing and co-operative and made good contact with his environment.

Before outlining the treatment for this hysterical reaction, we tried to obtain a better understanding of the setting of the personality. The patient was of good intelligence, his abilities along practical lines, but he was well able to understand the discussions of his life problems. Since childhood he had always been bashful and backward socially. There had been a tendency to be concerned about others' opinion of him. Although dependent on others and often easily led, he readily became obstinate. In dealing with his superiors he was very shy, but very domineering in regard to people under him. He was ambitious in his work but lacked confidence in himself. He was always reserved and confided only in his mother. He was therefore unable to discuss sex life and obtain advice for which he had a marked need during adolescence. From 15 to 17 he practiced masturbation and afterwards had intercourse with prostitutes until he married two years ago. The patient was anxious to discuss his married life but discussion always remained on the surface. He said that he and his wife had had frequent difficulties; both were quick tempered and she was often late in preparing meals, a fault which he did not like. He also stated that a physician had advised marriage because it might help overcome his nervousness. We did not get much information about the patient's ambitions and imaginations, but his brief personality outline was sufficient to direct our treatment. We then tried to get a better understanding of the development of his illness. He said that the feelings of constriction around his neck came on quite suddenly and that they showed marked variations. He felt that he would have an attack if he were to button his collar. His face usually became drawn to one side when he did. We tried to find dynamic factors through a psychogalvanic test. The history which we had obtained up to then presented a few topics which we wanted to clear up as soon as possible. There seemed to be a marked difficulty with regard to the family situation and his married life. The patient and his wife were living with his parents. We were interested in the reason for this and also in the relationship between his wife and his mother, to whom he was very devoted. Possible dissatisfaction with work was never clearly brought out. All these topics were discussed with the patient but very little information was obtained. The psycho-galvanic test showed numerous responses. He reacted especially to questions with regard to sexual life and to physical make-up and work. A discussion of his reactions brought out the fact that he had always been very concerned about his height and his family was afraid that he might have tuberculosis. On the trip to meet his fiancée's relatives, an uncle of his wife made a jocular remark about his height, and the patient resented it very much. The patient did not offer much with regard to difficulties in his work. He dodged questions concerning sex and resented being asked intimate questions.

He was not urged much for another week, and began to improve gradually. He had fewer sensations around his neck, but still had to keep his collar open. When several carious teeth were removed, the twitching of the jaw stopped. The patient explained the twitching as caused by "pus in the gums." With regard to the cure of this symptom, we dealt partly with a suggestive mechanism and partly with the removal of a somatic factor. We reassured him that the masses in his neck had nothing to do with his neck condition, but he was unable to understand this. He still insisted that a physical basis was the cause of his condition. Reformulating the case for ourselves (in early November), it became apparent that the married life and sexual problem should be investigated, and that the patient showed marked sensitiveness with regard to his physical make-up. We also realized that we knew very little about his real ambitions and desires and that it was necessary to arrive at an understanding of them. His married life was then analyzed and it was found that the patient married a Catholic girl, to whom his father was quite opposed. The patient made frequent remarks about her grouchy behavior towards him, and the wife was asked to come for an interview. She offered little with regard to the development of the present illness except that members of her family had made remarks about his tall figure, and after his "collapse" in 1922, they had advised strongly against the marriage because of the possibility of tuberculosis. She dated the onset of the present illness from the attack in 1922 and said that a year later, in 1923, the shaking of the shoulders started and that the patient had kept his collar open ever since. He began to refuse to go out with her but liked to go to the poolroom by himself. In 1924 he began to have his neck sensations, and he centered his attention more and more on that symptom. The wife was a rather aggressive, self-centered, and self-assertive person, very quick tempered and easily hurt. She told us that she was never able to stand any teasing from her fiancée and she often abused him and hit him in the presence of others. She first wanted to marry a friend of his and accepted him a year later as second choice. She said that she was anxious to have children but they had had to practice birth control because she had to go to work. In the beginning of their married life they had a Ford, which they had to sell later, because of financial reasons.

We discussed these statements later with the patient. He told us more about the treatment he had received during his present illness, and how he had spent all his money on physicians. He became definitely worse with these many attempts at treatment. There was still a marked reluctance to talk on the patient's part when his married life was discussed; he would say that he had already told us all. He now blamed everything on his own family situation and on the remarks and attitude of his wife's relatives. During October there had been a marked general improvement. The patient was now able to keep his collar buttoned. He always seemed to be quiet and cheerful but on one occasion he had a marked outburst of temper, which showed us that we were dealing with a rather superficial improvement. He began to discuss his early youth and brought out that he always resented having been the oldest in the family. He felt that the position of the oldest child caused him to be left alone more. This resulted in his shyness and bashfulness. It had been a handicap all his life. In carrying on his business affairs he had always been easily upset, and on such an occasion the dizzy feeling started two years ago.

We decided that it was now very important to urge the patient to give more information with regard to his sexual life, and he began to discuss it more thoroughly. Thus we were able to reformulate the case to ourselves at the end of November.

The patient had a period of masturbation from 15 to 17. Since 17 he had had sexual intercourse regularly with friends and prostitutes. He had known his wife five years previous to his marriage but did not stop his heterosexual experiences until a few weeks before his marriage. Because he felt that it was not healthy, he did not have intercourse more than once a week after his marriage. In his previous life he had usually had intercourse twice a week. He practiced birth control by the use of condoms and by withdrawal. He never received pleasure from such intercourse, and withdrawal was always a very great effort to him. In the periods between intercourse the patient indulged in much frustraneous sexual excitement with his wife. He was a person who found definite pleasure in exposing himself and gazing at his wife. She objected to this, but it often gave him more pleasure than intercourse.

We tried to obtain some dream material from the patient and an understanding of the variations of his sexual cycle while he was with us. The result was poor. There were obtained only a few dreams which presented interesting material. In one of these dreams he was with a girl whom he had known before he was married, but he insisted that this girl did not mean much to him any longer. We tried to give the patient advice with regard to sexual hygiene (against withdrawal and frustraneous sexual excitement), and we also tried to explain his wife's point of view with regard to his gazing desire. We had a discussion with his wife again, but she did not show much understanding and we realized that she, as well as her husband, was in need of advice. It was interesting to note that the patient often had to open his collar again after discussions of his sexual life. We also discussed the family situation and the patient began to talk about his father's drinking. He also pointed out that he had always been very shy in dealing with girls in his boyhood and that he shrank from kissing his mother. Such sexual shyness in childhood is interesting in the development of this rather passionate person. After these discussions (at the end of November), the dizzy spells passed away entirely and the patient was able to keep his collar buttoned all day.

He volunteered information about his work. Three months before his attacks in 1924, he began to have a tired feeling when he was at work. At that time his job was changed and he was worried about working a new machine. Ten months after the attacks he began having to keep his collar open. A pressure in his forehead and the stiffness in his face, as well as the dizziness, became marked for the first time six months after his marriage. He connected it with the attitude of his boss, a rather rough and snappy person who made remarks about his father's drinking, which caused the patient to leave his job. He then admitted that his wife had really wanted to have children but that he had practiced withdrawal because of financial difficulties. At this time the patient seemed to be very tense and finally he volunteered the statement that he not been honest with his physicians here. He had had sexual relations with his wife two and one-half years previous to his marriage. The last year intercourse took place twice a week, and he had always worried very much about it, feeling that he was being unfair to her. Previously, since the age of 17, he had frequently attempted intercourse with prostitutes but had always felt ashamed and, although greatly excited, had always been impotent. In the spring of 1925, after having considered himself engaged to his present wife for over a year, during which period he indulged in frequent frustaneous sexual excitement with her, he began having regular intercourse with her. He always took the aggressive part in inducing intercourse; his fiancée objected for ethical reasons. In the fall of 1923 he had intercourse also with another girl who was visiting in town for two weeks. He had known this girl in 1922. The patient had considerable scruples concerning this experience, especially as he felt morally bound to his fiancée because of their sexual relations.

After this discussion the feelings of pressure in his head disappeared rapidly, but the stiffness in his neck persisted. This was the time when he began to see the relation of his symptoms to personality difficulties and past life experiences. He now became interested in the analysis. He pointed out that the attachment to his family might have something to do with his illness. As the result of studying a marked emotional reaction produced by his not being allowed to spend Christmas with his wife and mother, the patient saw that he was not only very dependent upon his mother, but also upon his wife who dominated him. He had always been a person who showed marked aversion to certain people and who had been unable to make an adjustment to this.

In the beginning of December we gave a Jung's Association Test to the patient. He showed fewer and less marked reactions than in the psychogalvanic test. The outstanding topics were concerned with money, his social relations, family, and pride. We analyzed his answers very carefully with him. It led to a further discussion on sex. The final picture which we obtained of his personality was that of an individual who had always been very proud and sensitive about others' opinion of him. He was jealous of his younger brother who presented the ideal personality to him, a sociable, handsome, and well liked person. That brother also went ahead easily in life and holds a position which the patient would have liked to have himself. The patient had early heterosexual play experiences from the age of 7 to 10. They made a deep impression on him, making him feel that he had done something which was not honest. There have never been any religious worries, but pride has been an outstanding feature. Lack of money played a role, because he would have liked to have a car, children, and his own home. His ambition was to be independent in business. His pride was badly injured by his father's alcoholism and the unhappy family situation at home. This sensitiveness caused him to keep away from others. He formulated his present illness, relating his personal and marital difficulties to his symptoms. The whole development became clear to him. He now showed perfectly normal behavior.

Reformulating the development of his illness, the patient was then able to give a clear statement of the setting in which his illness had occurred. Since adolescence he had been greatly sensitive about his body, his height, and general appearance. Around 15 he became aware of sexual desires but, although indulging freely in imaginations, refrained for ethical reasons from actual experiences. From 16 to 20 (1918-1922) he frequently visited prostitutes but was always impotent. At 17 he began to go with his present wife. He was attracted to her but had frequent quarrels with her, which have persisted since. Around the spring of 1922 they began to indulge in frustraneous sexual excitement with much remorse. He considered himself engaged to her, although doubting whether, because of their impulsive personalities, they would be able to get along well. His engagement met marked opposition from his mother, to whom the patient was very devoted. His fiancée was sensitive about the patient's appearance and to others' teasing him about it. When visiting his fiancée's relatives for the first time the patient felt ill at ease, and restless, and anxious to make a good impression. They teased him about his height and nervousness. In this setting the patient had his first symptoms (fainting attack). Restlessness increased gradually and in the winter of 1921-22 he developed his neck symptoms. They increased with the initiation of intercourse with his fiancée, followed by remorse, and especially after a brief sexual experience with a former friend in the fall of 1923. (This girl appeared in a dream during treatment.) All these experiences were physically successful but rarely yielded full pleasure and relaxation. Work became more irksome because of an irritating superior. While developing increasing sexual dependence on his wife and being urged by her into marriage (1924), dizziness and pressure symptoms in the head started. He rationalized his marriage (1925) by convincing himself that it would help his nervousness. In 1924 he was promoted to a new position in which he had contact with high officials of his firm. Whenever this self-conscious and conscientious man had dealings with them his symptoms increased. His adjustment to marriage was poor. Dissatisfaction with work increased. Failure of sufficient advancement was blamed on his illness. Emancipation from his mother proved difficult. Financial handicaps did not allow the acquisition of a car and a pleasant home, which he craved primarily in order to be able to show others that he was successful.

In January we finished our treatment by trying to give him a constructive idea of his personality. For this purpose we administered a personality outline in the form of a questionnaire. The answers were carefully discussed with the patient and he obtained a clear understanding of himself. He began to realize that he could not have everything at once, and that he would be able to have children if he were willing to make sacrifices which would allow financial saving. He arrived at the conclusion that it would be best not to have a car, nor to buy much furniture, but to be satisfied with a modest home. We discussed with him his record at work and his ambitions. He pointed out that he would like to have a business for himself in order to be independent. This striving for independence was a characteristic feature of his personality. Therefore he resented his brother's success in life and also the fact that he had not been able to go through high school because he was the oldest son and had to start work as early as possible. He was still sensitive about his failure in his first job and about the unhappy family situation (alcoholism of father). He understood that he showed a lack of emancipation from his mother and that to some extent he had substituted his wife for his mother.

We tried to give him a better understanding of what is called will power. He believed that will power alone would enable him to gain his goal and he mistook obstinacy and a certain aggressiveness for will power. We tried to desensitize him with regard to his personal appearance. This final study of the personality was the synthesis of our analysis and the patient obtained an understanding of his personality and of how he reacted to various situations in life. He began to see where he could make adjustments. Letters which we have received since his discharge report that he took up his work immediately after his return home and that he feels well. One doubtful factor is the attitude of his wife. She, unfortunately, did not get as much understanding through our discussions as we had hoped she would.

We purposely did not attempt a thorough analysis of every feature mentioned. It did not, for instance, seem necessary to study very carefully his pleasure in sexual gazing. This feature never played an important role and was dealt with only in the course of the discussions on sexual hygiene. We felt that unnecessary material should not be brought into discussion, as the patient would hardly have been able to understand or benefit by a far-reaching analysis. A good adjustment in the six years following discharge supports our assumption that he had obtained a sufficient understanding. A follow-up in 1947 showed that the patient has remained in good health.

Distributive analysis, by submitting questions and problems to the patient, can be utilized for any kind of disorder. It requires plasticity on the physician's part and his willingness to utilize all possible psychotherapeutic methods which have been found practical and scientifically correct. He should select the procedure according to the actual problem. Sometimes he will depend entirely on psychotherapy in the narrow sense; at other times social and occupational adjustments may be more important. Pitfalls in the procedure occur if a physician is set in his own make-up and unable to change the plan of procedure if it should be necessary. A frequent mistake the physician makes is to ask pointed questions which require an answer instead of submitting the problem to the patient for his consideration. The direct distributive-analytic approach easily leads to superficiality if the physician does not have sound psychiatric knowledge and a healthy imagination to utilize in the treatment. It is no doubt easier to follow a definite method than to use a plastic procedure. Frequently the physician errs by trying to bring out dynamic factors through aggressive questions. Or he may be too readily satisfied with a superficial understanding of the dynamic factors and turn to social adjustment or to re-education. Many offer advice too freely instead of leading the patient to find his own solution.

There has been much discussion about whether the patient should face the physician sitting in a chair or whether he should lie on a couch, the physician sitting behind him. In the average case the usual way of carrying on a conversation is no doubt most advisable and less perplexing to the patient. There are patients, however, who constantly watch the physician in order to gain an understanding of his reactions to their discussion. In such a case it may be desirable to have the patient lie on a couch, the physician sitting behind him.

In the indirect approach with the use of free association along a distributive line, the physician is a guide who participates actively (see p. 130). The following case illustrates this procedure. A Jung Association Test was offered in the beginning to gain additional understanding of the factors involved because the patient's complaints were primarily symptomatic, but the test was not used for specific guidance. In this young girl who suffered from phobias, the sexual discussions assumed an important place in the beginning of the treatment. The patient needed this opportunity for the release of what was most puzzling and disturbing to her. Whatever was mentioned was brought into relationship with the setting of her whole personality, and sexual desires and difficulties gradually became a less central issue and were viewed in a broader way. The treatment led to a subordination of this issue to that of the personality as a whole.

Case 4:

An 18 year old, unmarried girl developed attacks which impressed the physicians as anxiety attacks in the summer of 1930. Under reassurance, with the help of a special nurse, she was able to lead a guarded social life. She improved considerably while treated by a neurologist, who gave her an interpretation of her symptoms with a great deal of authority. This was a successful suggestive treatment because the girl was of a suggestible make-up with submissive tendencies and a need for self-assertion. After treatment, she was well for three weeks, but had another attack when invited to the home of a family where she felt socially somewhat ill at ease. Another attack occurred after a large coming-out party. In addition to these "anxiety attacks," she developed fear of committing suicide, especially when seeing a pair of scissors, and fear that her father might commit suicide. She developed many other fears, such as fear of driving her car, because she might have some kind of accident, fear of passing churchyards, and fear of insanity. Superstitious tendencies increased considerably. All her symptoms were worse during menses when "everything seemed futile." The problem of death assumed large proportions. She was overwhelmed by the thought of the futility of life and of becoming nothing through death.

At the beginning of March 1931, she came for treatment which lasted four months, requiring three hours a week. The patient had great difficulty in discussing her personality as far as imagination was concerned, but gave with ease a fairly good description of the main features of her personality. During the questioning she always watched the physician carefully for the impression she made on him. She described herself quite correctly as a cheerful girl who was inclined to worry over details because of great conscientiousness and a perfectionistic attitude. She was sociable, but shy and self-conscious, and felt socially inadequate. She felt this especially in her own crowd and with people who were attractive to her and got along much better with older people, who enjoyed her intelligent conversation and early maturity. She had always had great difficulty in adjusting to failure, and a tendency to worry about remarks she made in social life, wondering whether they might have been considered tactless. She was sensitive to criticism, sympathetic toward others, but with a marked tendency to self-pity, easily confiding and frequently regretting it afterwards. In recent years there had been an increasing fear of failure. Physically, she was quite attractive.

Many factors in her environment which were elicited in the first few discussions were not quite satisfactory. Her mother was a highstrung, excitable person, who lacked control of her emotions, constantly anticipated difficulties, and was easily worried over finances, which she and her husband had discussed frequently in the last few years. Her father was a cheerful and sociable man, who as a result of financial strain, had been increasingly irritable in the last six months. The patient was the oldest of four children. One sister was one year her junior, an attractive and socially successful girl. Another sister was 14 and a brother 12, both in the adolescent spite stage.

The patient had always been in good health. Menses had been regular and without much pain until the previous year, but she and her mother paid a great deal of attention to it and her physician advised her to take paregoric whenever pain occurred.

Because of the difficulty in discussion, a Jung Association Test was given. This revealed marked reactions to words referring to death and cessation of life, security, sin, nudity, lying, pride and anger, sister,

narrow, town, ridicule, and pity. A brief discussion of these points did
not lead far and free associations were therefore started. The Jung
Association Test and dreams, as well as problems which otherwise
seemed of importance, were used as a guide for the distributive analysis.
With the help of free association, the patient learned to offer her
material without constant self-criticism. Before, she had always tried
to formulate her answer and smooth over the most important factors.

The facts which came to the foreground when discussing her fear
of death and her protection by superstitious activities were her inability
to accept the loss of individuality with death and her being bewildered
by the concept of eternity. This led to a discussion of sin and the question of punishment hereafter for immorality. Under immorality she
mentioned sex, stealing, and drinking. Usually patients mention their
symptoms in the order of their importance or the reverse. It became
obvious later that the group which she mentioned centered around sex.
For two years she had suffered from "guilt feelings" because of sexual
thoughts which had gradually occupied her imagination completely.
She began to wonder in social life whether girls were pure and whether
they had sexual relations and enjoyed them. Walking on the street
and driving her car, she began to look at strangers with similar thoughts
in mind. She began to mention that death was especially terrible for
young people and even more so for unmarried people. This was explained by the fact that old people had obtained from life what they
could expect, young people had not, and unmarried people had not
even had a chance to have sexual relations. There was a constant wondering whether life hereafter allowed sexual relations. Dreams of nude
men, especially when taking a course in art, had upset her greatly.
In discussing her art course, she mentioned a classmate who had been
considered slightly homosexual, and that the girl had held her hands.

The discussions of her heterosexual interests and desires occupied
about a month, but other problems were discussed in connection with
them. Frequently, when the patient was unable to proceed along a given
line, I changed to a different topic which seemed related to the discussion, returning to the first topic after some progress along other
lines had been made. This is one of the outstanding features of distributive analysis. Many times problems were left more or less unsettled
at the end of an hour, and they were often formulated as a question
before the patient left. This procedure, although the patient tried not to
think about treatment between consultation hours, stirred up some of
the dynamic factors and the next hour the answer to the question was
often easily obtained. Related topics were her sister's easy social attitude, and the fear that she might develop into a "wild girl" as some
girls of her social set were supposed to be. The patient stressed her
fear of drinking because it would diminish her resistance to her sexual

desires. The problem of stealing, which she had mentioned previously in connection with immorality (sex, stealing, drinking), was of more general importance and was apparently used in her formulation of her complaints primarily as a cover to conceal the importance of the other two complaints.

In the middle of April the patient was asked to give associations to "holding hands" which, as she had revealed some time previously, had to her a marked sexual meaning. The touch of the hands produced a local sexual sensation. At an age of about 13, when holding hands with a boy she had felt the first sexual stimulation, which had upset her greatly and induced a fear of being pregnant. She often since then has thought about sexual assault. The fear of this, which she gradually began to recognize as a wish, caused her fear of the dark which had been present since the onset of puberty.

Discussing the drinking of her parents (in the middle of April) led to an understanding that she was afraid of sexual misdemeanors by her father when under the influence of alcohol. She had noticed that he occasionally held some attractive woman's hand on such occasions, which to her meant that he would obtain the same sexual pleasure from it as she did herself. She also was greatly worried over the possibility of social misdemeanors in such circumstances and felt that the ideal which her father represented to her was lowered by his drinking. Her mother's drinking played a less important role, but there were some fears of sexual misdemeanor, especially with the family physician, who apparently paid a great deal of attention to her mother when he called on the patient. This physician was physically, and partly in behavior, rather similar to her father, but the patient did not make such a connection until much later in the treatment. Cardiac examinations, which he frequently repeated, stirred her sexually.

Soon after these discussions, i.e., after about seven weeks of treatment, the problem of her relationship to her father and the question as to whether the fear of his death might be the expression of a wish were put for consideration. Similar suggestions had been offered by the neurologist and had been repulsed, but now the patient was interested in the problem, having gained much understanding of the possibility of dynamic factors working in herself. Within an hour, she obtained a good understanding of this phobia with regard to death, which expressed her wish that death might prevent her father from social ruin, alcohol, and promiscuity. It also expressed, as was seen a few days later, a marked resentment to their present precarious financial situation, during which she was forbidden to buy attractive dresses, whereas her parents spent a considerable (to her, while in reality it was apparently negligible) amount of money on drinks. She discussed her resentment to her mother because of her interference and became aware of a certain jealousy with regard to her father. This point was not pushed much further, as the patient showed great difficulty in producing associations. There seemed to me other urgent topics which needed discussion and that we might return to the father-daughter relationship later.

A brief therapeutic rest was given for two weeks in May by turning the discussion to less stirring problems, such as her social adjustment and her need for self-assertion. In boarding school, she had been quite disliked because of her aggressiveness and her highly ethical attitude. During the last two years her need for "superiority" had augmented with increasing doubt of her own value. To appear above prejudices, she had suggested that a girl who had been considered a "fairy" by others share her room. When this was first mentioned, the patient did not pursue it further. About three weeks later (at the beginning of June) she returned to it, stating that she had felt quite attracted to the girl and that when holding her hand she received a similar thrill as when holding hands with boys. One night she had crawled into the girl's bed during a thunderstorm, but she later wondered whether it had not been due more to sexual attraction than to fear and whether she might not be homosexual. Discussion of this problem led to an understanding of the possibility of homosexual attraction, especially in adolescence, and its distinction from homosexuality as a life problem. Until the end of treatment, the patient occasionally came back to this problem and one was able to see an increasing ease in discussion of it. She also realized that besides physical attraction, her desire for affection and sympathy caused her to crave such physical contact. She never received it at home except from her father.

Her "great desire to be infinitely better than anybody else" caused her to be overnice to people, for which she had often been criticized. She was very sympathetic and kind-hearted. In marked contrast to this, was her belief in, and urgent defense of, capital punishment. This was due to a cruel streak which she had always hidden successfully but which was fostered in dramatic monologues. Recently her fears had centered about the possibility of her father's suicide when she had noticed a pistol in his car. She tried to justify suicide on the basis of depression or financial difficulties or in the case of extreme immorality on the part of a girl. This to her meant loss of virginity.

The problem of virginity had preoccupied her greatly and she had puzzled over the question of the Immaculate Conception (the patient was Episcopalian). During the last year, her sexual preoccupations had increased so that she was unable to keep them away for any length of time. Her whole thinking was dominated by it. Observations of her childhood, which she had long forgotten, came back with great force, such as those regarding male genitalia which she had noticed in her brother when he was an infant seven years ago (at 11), and she began to wonder greatly about the sexual relations of her parents. She had marked guilt reactions to such thoughts. As with increasing age admiration of her father grew, she became more aware of the physical factors. The analysis of her fiancé showed that he was to some extent like her father in physical build and his interest in books, politics, and his whole ethical attitude. She did not like his not being tall like her father. With the progressing treatment and the increasing emancipation from her father, she began to love her fiancé as an individual and to like the features in which he was different from her father as well as the similarities. She began to realize that her antagonism to her mother was to some extent based on jealousy and not only due to her mother's self-assertiveness. (This material was obtained in June.)

Her emancipation from simple childhood beliefs, the development of her own life philosophy and a religion which fitted her own personality developed during a discussion of her grandmother, who was narrowly religious and played a dominant role in the girl's life. Reward and punishment were the basis of the patient's religion. Her interest in capital punishment was not only based on a cruel streak but also on a desire for retaliation and a feeling that she would deserve death for having had those sexual wishes and death wishes for her parents. This horrified her because death would include eternal punishment. Together with this, she dwelt on thoughts of being a martyr. The problem of reincarnation puzzled her greatly. She pictured herself being re-born as a "wild girl" (predestination would then excuse immorality), or a man (men have the right to be promiscuous).

Closer analysis of her interest in her own hands and the use of perfume revealed a great interest in her own body. She wanted to be feminine in order to be admired. The leading image was a paternal aunt who was quite beautiful, who attracted a great deal of attention, and was said to be flirtatious. The influence of this aunt dated back to an age of about seven, but had increased during puberty. Her envy of her sister was based on the same exaggerated interest in her body. On the other hand, there was also the desire to be proud of masculine features in make-up and behavior because it would indicate independence and healthy self-assertion. The same exaggerated attitude which she had to her body also played a role in her own ethical evaluation, leading to wishes of being a leader, to be fully appreciated for her intellect and especially for her ethical purity, and to many dramatizations along this line.

Further analysis of her fear and her desire to be masculine (in July), showed clearly the multitude of factors involved — the fear and desire to be homosexual, the desire to appear independent, especially in sexual and social life. The patient obtained an increasing understanding of her personality and was able to see how some of the features of her make-up, which had developed in definite directions during life, could be modified. She saw, for instance, that her tendency to be too confiding in others was based on her constant need for dramatization; her tendency to be snobbish and patronizing was an increasing need for being appreciated. On the other hand, lacking confidence in herself, she constantly had to assure people that everything and everybody were wonderful, although she had a great desire to be frank and tactless, telling them just how she felt about it. Conscientiousness led to over-conscientiousness and anticipation of difficulties because of a lack of genuine self-confidence. Her desire to please others frequently led to impulsive promises which she had difficulty in keeping. Although previously tidy in her thinking and actions, she became untidy because she wanted to do too many things, never finishing a task completely and putting it off. She recognized that she had marked sympathy for the suffering of others and wanted to help, but that much of her present desire to be generous was based on a desire for superiority and a need for being admired. Her attitude to her future had been based on her great desire to be a success as a personality as a whole, but especially socially and culturally. She had wanted to go to college, but this had been refused by her mother who did not believe in a college education for girls. She thought constantly about becoming an ideal wife and bringing up a family. Her sexual preoccupations were less of a definitely topical nature than of this more general type. The patient began to integrate her various strivings which she had previously developed independently without attempting to adjust them to each other. At the end of the treatment she was aware of the need for the integration of her intellectual capacities and needs with her spiritual and material, sexual, and bodily interests. She understood the danger of developing isolated tendencies to perfection. Her attitude to her own body, to appearances, and to the social group changed greatly and she was able to feel more at ease at social gatherings. She began to learn not to indulge unduly in imaginations, guarding especially against sexual preoccupations and self-dramatization. Her menses, which had been irregular for the last year, became regular and were no longer painful. She had no need for superstitutions and lost her fears completely. In the last few hours, we investigated a few of the symptoms which had not been discussed before, such as her fear of a pair of scissors, which was based on her desire to stab her father when he was imbibing alcoholic beverages. Her fear of heights was based on a fear of being unable to control suicidal wishes. These wishes were not only the expression of feeling desperate and nearly panicky about her fears, but were also due to a tremendous curiosity about death. The factors which had been indicated by the Jung Association Test had all been cleared up.

During the whole treatment no attempt was made to break through resistance, but the treatment was directed along other lines, and the patient prepared for a discussion which had previously been impossible. It seems to me that the exaggeration on the part of some authors of the value of resistance and of breaking through resistance is a remnant of the influence of catharsis. This is of very doubtful value.

The reactions of fear in this patient were based on many factors, the most important of which were her need for self-assertion and fear of losing her individuality in eternity; the sexual upheaval of adolescence with its heterosexual and parental relationships and the fear of cessation of sexual life with death; her relationship to her father and her mother; her changing religious and ethical beliefs and her great curiosity about death; the desire to be appreciated (death of members of her family would make her important in her own family), and her great interest in her own body. There developed a general insecurity which might easily have led to slight panic reactions, as was indicated by her desire to scream at night. The patient has been in good health for 15 years and has led a successful life as wife and mother.

BIBLIOGRAPHY

DIETHELM, O.: Investigations with Distributive Analysis and Synthesis. *Archives of Neurology and Psychiatry*, 35, 1936.

Chapter VII

THERAPEUTIC ACTION OF VARIOUS PHYSICAL AND CHEMICAL AGENTS

ATTEMPTS to influence excitements and other marked psychiatric disorders by somatic procedures have always been made in psychiatry, depending on the status of the knowledge of physiology and psychopathology. It is important that one assume a critical attitude to such therapeutic proposals which are not supported by sound theories. On the other hand, one must guard against a timid conservatism which stultifies scientific imagination. A sound knowledge of physiology and psychopathology will prevent us from going too far afield therapeutically. With such an attitude one should consider the great strides which have been made with somatic procedures during the last fifteen years.

In this chapter, I shall limit the discussion to selected physical and pharmacological procedures and omit a discussion of the specific topics of diet, endocrinotherapy, and cathartics. They belong to the field of internal medicine and a knowledge of them is to be expected in a well-trained psychiatrist. Whenever there is a well-defined medical indication, these somatic treatments should be used in their proper form. In later chapters I shall refer to these somatic procedures in discussing the treatment of special psychiatric disorders.

1. CONVULSIVE THERAPY

After a period of several years during which convulsions were produced therapeutically by means of metrazol and considered a specific therapy for schizophrenia, the procedure was greatly improved by effecting convulsions through application of an electric current. It was found that best results are obtained in affective disorders especially when intense resentment is present. These psychopathologic reactions are outstanding in late-life depressions (the involutional melancholia of the older authors). The results are surprisingly good even in those cases where rut-formation or catathymic harping had made the prognosis poor. Paranoid and paranoic projections and systematizations and aversion reactions which are connected with affective features yield well to convulsive therapy. In depressions in young and middle aged persons good results are obtained if convulsions are administered after signs of improvement become noticeable. The results are less satisfactory and frequently discouraging in schizophrenic illnesses, especially when the illness became manifest after the prolonged presence of psychoneurotic symptoms. In anxiety neuroses and hysterical and compulsive reactions the results have not been satisfactory. The presence of marked hypochondriacal symptoms is considered unfavorable but the results may be good if convulsions are administered after a period of prolonged psychotherapy.

Satisfactory explanations for the results of this treatment are lacking. It is, however, worthwhile to keep in mind that affective illnesses in epileptics are accompanied by intense resentment and paranoid projections. These illnesses as well as prolonged periods of intense resentment may be terminated abruptly by the spontaneous occurrence of convulsions.

Indications for the treatment are the above-mentioned illnesses. In every case convulsive therapy should, however, be considered of only symptomatic value and therefore should always be offered in the setting of well-planned psychotherapy. When convulsive therapy leads to recovery through repression of the essential dynamic factors and is not accompanied by their psychotherapeutic adjustment, the prognosis for life must remain uncertain. Fortunately, even then the majority of the patients remain in good health. Little is known yet at what phase of the illness the treatment should be started. In contrast to general belief, it does not seem possible to stop the development of a depression by giving convulsions at the earliest onset. The number of depressed patients who are admitted to psychiatric hospitals after having received unsuccessful convulsive therapy is high. There are no publications which present conclusive, or even likely, evidence that acute depressive episodes which cleared up after a few convulsions would have had a prolonged course without the treatment. Ambulatory treatment in the physician's office does not permit a careful observation of the changing psychopathology.

Contraindications for convulsive therapy are organic cardiovascular disease, acute tuberculosis of the lungs, advanced arteriosclerosis, and pregnancy. One should also hesitate in starting treatment in the presence of febrile diseases or abnormal laboratory findings in blood and urine until the underlying causes can be recognized. Contraindications are always relative, and the physician should evaluate whether the convulsion or the subjection to chronic illness presents the greater hazard.

The most frequent complications are fracture, especially compression fracture of the spine, and dislocation of the jaw. The latter can be readily corrected immediately after it has occurred. The use of curare has decreased the danger of fractures in elderly and poorly nourished people. One must always be prepared for the occurrence of respiratory distress (apnea). Cardiovascular complications are rare but they are probably largely responsible for the occasional death (the death rate is estimated at 0.06%). There is no doubt that cortical damage may also occur in the brains of young patients. One is then dealing most likely with postconvulsive hemorrhages. The resulting retention difficulties are usually minor but cases of a prolonged, or Korsakow, syndrome have been observed. A permanent marked retention disorder is no doubt rare.

The course of treatment depends on the psychopathologic findings and the patient's reaction to convulsive therapy. In the average patient, a total number of 6 to 10 convulsions is sufficient. It seems desirable to administer two to three convulsions a week. The spacing of the treatment over a three-week period permits an active psychotherapy which will insure the psychodynamic adjustment. In schizophrenic patients, except in acute excitements, a course of 20 convulsions seems desirable. In cases of relapse, another 10 convulsions are indicated. When in the course of treatment psychopathologic symptoms which suggest structural damage (confusion, marked retention disorder, impulsive outbursts of anger, and combativeness) occur, the treatment should be discontinued. Literature presents evidence that in excitements desirable results may be obtained by the administration of one or even several convulsions a day, as well as a higher total number of convulsions during the period of treatment than suggested above. The evidence presented does not permit definite conclusions as to whether or not such changes are indicated and under what conditions.

The technique is simple and can be readily mastered. The preparatory examination should include a complete physical examination, routine urine examination, complete blood count, blood Wassermann or comparable test for syphilis, electrocardiogram, posterior-anterior x-ray examination of the thorax, and lateral x-ray picture of the entire spine.

The psychologic preparation of the patient should be suited to the individual case. Adequate sedation may be given as indicated on the night before treatment. A very light breakfast is permissible. The patient voids and defecates, if possible, and then is sent to the treatment room clothed in pajamas or nightgown, bath-robe, and slippers. Dentures, chewing gum, hair pins, etc., are removed before treatment. Preliminary medication of atropine sulphate in a dosage of 0.0006 gm. ($\frac{1}{100}$ gr.) may be given orally one hour before treatment in patients who tend to salivate excessively during the convulsion.

Equipment of the Treatment Room — Treatment may be given on any relatively firm surface, such as a hospital bed, or a sturdy treatment table covered with a waterproof mattress. The source of current may be any one of a number of electro-shock machines produced by a reliable concern. The machine should permit regulation of the A-C voltage and the time during which it is applied to the patient. Any other controls or measuring devices are superfluous. Disc electrodes, held in place by a wide rubber strap are the most satisfactory. A loop of rubber tubing wrapped in gauze makes a satisfactory mouth-gag.

Supplies for the treatment of emergencies can be minimal. Facilities for the intravenous and intracardiac injection of adrenalin should be available in the event of circulatory collapse or cardiac arrest. Chemical stimulants of respiration are useless. Respiration can be stimulated by turning the patient's head to one side, by squirting ice-water on the face, and, if necessary, by prone pressure artificial respiration. A moulded rubber air-way should be on hand in the event that undue relaxation of the tongue results in respiratory obstruction. Respiratory difficulties caused by accumulation of mucus and saliva are best treated by postural drainage. In the event that curare is employed, the antidote, prostigmin, should be available for immediate injection. Status epilepticus is best treated by intravenous sodium phenobarbital (p. 348).

Administering the Convulsion — The patient lies supine, with moderate hyperextension of the mid-dorsal spine secured by the suitable placement of a sandbag or small firm pillow. A small pillow is placed between the knees. Assistants provide moderate traction on the humerus, moderate resistance against violent ventral jerks of the shoulder, and sufficient pressure to prevent flexion of the legs at the hip.

The temporal region of the patient's head is rubbed with electrode jelly to produce mild erythema. Electrodes are moistened with saline and applied to the prepared area, and any excess fluid or jelly carefully wiped off. The operator puts the mouth gag in place and holds the jaw closed with his left hand; he presses the treatment switch with his right hand, and immediately places his right hand under the patient's chin so that he may use both hands to resist the forcible opening of the patient's jaw that occurs during the tonic phase of the fit. This safeguards against dislocated jaws. During the clonic phase, the operator prevents violent side to side jerking movements of the head. When twitches cease, the operator assumes responsibility for the restoration of respiration. If the patient is moved from table to bed, the operator is responsible for maintaining the head and neck in proper alignment with the trunk.

The patient recuperates in bed. He should be turned on one side with the head in a position to promote postural drainage. Any unnecessary manipulations promote motor excitement and should be avoided. If the patient is restless, it is best to allow him to move about at will, using pillows to prevent him from injuring himself. Only in the most violent excitements is forcible restraint indicated. A period of at least 30 minutes' rest in bed is desirable following the fit.

The dosage of electricity warrants some discussion. It appears most desirable to produce a grand mal convulsion with a tonic phase as well as a clonic one. A dose which is too small may cause severe discomfort without loss of consciousness. A somewhat larger dose produces loss of consciousness with some tonic manifestations. This is undesirable because the patient experiences considerable discomfort, probably as a result of tension, during the rest of the day; confusion after treatment seems to be more severe and prolonged than with a larger dose, and respiratory and cardiac complications are more apt to occur. It appears that this incomplete sort of seizure is less efficacious therapeutically. A dose which is too large throws the patient violently and immediately into a clonic fit, and it is likely that more fractures occur with this type of induction. The ideal dose produces a brief tonic phase which passes smoothly into the clonic phase. A reasonable starting dose is 110 volts for 0.1 seconds. Subsequent doses are judged by the response obtained.

The operator can best judge what is happening by watching the eyes of the patient. Should the patient fail to lose consciousness, he immediately begins to look around the room, and usually to talk. In this case, the time should be increased by 0.1 seconds and a second shock might be given immediately. If there is a delay of more than 5 seconds between shocks, the brain will be refractory, and no convulsion will result. If the first shock produces loss of consciousness and some tonic manifestations, it is probably just as well to omit the second shock and to increase the dose the next treatment day. Tonic phenomena can be seen earliest in the eyes, which show, after an initial blink, a tonic opening of the eyelids, conjugate deviation, and dilatation of the pupils. The presence of these tonic eye phenomena indicates loss of consciousness and amnesia for the treatment experience.

Use of Curare — Violent muscular contractions can be prevented when the physical condition of the patient makes it necessary by intravenous administration of d-tubocurarine chloride (Squibb), in doses of 1 cc. per 40 lbs. body weight. This drug is injected intravenously at the rate of 2 cc. per minute. Muscle weakness reaches its maximum 2 to 4 minutes after the completion of the injection, and at this point, the convulsion is induced. Immediately after the fit, a moulded rubber airway is routinely inserted to insure unobstructed breathing. Unusual delay in the resumption of respiration is treated by artificial respiration plus the intramuscular or intravenous administration of prostigmin. Artificial respiration is by far the more important of the two measures. Where artificial respiration must be carried out for more than a few seconds, it is desirable to administer oxygen simultaneously.

2. INSULIN THERAPY

The therapeutic use of insulin in psychopathologic disorders has become well established. The originally rigid and elaborate procedure has been adjusted to the varying needs of the individual patient. There is considerable evidence that an insulin reaction above the comatose level is efficacious and that in moderate cases of anxiety even ambulatory treatment by small amounts of insulin can give the desired results. Our very satisfactory results have been obtained exclusively by subcomatose treatment. The best results are obtained in acute psychopathologic conditions with marked anxiety present, catatonic and other schizophrenic excitements, panic reactions, and intense anxiety in psychoneuroses. Manic excitements with varying degrees of anxiety react well, while less satisfactory results are obtained in depressions.

There is no adequate explanation for these therapeutic results. It seems that the essential benefit is exerted on anxiety but the physiologic links are unclear. Coma presents a special type of psychobiologic experience and its psychopathologic and therapeutic implications should be studied separately from the effect of insulin. Such discriminative studies have not been undertaken as yet.

Indications for the treatment are the above-mentioned illnesses. As in convulsive therapy, its symptomatic value must be stressed. Psychotherapy, which is essential, should usually be given in the afternoon while the patient is undergoing a course of insulin therapy. In some patients it may be wiser to delay analytic investigations. In difficult excitements insulin therapy should be started as soon as a thorough psychopathologic and physical survey has been done. In cooperative patients one is justified in waiting to observe the results of psychotherapy, occupational therapy, and the efficacy of sedation. This somewhat conservative approach may prevent the inception of a prolonged and cumbersome procedure in brief excitements and in the average panic reaction. The judicious use of insulin treatment changes the picture of a ward for excited patients and is one of the main ways of treating the vast majority of these patients. In refractory cases or in chronic excitements insulin therapy should be followed by repeated convulsive therapy. Some authors (Kalinowski and Hoch) also advise combined insulin-convulsive therapy.

Contraindications are cardiovascular disease, pulmonary tuberculosis, unclear febrile diseases, acute and chronic diseases of the liver, kidney, pancreatic, thyroid and adrenal glands, and diabetes. Death with insulin therapy is negligible if these contraindications are kept in mind and especially if one watches most carefully the cardiac reactions in patients over 45 years of age. If one uses a procedure in which coma is produced the dangers increase considerably, especially when irreversible coma occurs.

The technical procedure varies. The most essential distinction is between that in which a hypoglycemic coma is avoided and that in which it is produced purposely and maintained for a definite period of time. In either case the preparatory examination, the equipment of the treatment room, and the precautionary measures are the same.

The preparatory examination should include a complete physical examination, routine urine examination, complete blood count, blood Wassermann or comparable test for syphilis, posterior-anterior x-ray examination of the thorax, and electrocardiogram. A sodium amytal interview, which is frequently conducted to determine the patient's reaction to relaxation, is not essential nor is an electro-encephalogram or an insulin test with repeated blood sugar determinations.

The psychologic preparation of the patient should vary individually and be directed mainly toward obtaining the patient's cooperation by explaining the purpose of the treatment, and alleviating anxiety. On the day of the treatment, breakfast is withheld. Artificial dentures are removed.

Equipment of the Treatment Room — It is desirable that the room be darkened and that loud noises be eliminated. Small dormitories of three to five patients are suitable, with screens separating individual patients. Larger dormitories are usually undesirable if one wishes to be in a position to offer adequate nursing care at any given moment. An adjoining bathroom is desirable. A nurse should record regularly every 15 minutes pulse, respirations, and general observations (twitchings, convulsions, disorientation, emotional outbursts, onset and depth of coma). A small table should contain supplies for the treatment of emergencies — a gavage tray with 40% solution of glucose, and a 50 cc. syringe and needles with supplies of 50% glucose for intravenous administration.

Administration of subcomatose treatment — At 7 A.M. the

patient, who is resting in bed, is given the appropriate dose of insulin subcutaneously. Regular insulin (as distinguished from crystalline or protamine zinc insulin) is used. Starting with a dose of 25 units and increasing ordinarily by 10 units, the dose for each day is determined by the physician from the preceding day's reaction. Apparent increasing and decreasing sensitivity to insulin influences the dosage. The goal is to obtain a prolonged hypoglycemic reaction of drowsiness or sleep which is terminated after 1 to 2 hours. Indications for earlier termination are the occurrence of convulsions, marked excitement, or coma. Coma from which the patient cannot be aroused is usually preceded by marked clouded consciousness and evidence of sympathetic nervous system overactivity (pupillary dilatation, increased pulse rate, and perspiration). Changes in the patient's behavior will determine the daily dosage as seen in his total reaction and in the signs of impending coma. The guide to the amount of insulin necessary should be the changing psychopathologic picture. A full course of treatments has been set arbitrarily at 50. This number should be revised considerably if psychopathologic changes indicate shortening or lengthening. In acute panics, 20 treatments may be sufficient; in some excitements, 70 to 80 treatments may finally give the desired results. At times, a lowering of the dosage by 10 or 20 units may be indicated; at other times an increase of 5 units is sufficient to reach the right dosage.

Termination is routinely effected by the oral administration of 400 cc. of lemonade containing 160 grams of glucose. In the event that the patient cannot drink this mixture, 400 cc. of 40% glucose is administered by gavage, or, preferably, 10 to 50 cc. of 50% glucose is given by intravenous injection. Patients should remain in bed until return of full consciousness; then a shower is given and the noon meal taken. Care should be taken that the meals later in the day are eaten, and that glucose solution is available for patients who may suffer a delayed hypoglycemic reaction in the afternoon. The repeated occurrence of convulsions can be prevented by the administration of phenobarbital 0.06 gm. (1 gr.) at 7 A.M.

Administration of insulin therapy producing coma—Whereas previously the aim was to produce coma with the smallest possible dosage, in recent years efforts have been directed toward prolonging the coma, regarding convulsions desirable. The advantage of this type of insulin treatment over the one previously described is not clear from the literature on the subject. The danger of death is a definite concern and seems to be related to the occurrence of prolonged or irreversible coma, respiratory and circulatory complications, and intracranial hemorrhage. In order to obtain coma one may start with 25 units, increasing by 20 units each day until brief periods of coma occur; from then on, an increase of 10 units a day is advised. If, however, no coma occurs with a high dosage of insulin, one may increase by 30 to 40 units a day. When a definite comatose reaction has been obtained, one should determine the lowest amount of insulin by which the coma can be maintained. The length of the coma is increased gradually from a minimum of 15 minutes to the maximum duration which can be reached without danger (one hour). The signs which necessitate termination are fall in blood pressure below 100 mm., poor peripheral circulation, and a drop in pulse rate to below 55. A dangerous stage of coma, but one recommended as therapeutically desirable for a maximum of 15 to 20 minutes, is deep coma characterized by contracted pupils which do not respond to light, absent corneal reflexes, pulse rate between 50 and 60, respiratory irregularities, and muscular hypotonia. The average daily period of coma is about 30 minutes. Coma should be interrupted by the administration of glucose given by nasal tube. In case of danger, glucose must be given intravenously. Treatment may be successful after two weeks or may take a much longer period of time. If satisfactory results are not obtained by the end of three months, treatment should be terminated.

3. PROLONGED SLEEP TREATMENT

In seeking a treatment which would allow the easier handling of excited patients and a forceful adjustment to reality, a continuous sleep of about 10 days' duration was induced by means of barbiturates. This treatment is little used in this country but has remained an important therapeutic tool in European psychiatry.

In prolonged sleep treatment one attempts to produce a more or less deep sleep with various drugs. The assumption that certain drugs produce a central anesthesia has been given up. Many authors now feel that it is more important to produce a somnolent (twilight) state than a real narcosis. In this protracted state, and for one or two days afterwards, the patient feels tired and exhausted. His thoughts and imagination become less clear and less active, and motor expression diminishes. Hallucinations may not disappear entirely, but the patient develops a more distant attitude to them and to other psychopathologic experiences. He is able to ignore them or to fight against them. Autistic withdrawal is lessened and the patient develops a better rapport with the environment, appreciating the help of the physician and nurses. His need for self-preservation is aroused, bringing him back to better contact with reality. Sleep treatment, especially psychiatric treatment following the prolonged sleep, allows the physician to meet the patient on a ground which he is willing to accept, i.e., his physical welfare, and to form a more or less lasting rapport. All this points to the need for intensive psychotherapy before and after termination of treatment. Schizophrenic patients frequently come out of the sleep treatment with a feeling of clearness and while still under the influence of the somnolent state, are ready to accept the environment. They are emotionally freer. Manic patients, according to Oberholzer, remain somewhat drowsy for about two more days. When they are clear, they are better able to utilize their emotions for an adjustment to the environment. On the whole, the results are satisfactory rather than brilliant, especially in distressing schizophrenic excitements with much combativeness and smearing of feces, where one is unable to gain rapport by any other means. It is psychotherapeutically important at the termination of the treatment to remove the patient to a quiet ward, to put him immediately into full routine, and to cultivate the rapport which has been gained and the interest in reality. The patient should be urged to neglect any persisting hallucinations. More thorough analytic-synthetic treatment should be delayed until a sufficient stability of the personality has been achieved. Many physicians utilize this rapid improvement for an early discharge. This seems to me advisable only if one is convinced from previous hospitalization that the patient is not able to gain from further attempts at a more thorough adjustment.

Intravenous somnifen, which was used in the initial development of sleep treatment, is still considered favorably in British psychiatry. On the European continent this drug has been substituted by intramuscular or rectal administration of dial Ciba. Other barbiturates have been recommended. I shall present here the rectal dial Ciba and the intravenous somnifen treatment because I have used both methods. Psychiatric literature does not yet present enough evidence that the newer methods are superior to these two. In all these methods, the mortality rate is still discouragingly high.

Sleep treatment is advised in the various acute and subacute schizophrenic excitements, autistic and negativistic withdrawal, markedly hallucinatory phases, and in pronounced stereotypes, especially in stereotyped thinking. Catatonic reactions with marked affective admixtures are considered especially suitable. Deteriorated and paranoid patients react poorly. Some authors use it for the treatment of manic excitements. The results in manic cases seem to be good, but I would hesitate to advise it because considerable danger is involved in sleep treatment and I do not feel justified in subjecting a patient to it when he suffers from a psychiatric disorder which will terminate in any event in a reasonably short time. Patients suffering from depressions, especially when accompanied by marked anxiety, do not respond well. Sleep treatment in order to facilitate morphine withdrawal is not desirable. Definite contraindications are infections of the respiratory organs (colds, bronchitis, tuberculosis), kidney disorders, cardiac weakness, metabolic diseases, and marked undernourishment. Treatment is avoided during menses.

The administration of dial by rectum has been recommended because the rectum absorbs the drug well and without irritation. The effect is strong enough to produce a somnolent state. Administration by rectum permits rectal feeding at the same time, thus avoiding the danger of aspiration, which has frequently been blamed for the development of pneumonia. The symptoms which accompany sleep treatment are slight tachycardia, rise in temperature, and slight oliguria. Serious symptoms which necessitate immediate termination are beginning collapse, usually recognized by a drop in the systolic pressure with unchanged or increasing diastolic pressure, and change in pulse quality and frequency; lobar pneumonia, and insufficient urinary output. Cardiac complications are the most frequent danger. Some patients develop a delirium in which psychogenic factors play a leading role. Most of these patients can be urged to take care of urination and bowel movements during their somnolent stage.

In carrying out this treatment, the physician should adhere closely to the rules until he has gained extensive experience with this type of procedure. Lack of success and the high number of complications which have been stressed by several authors are probably largely due to improper technique or insufficient care in the selection of cases. No nourishment or fluids are given by mouth during the treatment, which is carried out in a darkened room. Special nursing attention is necessary. The evening before treatment is started, the bowels are thoroughly evacuated with a high enema. During the whole treatment, every three or four hours, day and night, 400 cc. of 5% glucose is given rectally by the Murphy drip method. Once in twenty-four hours, the glucose is replaced by the same amount of normal saline. The patient should receive 2000 to 3000 cc. of fluid in twenty-four hours. Catheterization may be necessary. If the bowels do not move over a two-day period, an oil enema is indicated. For irregular pulse, strophanthin 0.00025 to 0.0005 gm. ($\frac{1}{240}$ to $\frac{1}{120}$ gr.) or intravenous glucose administration (20 to 40 per cent) is advised. In case of collapse, oxygen inhalations help promptly.

It is best to start with a hypodermic injection of scopolamine 0.001 gm. ($\frac{1}{60}$ gr.) together with morphine 0.015 to 0.02 gm. ($\frac{1}{4}$ to $\frac{1}{3}$ gr.) which produces sleep or at least rest, and allows the dial to work more efficiently. Scopolamine-morphine may be repeated after twenty-four hours. The amount of dial varies individually and should be kept as low as possible. One should keep in mind that the first symptoms of intoxication may be increased restlessness and poor sleep. It is then of vital importance to decrease the medication. In the average, well-nourished case, one may administer 0.6 to 1.0 gm. (10 to 15 gr.), repeating this when sleep becomes more superficial. This would usually mean one to two rectal administrations in twenty-four hours. In recent years, smaller doses have been found more advantageous; i.e., 0.2 to 0.3 gm. (3 to 5 gr.) offered whenever the patient wakes up. During the period from the second to the fifth day, in which intoxication occurs frequently,

0.2 to 0.3 gm. (3 to 5 gr.) may be sufficient in twenty-four hours. The duration of successful treatment is between seven to ten days. The total amount of dial reaches about 12 gm. in men and 10 gm. in women.

The intramuscular administration of somnifen should be preceded by an enema, which should be repeated every second day if indicated by unsatisfactory bowel movement. Fluid intake and urine output must be charted so that urinary retention can be detected early. Urine should be tested for ketone. Large fluid intake should be stressed. It has been suggested that the patient be offered 3000 cc. of water containing glucose in 24 hours. Recently, the giving of 10 units of insulin twice a day has been advised. A careful pulse and blood pressure chart are necessary. The patient should be treated in a darkened room.

An hour before the first somnifen dose is administered, the patient receives an injection of hyoscine 0.0006 gm. ($\frac{1}{100}$ gr.) and morphine 0.015 gm. ($\frac{1}{4}$ gr.). The patient should be kept in a somnolent state by the smallest amount of drug possible. One should start with 2 cc. of somnifen morning and evening. The dosage may be varied slightly according to the patient's reaction but 4 cc. in 24 hours should be considered the average maximal dosage. The injections should be spaced so that the effect begins to wear off at mealtime which will permit the patient to be fed. The usual duration is about 10 days. Earlier termination is indicated if fever or respiratory difficulties or signs of cardiovascular collapse threaten. In such a case 10 cc. of picrotoxin solution (1 mg. to 1 cc.) should be injected intravenously at the slow speed of 1 cc. a minute. In addition, 100 cc. of glucose (33% solution) should be administered intravenously. Urinary retention requires catheterization. Fever, caused by dehydration, will clear up fast with increased fluid intake. Fever gives early warning of the development of pneumonia as well as the possibility of minor local infection. The dangers of somnifen treatment are dependent on the physician's knowledge of internal medicine, on careful physicial observation, his acquaintance with toxic effects of barbiturates, and his willingness to discontinue the treatment rather than to force it by increasing dosage or adding other drugs to enforce sleep.

4. SURGICAL PROCEDURES ON THE BRAIN

With the development of brain surgery attempts have been made to use this knowledge for psychiatric treatment. Surgical operations on the brains of epileptic patients may be important for the control of convulsions but have not shown any influence on the psychopathology of deterioration. In the last ten years prefrontal lobotomy, which was introduced by Moniz, has attracted much attention. The operative procedure, if carried out by a skilled brain surgeon, is simple and mortality is low if patients who are in good physical condition are selected. The possibility of permanent brain damage is difficult to evaluate because of our limited knowledge of the relationship of psychologic functions to brain localization. It is certainly necessary to obtain a year's postoperative observation to evaluate the results and to determine what psychopathological symptoms may develop.

Indications are unclear, but some general principles have evolved. Surgical treatment should be advised when there are very distressing psychopathologic syndromes which have not yielded to any other psychiatric treatment administered with the necessary skill and over a sufficient length of time. Special psychiatric illnesses cannot be considered an indication. The factor of chronicity is indicated by the duration of the illness or by psychopathologic signs of permanent deterioration. It is obvious, however, that one should guard against accepting signs of permanent deterioration in cases of short duration. The patients who seem to react favorably are those who suffer from strong emotional disorders leading to persistent attempts at self-mutilation or suicide, and aggressive outbursts which are dangerous to others. These psychopathologic reactions may occur in schizophrenic, affective, and organic psychiatric illnesses. Patients with unmanageable habit-deterioration should be considered if there is evidence of the destructive role of affective factors. Not enough is known yet about the possibility of modifying or eliminating the impulsive outbursts of structurally damaged brains (idiocy, post-encephalitic, arteriosclerotic, and traumatic conditions). Persistent hallucinatory and delusional experiences as well as compulsive behavior may be alleviated if emotional factors play a leading role. In this group one should further consider to what extent these psychopathologic reactions interfere with a suitable adjustment outside or within a psychiatric hospital. One should never forget that life in a psychiatrically protected environment may offer the asylum which some patients need to lead the most satisfactory life in our present civilization.

The operation has undergone considerable modification. Besides the cutting of brain tissue (lobotomy, leucotomy), the removal of brain substance is also recommended. Most surgeons operate on the prefrontal area but some recommend attacking the frontal lobe. This uncertainty in the choice of technique and localization in the brain is an expression of therapeutic insecurity which should exert a strong critical hesitancy on the part of the clinician who is considering surgical procedure.

5. USE OF SEDATIVES AND HYPNOTICS

In considering the use of sedatives and hypnotics in psychiatry, one can distinguish between their therapeutic value in alleviating anxiety and tension, in producing sleep, and in controlling marked behavior disturbances. Obviously, in a patient, all these difficulties may be interlinked. Anxiety may frequently be the main factor in a sleep disorder and in excitements, and its alleviation by chemical or psychotherapeutic means leads to a marked change in these difficulties. The discussion is therefore primarily orientative and the actual application will be discussed in later chapters.

There is, on the whole, a tendency to administer drugs too freely. It is best for the physician to be thoroughly acquainted with a few hypnotics and sedatives and to use them individually, or in combination, if desirable. He should refrain from using patent medicines. Otherwise, there is considerable danger that he will not be clearly aware of the specific factor of the drugs and of their combined influence. Such treatment would be haphazard, leading to frequent changes in medication in an effort to find the most suitable drug without clear awareness of the indications and contraindications, susceptibilities, and toxicity.

Sedatives are used to alleviate anxiety and tension. Small amounts of barbital 0.15 gm. (2½ gr.), three to four times a day, have proved to be most satisfactory. It is important that, with improvement, the sedatives be diminished gradually by omitting one dosage one day, and a few days later another, otherwise tension may increase rapidly if the patient is not as well as he seemed. Small amounts of phenobarbital 0.06 gm. (1 gr.) twice to three times daily seem to give less satisfactory results. Sodium amytal 0.2 gm. (3 gr.) has a briefer action and is therefore not to be recommended for continuous sedation.

According to their points of attack, hypnotics are grouped into cortical and subcortical drugs; the former are used to overcome difficulties in falling asleep, the latter for producing a prolonged sleep. In their use, one must be guided therefore by the clinical picture of the sleep disorder as well as by the empirically determined susceptibility and the person's sleep type.

There are two normal sleep types: some persons feel tired rather early in the evening, fall asleep soon, and the depth of sleep reaches its maximum soon with gradual diminution; others feel fresh until late in the night. Their sleep reaches its maximal depth towards the morning until they are refreshed by a bath or get started at work. These constitutional differences should be considered as well as the average amount of sleep needed, with due consideration, however, of the total situation. Many patients have the erroneous belief that the amount of sleep they need is either more or less than corresponds to their constitutional make-up.

Susceptibility to drugs varies greatly. The average amount may cause toxic symptoms in some and be without practical effect in others. This, as well as the individual possibilities of addiction, is discussed in the chapters on delirious reactions and drug addiction. Alkaloids and alcohol should not be used for the treatment of essential sleep disorders. One only needs morphine and opiates when the sleep is disturbed by pain. Alcohol, e.g., in the form of beer, is frequently offered to older patients. It seems to me essential that we keep in mind the difference between a patient who suffers from a personality disorder and therefore needs help, and a person who uses alcohol because of its taste and minor psychologic effects. The danger of habit formation when offering alcohol to a depressed patient, to persons who suffer from minor or major personality disorders, and from diminished resistance in old age cannot be stressed enough.

Clinically one distinguishes between sleep disorders on a structural cerebral, and a functional, basis. To the first group belong many of the encephalitic, general paretic, luetic, cerebral arteriosclerotic, pre-senile, and senile sleep difficulties. They may manifest themselves in a craving for sleep and an increased amount of sleep, in reversed sleep, and in complete inability to sleep. The possibilities of correction or modification through re-education and drugs are discussed in Chapter XIII. To the functional group, in its broadest sense belong the delirious disorders (especially drug deliria), toxic disturbances (caffeine, cocaine), somatic illnesses, and various psychiatric disorders (especially affective and schizophrenic illnesses). They are the main field for the use of drugs. Functional sleep disorders, in the narrower sense, are part of the psychoneurotic reaction set, especially hysterical, hypochondriacal, and anxiety reactions. In these cases drugs are contraindicated, and psychotherapy should be used exclusively. Transient sleep difficulties occur as a result of somatic factors (pain, cough, gastro-intestinal complaints) or worry, sorrow, anger and annoyance, or unsettled problems. According to the factors involved, hypnotics, analgesics, psychotherapeutic procedures, or regulation of general life hygiene are indicated. In dealing with any sleep disorder, the personality setting must be considered and attempts at correction of the fundamental factors be made before one resorts to the merely symptomatic treatment by drugs.

Difficulties in falling asleep are best influenced by paraldehyde and chloral hydrate. Paraldehyde works fast if given in amounts of 2 to 6 gm. (2 to 6 cc.) but has a disagreeable taste and, being exhaled through the lungs, is undesirable for patients who lead an active group life. Its use is therefore restricted to patients who need to be more or less isolated or who are on the disturbed ward of a psychiatric hospital. Some authors warn against the use of chloral hydrate in patients with myocardial damage. The fear of cardiac danger has, however, been greatly overemphasized and the use of chloral hydrate as a valuable hypnotic has been unjustly neglected. The dosage varies from 0.5 to 1 gm. (7½ to 15 gr.). Some patients show a sensitivity to it (exanthema, indigestion, excitement). Through hypodermic administration of soluble hypnotics (dial, amytal), sleep can be forced but this procedure is not practical in sleep disorders of long duration. The slight hypnotics and sedatives that are frequently used are only helpful in combination with other sedatives or as a means of preparing the patient for sleep by producing relaxation. They are not strong enough to be used in serious sleep disorders. To this group belong bromide and its many combinations.

Broken sleep and sleep of short duration with the inability to go back to sleep are best treated by barbiturates, the most effective among them being barbital (veronal), phenobarbital, and amytal. There are many others which have slight advantages along various lines but which are not essentially different. Barbiturates produce sleep after one to two hours. Some patients are susceptible to them and easily show symptoms of intoxication (dullness of thinking, especially for two to three hours after awakening; fatigue, or slight ataxia), while others react with definite idiosyncrasy (exanthema and kidney irritation). In serious insomnia, such as in a depression, barbital 0.5 to 1 gm. (7½ to 15 gr.) is frequently sufficient to produce only a few hours' sleep. Phenobarbital (luminal) 0.2 gm. (3 gr.) helps in senile sleep difficulties. It is usually used in combination with barbital, forming an effective combination. Dial 0.4 gm. (6 gr.) can be administered by mouth as well as rectally. Amytal 0.4 gm. (6 gr.) works faster than the other barbiturates and seems to produce less after-effect, but may depress the heart action. It is also unsuitable for prolonged periods of treatment because it is definitely habit forming. Among newer drugs pentobarbital sodium (nembutal) and propyl-methyl-carbinyl allyl barbituric acid (seconal) have proved to be valuable hypnotics, both given in the amount of 0.1 gm. (2 gr.).

Combination of hypnotics and sedatives is frequently desirable. A combination of paraldehyde or chloral hydrate with barbital may be advisable to induce sleep rapidly and sustain it over several hours — paraldehyde 2 to 3 gm. (30 to 45 gr.), or chloral hydrate 0.5 to 1.0 gm. (7½ to 15 gr.) with barbital 0.5 gm. (7½ gr.). In many cases sodium bromide 0.5 to 1.0 gm. (7½ to 15 gr.) with barbital will be successful in restoring greater ease and will allow the barbital to be more effective. The addition of aspirin or phenacetin to barbital not only helps to prevent dull head sensations in the morning, but also increases the hypnotic effect. Scopolamine (hyoscine)-morphine should not be used as an hypnotic but reserved exclusively for the treatment of excitement. The combination of hypnotics (phenobarbital) with opium may be helpful in depressions with marked anxiety. It should not be carried out for any length of time because of the danger of addiction. In mild sleep disorders sedatives may be sufficient, e.g., bromide, or small amounts of phenobarbital or barbital. Where such a mild sleep disturbance persists over a long time it will be wisest to omit drugs and depend on psychotherapy and adjustment of the routine with or without the help of hydrotherapy (continuous baths or cold wet packs). In older patients one should always investigate blood pressure and blood sugar late in the evening. It is frequently possible to produce satisfactory sleep, with or without some hypnotic, by raising the blood pressure (through a cup of coffee) or by correcting a slight hypoglycemic reaction through candy or a drink rich in carbohydrate. Mild hypoglycemia occurs also in tension reactions. A warm drink, such as milk or chocolate, has a definite sedative influence. Dietary management should always be included in the treatment of insomnia (time, amount, and type of evening meal). Coffee or tea may prove too stimulating. The hours before retirement should be spent in recreational activities which do not stimulate or excite. Physical exertion and too great physical fatigue prevent sleep. As a rule, any therapeutic discussion should take place before 6 P.M.

One should never use hypnotics exclusively and neglect psychotherapy. The patient needs to be encouraged or taught to assume a passive attitude to his body as well as his thoughts, including the present (effort to sleep and waiting for sleep), past (guilt), and future (planning and anticipation). In broken sleep one should investigate dreams which may indicate a psychodynamic or toxic (drug) basis which needs to be corrected. In recovering depression in the male, erections which may be disturbing in the early morning hours are frequently due to a full bladder, and the patient can fall asleep again after urination.

6. INTRAVENOUS ADMINISTRATION OF BARBITURATES FOR PSYCHOTHERAPEUTIC INTERVIEWS

The value of producing periods of relaxation, which can be used psychotherapeutically, has long been recognized and attempts to achieve it have been made by hypnosis and by drugs. In the last

20 years, and especially during the recent war, sodium amytal and later sodium pentothal have been found most useful for this purpose.

In using this type of interview one has to be guided by the individual psychopathology. These treatments belong in the hands of psychopathologically well-trained psychiatrists who can recognize, evaluate, and treat emergency suicidal dangers and paranoid projections. In some patients incoherence of thinking, e.g., in acute catatonic patients, may not only prevent a constructive discussion but increase the thinking disorder by the strong emotions which accompany an emotional catharsis. Instead of relaxation, increased anxiety may occur because of the freeing of such emotions.

The main indication is to offer the patient the opportunity to discuss suppressed material. The effect of the drugs diminishes the unpleasant emotion and enables the patient to talk of unpleasant experiences. It is the unusual case in which much repressed, i.e., dissociated, material is obtained. Whenever this occurs one must evaluate the possibility of a disorganizing process. Whatever is presented should be used for psychotherapeutic discussion either during this interview or in later interviews without the use of drugs. Repeated interviews under the influence of these drugs without progressive psychotherapeutic discussions exclusive of drugs have, in my experience, been unnecessary and undesirable. The factor of emotional catharsis is important in connection with recent acute traumatic experiences. Excellent results can therefore be obtained in recent war experiences but rarely in the reactions to problems of ordinary life. The value of catharsis is also highly limited in the discussion of war experiences which are no longer acute and have become part of the individual's developing psychopathologic reaction. One should, however, avoid provoking confessions and, if they occur, consider them a serious traumatic experience. The catharsis of resentment is desirable as relief, but should be repeated only if the dynamic factors involved become adjusted. Under the influence of these drugs, the dynamic relationship with the physician is strengthened. The combination of planned suggestion and of hypnosis with intravenous administration of barbiturates may have advantages in reaching repressed material.

Contraindications for this type of treatment on a one-trial basis do not exist if the patient is cooperative. (However, one should take into consideration any drugs which the patient might have previously received.) The treatment should not be forced on frightened or antagonistic patients. Repeated administration should not be used if the patient's thinking disorder is too marked for him to make constructive use of the discussion, if suicidal urges increase, or if paranoid projections develop. In erotic schizophrenic patients an undesirably strong transference may develop. This attachment necessitates termination of these interviews.

The *technique* can be learned readily. The amount of 0.5 gm. (7½ gr.) of sodium amytal, diluted in 15 cc. of water, is injected intravenously over a period of at least 10, and usually 15, minutes. The patient is asked to state when he first feels drowsy or flushed in the face. If nystagmus, slurring of speech, or excessive drowsiness appears, the speed of injection is slowed down or discontinued before the full amount is given. The patient is questioned rather steadily, or conversation is kept up during the injection, so that the patient does not fall asleep. Ordinarily, marked talkativeness starts after the first 5 cc. have been given. An interview may last from 30 to 60 minutes, followed by a sleep of several hours' duration. The sleep can be shortened if one gives the patient a cup of coffee at the end of the interview. Some patients remember the whole conversation while others have to be told. It may be therapeutically wise not to force some patients to become aware of what has been discussed.

The complications which may arise are respiratory difficulties and cardiovascular collapse. In cases of respiratory difficulty, one should immediately discontinue injections, use artificial respiration and infusion of saline. The action of the drug is short and the above treatment will carry over the immediate difficulty without resort to stronger stimulants. In case of threatened cardiovascular collapse epinephrine, metrazol, or picrotoxin are of value. The drugs are given in small doses, repeating until the patient recovers. (The patient should be watched carefully for signs of overdosage.) It is rarely necessary to resort to these drugs if the injection is given slowly. If a state of shock develops, transfusions or infusions of fluids are indicated. It is essential that the preparation of treatment include all the drugs and means which are required in an emergency.

Sodium pentothal has the advantage of faster action and shorter duration. It is therefore especially suitable for ambulatory treatment. On the other hand, the sleep which follows a sodium amytal interview may have a beneficial effect. It permits the patient some unconscious adjustment of the emotional upheaval which may have occurred. From the point of psychopathologic consideration, sodium amytal interviews are safer than those with sodium pentothal.

Sodium pentothal is administered intravenously in the amount of 0.5 gm. (7½ gr.), diluted in 10 cc. of water. It is injected slowly over a period of 5 minutes. During this period, the physician must watch the patient constantly for any toxic signs. He should carry on his psychotherapeutic questioning from the beginning of the injection, the effectiveness of which will disappear rapidly after about 30 to 60 minutes.

In ambulatory treatment all the above requirements are necessary. The return to normal alertness will be hastened by the administration of caffeine benzoate 0.6 gm. (10 gr.) or a cup of coffee at the termination of treatment. The patient should not be permitted to leave for two hours after termination of sodium amytal treatment and for one hour after sodium pentothal treatment because of possible delayed respiratory reaction. Whether he can be permitted to return home alone or even to work depends on his psychopathologic, general physical, and neurologic status, and on the patient's task ahead.

7. HYDROTHERAPEUTIC PROCEDURES

Although in recent years there has been a considerable disregard of hydrotherapeutic procedures in many hospitals, its well-established value deserves to be kept in mind. Its importance for the treatment of marked excitements has diminished greatly but not for the alleviation of anxiety and tension and its many somatic expressions. Continuous warm baths and cold wet packs diminish motor restlessness and produce rest and sleep by their influence on the cardiovascular system. In addition, these hydrotherapeutic measures stimulate respiration and general metabolism and exert a definite influence on peristalis. For practical reasons, I shall discuss separately and at length continuous baths and cold wet packs, mentioning briefly cold sitz baths and general hydrotherapeutic procedures.

The continuous bath treatment utilizes the sustained influence of moderately increased warmth. This produces a hyperemia of the skin and thus decreases the blood volume of the central nervous system. It leads to freer circulation. Disturbing stimuli are kept from the skin. The result is a physical relaxation which is recognized in the deep and slower respiration, diminished muscle tonus and reflexes, lowering of the body temperature, diminished blood vessel tonus, and slight decrease in blood pressure and pulse rate. These physiologic reactions produce a feeling of fatigue. Of importance is the psychobiologic factor of relaxation, which causes an agreeable feeling, and together with all the above-mentioned reactions frequently leads to sleep. There is, no doubt, a strong suggestive influence — relaxation, fatigue, and a feeling of drowsiness accompany normal sleep, and these sensations make the patient feel that he is falling asleep. Well-directed and suggestive remarks by the physician may increase the hydrotherapeutic influence. It is doubtful whether we can go further at present in explanation of the hydrotherapeutic effect of continuous baths or whether we are justified in accepting Dastré-Moret's theory that there is an antagonism of peripheral and inner circulation. This may not apply to circulation in the head and brain. It has been demonstrated on a patient whose skull was open, that the vessels of the pia mater contract under the influence of continuous baths, but we cannot be certain that the vessels of the cortex and brain centers react the same way and that actual oligemia of the brain results. Recent investigations show that chronaxia decreases. This is one of the few proofs that hydrotherapy does produce a definite muscle relaxation. With further investigation of hydrotherapy, a better understanding of the results which are now known to us from practical application will be obtained, and indications for the use of this treatment can be better worked out.

Thus far, we know that continuous baths are helpful in the treatment of various kinds of excitement in producing relaxation and decrease of body stimulation. In contrast to some authors, I also urge its use in the various delirious reactions, with a need of careful supervision. Single tub-rooms are desirable for all excited patients. Where this is not possible a separation, in the form of a screen, will help to decrease stimulation of one patient by another. Patients who are tense, relax well in continuous baths, which should be administered according to the patient's need, e.g., in the morning for depressed patients who feel tense in the morning hours, and before retiring for patients who become tense in the evening. If given in the evening, it serves for sleep preparation and decreases the need for sedatives. Tension is outstanding in many depressions, in schizophrenic reactions, and in the various psychoneuroses. All patients suffering from these illnesses usually react well because of the general metabolic stimulation. Many patients with agitated depressions feel more at ease in continuous baths. We should, however, never insist upon them if the patient's fear cannot be overcome by repeated psychotherapeutic formulations. In some patients, especially in older age, the temperature has to be lowered by one or two degrees Fahrenheit (to 96.5 or 95.5 degrees). If we keep this in mind and watch the blood pressure, cerebral arteriosclerosis is not a contraindication. It is frequently difficult to treat the various excitements in old age and at the same time protect the patient from cardiac strain. The treatment of cerebral arteriosclerotics advised by some authors is a combination of hydrotherapy, diuretin three times a day, and powdered opium 0.03 gm. (½ gr.) at 8 P.M.

The most important contraindications are fear, great agitation, and excitements which cannot be managed in the bath. It would be wrong to keep a patient in the bath by force. Repeated attempts with well-planned persuasion, however, frequently lead to an acceptance of the treatment. It is occasionally helpful to give a sedative (barbital 0.5 gm. — 7½ gr.) half an hour before the bath is administered. This, however, should be done only a few times. Cardiovascular and renal disorders are rarely a contraindication if all the necessary medical precautions are considered. Otitis media or certain skin reactions such as eczema, trichophytosis and furunculosis may necessitate termination. Menstruation is not a contraindication except for aesthetic reasons in sensitive persons or in prejudiced patients.

The temperature of the water should be kept around 97.5 degrees Fahrenheit and the water should be constantly changing. The patient lies elevated on a canvas. He is more comfortable and relaxes better in this way than when lying directly in the tub. It is desirable to have a canvas cover over the tub so that the patient is not exposed. This decreases sexual stimulation and protects the patient's feelings. This cover, however, should not be used as restraint. With persuasion the patient is usually willing to stay, even though he may get out of the tub occasionally. Many manic patients splash a great deal and nurses should wear rubber aprons. The duration of the bath depends on the patient's need, and may vary from one hour once or twice a day to continuous treatment during the whole twenty-four hours. This is occasionally necessary for a few days in highly excited patients. Such patients usually sleep several hours a day in the bath. To make the patient more comfortable, an air-filled ring should be placed under his head. Ice water should be offered freely and a cold towel applied to the forehead. The nurses are requested to take the patient's temperature every fifteen minutes and to check the temperature of the water at frequent intervals. The patient's subjective feeling about the temperature should always be considered. If any disturbing cardiovascular reaction occurs, the treatment must be discontinued at once.

Cold wet packs have a much stronger hydrotherapeutic influence than continuous baths. The reaction is primarily based on the "hydrotherapeutic shock" which occurs when the cold sheets are applied to the body. This produces first a contraction of the cutaneous vessels and then marked dilatation, which leads to a flooding of the body surface with blood and to a pleasurable sensation of warmth. Through the dilatation of the vessels, a rapid circulation and interchange between the cold blood near the surface and the warm blood of the body interior is said to produce a "cardiovascular massage." This is considered highly desirable. After about fifteen to thirty minutes the patient should relax and feel comfortable, frequently falling asleep. The temperature of the sheets and the body surface is then the same. If no beneficial reaction has been obtained after one hour the patient should be removed but may, however, without drying, be immediately put in another cold wet pack. A sufficiently strong hydrotherapeutic shock may then be obtained and relaxation achieved. If the second pack is not successful, one should resort to bath treatment. It sometimes happens that a patient reacts favorably after a few days if one does not give up and continues to formulate the reasons for this type of treatment. Much of the success depends on our psychotherapeutic approach. We can hardly expect good results if we stir up fear or antagonism by using cold wet packs as a threat.

The indications for cold wet packs are the same as for continuous baths. Cold wet packs, however, can be used more freely in the psychoneurotic sleep disturbances. If the pack is well administered, there are practically no contraindications except consideration of the cardiac condition. The pulse must be watched carefully to prevent heat accumulation which might lead to collapse.

To administer a cold wet pack, a linen sheet is rinsed in tap water and wound closely around the body. The arms are pressed closely to the body (a towel in each axilla will prevent pain). Then, two woolen blankets are put around the body and the top sheet fastened with safety pins (many physicians prefer to omit pins, but this is hardly practical in restless and excited patients). To protect the bed the patient is laid on a rubber sheet. An ice bag should be applied to the head and ice water offered freely. The duration of the pack is usually two hours. The patient should then be dried and put in his warmed bed for further rest or sleep. Some advise a brief cold shower after removal from the pack, followed by hard dry rubbing. It is, however, not very practical in most excitements and therefore usually omitted.

In cooperative patients, the pack can be given somewhat loosely so that the patient can free himself from the sheet and blankets if he feels that he cannot stand it any longer. This is especially desirable in anxious and fearful cases. Most patients are then willing to remain in the pack for the desired length of time. Loose packs are always given if possible, but they should be tight enough to secure the hydrotherapeutic effect. In quiet, fearful patients half-packs can be given, i.e., the arms are left outside the blankets. This, however, greatly reduces the hydrotherapeutic effect, and the addition of wet towels and blankets as broad shoulder straps (three-fourth packs) does not increase it much. Both the half-pack and the three-fourth pack are used little.

With individual psychotherapeutic attention and the proper ward atmosphere cold wet packs are usually not resented or felt as torture by the patient. The unfavorable attitude of some German authors toward this method is probably due to the fact that they do not offer sufficient individual preparation or consider individual reactions which demand modification. It is essential that nurses and attendants be well trained in the application of various hydrotherapeutic procedures, and that all the preparations be carefully carried out before attempting to administer the treatment. The physician should be present when a difficult patient is put into the pack. He should see the patient frequently while in the pack and order removal not only for physical, but also for psychotherapeutic, reasons if it is desirable.

Warm packs do not produce the "hydrotherapeutic shock" reaction that is produced by cold wet packs. Instead of feeling comfortable and relaxed, many patients after a while begin to feel chilly and become restless. Dry packs are merely restraint. They may be indicated to prevent cardiac strain or as the most harmless and safest restraint during tube feeding. In the latter case, the pack should be removed immediately after the feeding has been finished.

In psychoneurotic sleep disorders, general hydrotherapeutic treatment is occasionally indicated. Strasser advises a cold wet pack for one hour in the morning, followed by a half-bath (85 degrees Fahrenheit) for five minutes, an hour's rest, and a long walk. In his experience, this leads to sleep education. Most psychiatrists, however, prefer to rely upon psychotherapy. The use of properly individualized hydrotherapy does not interfere with psychotherapy. Less can be said for the treatment given in the hydrotherapy and physiotherapy departments in many psychiatric hospitals. This treatment is mostly administered without the consideration of indications and physiologic effect, and merely produces a general stimulating effect. Such treatment has about the same value as the physical exercises in old-fashioned gymnasiums. Scotch douches (after preparation with a moderately warm shower, cold and hot jets of water under high pressure, are alternately thrown along the spine) have a most stimulating effect and help to increase sexual potency in men who are physically let-down and have not sufficient time for physical recreation. It hardly needs to be mentioned that such treatment should only be given after a regulation of the patient's life and an adjustment of his personality difficulties.

Cold sitz baths are of great value in reducing sexual tension. They produce an oligemia in the genital organs and for anatomical reasons are more effective in women than in men. The patient is advised to take a cold sitz bath in the morning and before retiring, sitting for five minutes in a half-bath of cold water (50 degrees Fahrenheit) with the feet in warm water. The time is prolonged by one minute every day until a duration of ten minutes twice a day has been reached. This, combined with psychotherapy, usually leads to prompt relief but the final result depends on psychotherapy. Sitz baths are indicated in marked sexual tension in various psychoneuroses and depressions, and especially with the increase of sexual desire at the involutional period. Sitz baths may also help relieve pre-menstrual sexual tension.

BIBLIOGRAPHY

1. KALINOWSKY, L. B., and HOCH, P. H.: *Shock Treatments and Other Somatic Procedures in Psychiatry.* Grune & Stratton, New York, 1946.
2. RENNIE, T. A. C.: Use of Insulin as Sedation Therapy; Control of Basic Anxiety in the Psychoses. *Archives of Neurology and Psychitary,* 50, 1943.
3. SARGANT, W., and SLATER, E.: *Somatic Methods of Treatment in Psychiatry.* The Williams and Wilkins Company, Baltimore, 1946. (Includes a discussion of prolonged sleep treatment.)
4. GILLESPIE, R. D.: Narcosis Therapy. *Journal of Neurology and Psychiatry,* 2, 1939.
5. BRODY, E. B., and MOORE, B. E.: Prefrontal Lobotomy. A Review of Recent Literature. *The Connecticut State Medical Journal,* 10, 1946.
6. Conferences on Therapy. Treatment of Barbiturate Poisoning. *Journal of the American Medical Association,* 1, 1946.
7. KRUSEN, F. H.: *Physical Medicine; The Employment of Physical Agents for Diagnosis and Therapy.* W. B. Saunders Company, Philadelphia, 1941.
8. MENNINGER, W. C., and CUTRER, M.: The Psychological Aspects of Physiotherapy. *American Journal of Psychiatry,* 93, 1937.

Chapter VIII

EXCITEMENTS

EXCITEMENTS are characterized by overactivity, with more or less marked mood and general behavior disorders. They may be essentially emotional disorders (manic excitements) or merely incidental to a more important delusional or confusional disorder, with fear, hate, and jealousy. In other excitements disharmony of affect and content are leading characteristics (schizophrenic excitements). The management of all types of excitement is guided by the same general principles, but one must take into consideration the characteristics of the reaction type to which the excitement belongs and the individual variations. The therapeutic approach should be modified accordingly.

The manic excitements belong to the affective reaction type; they have as outstanding features elated mood, overactivity, distractibility, and ease of stimulation, with corresponding disturbance in thinking and behavior. Psychopathologic studies indicate that anxiety, resentment, or depression may be hidden by the elated mood. According to the personality setting, less specific features may play a dominating role, especially in paranoic constitutions, psychopathic, and adolescent patients. Schizophrenic admixtures are relatively frequent. These excitements are of circumscribed attack form (with a well-defined beginning and end), often recurrent, and frequently, although not always, preceded or followed by depressions. Most manic excitements belong to the manic-depressive group. Schizophrenic excitements are phases of varying duration in a schizophrenic illness, with content disorder and complete withdrawal from reality into fanciful life. Less predictable catathymically-determined outbursts complicate the picture. In excitements caused by panic, fear of an imagined danger makes the patient desperate in his need to escape. These patients are violent because of their distress and they must obtain security from the environment. Such panics may occur as phases in schizophrenic and depressive illnesses and also frequently in delirious reactions, oligophrenic, and organic psychoses. Most toxic and organic deliria are states of excitement which present the main therapeutic problem except for the more specific approach. Oligophrenic manic patients are especially difficult to handle. In oligophrenic, psychopathic, and organic patients, brief excitements, usually in the form of anger outbursts and destructiveness, are frequent.

Constitutional factors are etiologically most important and specific treatment is possible only in symptomatic excitements. The claim of some that various chemical compounds have a specific influence in manic excitements and the claim of others for nonspecific protein therapy are based on insufficient proof. The hope has been abandoned that through sleep treatment the fundamental factors of the schizophrenic reaction would be influenced. Psychobiologic treatment takes into consideration the fundamental factors involved and is guided by them psychotherapeutically, although the personality analysis and adjustment should be delayed until the excitement has subsided. In dealing with excitement, it is essential to remove the patient from all exciting and disturbing influences. He should be interfered with as little as possible.

The treatment depends largely on the outstanding symptoms of the excitement and the patient's personality make-up. Generally speaking, the elated manic patient forms rapport easily and can be led to accept the restrictions which are necessary to prevent overstimulation and to protect him and others from acts arising from his elated mood and self-assertion. Dealing with the excited patient is more difficult in cases with self-assertive and paranoic personalities, or when the patient's judgment is affected by constitutional (oligophrenic) or acquired deficit (cerebral damage), when his grasp is limited (panics and delirious reactions), or when catathymic factors are important. Combativeness occurs easily and should always be carefully analyzed in order to reduce it or to prevent a recurrence. In manic excitement, combativeness is usually the reaction to interference and to obstacles to which the self-assertive patient is unable to adjust. He therefore reacts with anger. More difficult to handle is combativeness on a catathymic basis with which one may be frequently confronted in catatonic and paranoid reactions. Some of these outbursts are not predictable but, on the whole, skilled physicians and nurses should be able to detect signs of tension. Hydro-

therapeutic procedure, planned occupational therapy, and psychotherapy frequently restore ease. One should remove any objects
of value, or anything which the patient might use to injure himself
or others. Overactivity should be diminished to prevent constant
stimulation and physical exertion. Hydrotherapy and insulin treatment are the primary methods for quieting an excited patient. In
unmanageable excitements intensive convulsive therapy has been
recommended (see Chapter VII). Hypnotics or sedatives should,
if possible, be given only at night. Medication should be administered in high enough dosage to affect such a patient. Repeated
medication within twenty-four hours is usually undesirable as it
easily leads to toxic accumulation or to an insufficient persistent
influence which produces an irritable, and not a sedative, reaction in
the patient, making handling more difficult. Sedatives should never
be given to quiet noisiness and shouting in the day time. The patient
should be removed to a psychiatric hospital if the disturbance is
beyond toleration in a private home or general hospital. Such excitement can frequently be surprisingly well managed after transfer
because of diminished interference, omission of much of the sedation, and the use of hydrotherapy.

During the excitement most patients neglect personal hygiene
which requires tactful and persistent correction from nurses and
attendants. Continuous baths will help a great deal in carelessness
with urine and feces. Smearing is rare in pure manic excitement, but
it frequently presents a distressing problem in schizophrenic reactions. Many patients expectorate carelessly and refuse to be influenced by corrective remarks. These features necessitate frequent
cleansing of the room and washing of floors and walls. If this is
consistently done, and if patients are moved to other rooms when
necessary, it is usually possible to avoid the odor which characterized disturbed wards in the older hospitals. It is naturally essential
that the room be well ventilated both for hygenic reasons and for
the patient's comfort.

The somatic features which deserve attention are poor sleep,
loss of weight, and neglect of sufficient intake of food, constipation, and incidental wounds. No sedatives should be given during
the daytime, as they merely cause irritability and a feeling of being
held down. For the night's sleep the patient may be given high

amounts of paraldehyde (12 cc. by mouth or double the amount by rectum), amytal 0.4 to 0.6 gm. (6 to 10 gr.) intramuscularly, and only occasionally scopolamine 0.0006 to 0.001 gm. ($\frac{1}{100}$ to $\frac{1}{60}$ gr.) combined with morphine 0.02 gm. ($\frac{1}{3}$ gr.) intramuscularly around 10 to 11 P.M., according to the individual responsiveness. All these drugs have the advantage of being rapidly eliminated and the patient does not show any after effect in the form of headaches or sluggishness and irritability the next morning. These after-symptoms frequently make the use of barbiturates undesirable. In some cases, however, the usual amounts of barbital 0.5 to 1.0 gm. (7½ to 15 gr.) have a sufficient sleep- or rest-producing effect without these hangover symptoms. All these hypnotics should be combined with hydrotherapeutic procedures and should be dispensed with as soon as the patient's condition allows.

Most manic patients will take sufficient food and fluids. Tube feeding, as a rule, needs to be resorted to only in manic stupors and in manic patients with a marked aversion to the acceptance of illness and treatment. Aversion reactions occur in self-assertive or suspicious patients who often have definite delusions of persecution, and also in oligophrenic and psychopathic settings. It is more frequent in schizophrenic excitements. The diet in all these cases should be rich in carbohydrates and of high caloric value. Milk and egg-nogs, which patients will take well because they are thirsty, help to increase both the food and fluid intake. Diet should be varied as much as possible, and patients should be urged to eat. If such patients are not encouraged to eat, their weight loss may reach a marked degree as they do not pay much attention to hunger sensations. Unless they are well nourished, constant overactivity may lead to exhaustion. Moreover, a good physical condition will help the patient to endure his excitement better and to regain his health sooner after the excitement has subsided.

Constipation can usually be easily controlled with cathartics (see Chapter IX). Enemas will rarely be necessary. Most patients are willing to cooperate in the taking of pulse or temperature, especially if one does not insist on unnecessary rectal temperatures. Both pulse and temperature may remain within normal limits if they are taken when the patient is at ease. Tachycardia is found in irritable and angry patients. A rise in temperature should always indicate the probability of a physical involvement and should not merely be explained away by the excitement. It is often due to dehydration or to colds, but may also be the indication of beginning pneumonia.

Menstruation is occasionally disturbed in duration, flow, or regularity, but this does not need special attention except for psychotherapy. An increase of excitement at the menstrual or premenstrual period is frequent and can be diminished or prevented by more frequent hydrotherapy and sedatives and a modification of routine. In many cases the menstrual reaction is accompanied by an increase of sexual excitement, which can be adjusted by hydrotherapy and the elimination of certain visitors or other stimulating factors. Most manic patients are sexually excited. Therefore it is wise to restrict contact with nurses and to avoid opportunities for exposure. Frequently one has to guard against homosexual stimulation by nurses or other patients. This is usually more difficult on the female wards because nurses are frequently careless in expressing affection by putting their arms around the patient's waist or even kissing the patient as a spontaneous expression of sympathy. Patients should not be given magazines with erotic content. These patients usually express their eroticism in vulgar talk, songs, or gestures; it rarely happens that overt acts go beyond kissing. It is therefore quite possible to have female nurses take care of disturbed male patients. The fear of sexual assault which caused the older psychiatrists to have male attendants exclusively on a male ward, is unwarranted if normal precautions are taken and warning signals in certain patients heeded. It is to be regretted, however, that training schools are not educating more male nurses. Every nurse must realize that manic patients may use a great deal of vulgarity and learn not to consider them ethically undesirable personalities. She should learn to keep a healthy distance between herself and the patient and ignore his remarks without showing a prudish attitude. On the other hand, the physician should not expect the impossible from his nurses and should consider their individual sensitiveness. Erotic expressions from the patient should be dealt with psychotherapeutically. At quiet moments patients are usually willing to recognize the undesirability of their excited behavior and will make efforts to use more self-restraint.

From the above discussion, one can understand the need for constant psychotherapeutic efforts during an excitement. The whole ward atmosphere, the attitude of physician, nurses, and other patients should exert a wholesome influence. Discussions of minor, or more serious, disturbances should be adjusted to the patient's personality and condition at the time and should always end with a constructive formulation which points out workable possibilities. Argumentation and persuasion by reasoning will irritate rather than calm the patient. Reactions to visitors, to persons on the ward, and to letters can be analyzed advantageously. Outstanding personality traits may need analysis and study. Delusions and hallucinations deserve special attention. The patient's attitude to the illness, based on the available insight, to hospital treatment, and to the physician's interference are explained and modified. Analysis of the dynamic factors, however, must be delayed until the excitement has settled down and the patient has achieved sufficient stability to use constructive criticism.

Hospitalization is desirable in any excitement which lasts more than a few days. Correct treatment, especially hydrotherapeutic procedure, cannot be carried out well in a private home, even though financial means may allow far-reaching environmental changes. Most physicians and relatives delay too long and much money is spent unnecessarily because of prejudice against psychiatric hospitals or because they anticipate great difficulty in transferring the patient to a hospital. Both objections are unjustified. The dealing with excitements is now a planned and individualized procedure, devoid of the attitude of fear which formerly led to rigid and even cruel restraint. The understanding of many of the factors which cause and increase excitements has led to intelligent management, to the introduction of careful hydrotherapy and occupational therapy, and to the removal of many undesirable features. The disturbed ward in a modern psychiatric hospital does not resemble the wards of fifty years ago, with the fighting, uncontrolled behavior, or other dangers which contributed greatly to the prejudice against psychiatric hospitalization. A visit to the disturbed wards of the hospitals available in his community will, however, show the physician whether he is dealing with a well-equipped and well-managed hospital to which he can confidently refer his patients.

Taking an excited patient to a hospital should present little difficulty if the procedure is well planned. It is advisable to complete the necessary arrangements before informing the patient of the plan. The physician should be familiar with the available hospitals in his district and the possible expense involved, and with the commitment procedure in his state. In states in which the legal papers can be made out by practitioners, every physician should keep blanks in his office. In arranging for the commitment of a patient, the necessary permission from the authorities for admission to a public hospital should first be procured. A sufficient number of members of the patient's family, or close friends or neighbors, should be at hand to overcome any attempt at physical resistance. The police should only be called in if all other resources have failed, and then they should not be uniformed members of the force. Administration of morphine 0.02 gm. (⅓ gr.) and hyoscine 0.0006 to 0.001 gm. (¹⁄₁₀₀ to ¹⁄₆₀ gr.), hypodermically, will often diminish the patient's resistance and make transfer to the hospital a relatively easy task. In some cases it has proved helpful to give amytal 0.3 gm. (5 gr.) by mouth a half hour before the patient was informed of the proposed transfer. Having prepared everything carefully, the physician should inform the patient of the need for immediate hospitalization and the hospital selected. Lengthy arguments should be avoided, and the patient should be taken at once to the waiting ambulance or closed car and driven to the hospital. In an accompanying note, the physician should inform the hospital physician of the amount of hypnotics and sedatives which the patient has received recently so that no perplexity will arise at admission in regard to the pharmacologic effect of the drugs and so that the physician who will have to take care of the excited patient will know what he can administer.

The general principles of treatment can best be demonstrated with regard to manic excitements. The other excitements differ therapeutically along more specific lines which necessitate modifications in the psychotherapeutic approach.

MANIC EXCITEMENTS

For practical reasons, a distinction is made between the hypomanic and the manic phase, the difference being in the degree of the psychopathologic disorder. In the hypomanic phase, the patient is elated, overactive, and constantly making plans. His judgment is definitely impaired by his optimistic mood and self-restraint is usually considerably lessened. The increased self-confidence and self-assertion frequently lead to clashes with interfering persons. In the manic phase all these features are greatly increased and high distractibility leads to marked disorders of thinking. Delusions and occasionally hallucinations occur, their content in conformity with the dominant mood of elation. The recognition and treatment of hypomanic reactions is important because they are usually treated outside of the hospital and exposed to dangers which can be controlled only to a limited extent. There is also no doubt that the correct management of such cases will occasionally prevent the outbreak of a full-fledged excitement. There are, however, manic excitements which develop rather suddenly within a few days with a hardly noticeable prodromal phase. Most manic excitements end gradually and they may be a slow change (hypomanic phase) to normal.

In any patient in whom one deals with elation with a definite onset and accompanied by sleep disturbance, loss of weight, and constipation, one should treat the condition as hypomanic. Stimulation will increase the excitement and the patient's activity should be curbed. A study of the personality will indicate the factors and situations which stimulate the patient. In some, it may be work strain, in others, disappointments and friction in business or private life. Change in a vacation, or cutting down on responsibilities will decrease the stimulating factors for some; in others, removal to a more neutral environment is necessary. One has to keep in mind, however, that a vacation spent on a trip or at a resort will usually be detrimental because of stimulation. If such a patient can continue his usual routine, a schedule should be worked out with the patient and his family, which will include work and recreation. The suggested routine should utilize the patient's interests and make him feel the interference no more keenly than is absolutely necessary. Such a schedule should be elastic, allowing the physician an opportunity to give in on minor points if desirable, but the patient should understand that here are certain limits beyond which the physician cannot go.

The optimistic mood of these patients must always be taken into consideration. It usually prevents insight into the illness, and such a patient may take physical and financial risks which will cause irreparable damage. A spirit of recklessness may cause physical carelessness, such as reckless driving, exposure, or neglect of physical illness. Some patients become involved in ethical difficulties, signing worthless checks or taking part in illegal enterprises. These patients should never be allowed to carry full financial responsibility, and they need to be especially protected from unwise investments and financial schemes.

There are a number of other dangers against which such patients must be guarded. Their domineering attitude often makes them unbearable to others and their resentment to interference may lead to quarrels or actual fights. Increase of sexual desire, although with decrease of potency, frequently leads to serious involvements of this nature. The danger of promiscuity, with risk of venereal disease, and in women, the possibility of impregnation, must be kept in mind. Many young hypomanics have their first sexual experiences during their illness, and an adjustment to them afterwards is sometimes very difficult for persons with rigid ethical standards.

Alcoholic excesses are also frequent. If possible, a physician should prohibit all alcoholic beverages during the entire course of the illness because of their stimulating influence. Excessive smoking needs to be curbed. Ten cigarettes a day should be sufficient; in cases of very young people, or where there are physical complications, smoking should be prohibited. It is, however, not wise to be too strict with regard to smoking, as it is usually a minor point and some leniency along this line may induce a patient to accept other restrictions more willingly. Movies and shows are rarely advisable but can sometimes be used for easing the rapport (the physician should know the material to which he is exposing the patient and to prevent, for example, erotic stimulation). In the choice of companions, especially special nurses, one should be guided by the same principles. Considerable attention should be paid to physical factors, as stimulation of every kind should be reduced as much as possible. The great desire for activity has to be curbed. Otherwise it will lead to over-stimulation and not to the hoped-for fatigue. As a result of the illness itself, as well as his overactivity, the patient loses weight. Every patient should therefore be urged to eat a well-balanced diet at regular hours. Mild cathartics should be sufficient to regulate the bowels. The poor sleep, which the patient is inclined to pass over lightly, can be corrected by sedatives such as barbital 0.5 gm. (7½ gr.) around 10 P.M., but it is advisable first to try prolonged baths of one to two hours' duration before retiring. This can be well managed, if necessary, in a private home. In women cold sitz baths (see p. 177) diminish the sexual tension. Sedatives of any kind are contraindicated during the daytime. They are not felt as relief but as something which restrains the patient's ease of activity, and this may produce an irritable mood and reactions of anger.

Whether a hypomanic or a manic patient can be well managed depends to a large extent on the patient's personality. Irritable and self-assertive persons may need hospital treatment because of their inability to cooperate or because they are unbearable to their environment. Hospitalization, i.e., usually commitment, is also necessary if a patient is unable to cooperate along the fundamentally important lines, particularly when the patient's financial, physical, or ethical status is endangered.

Case 5:

A 35 year old salesman developed in 1930 a gradually increasing hypomanic reaction, characterized by overactivity and optimistic mood with carelessness in business transactions and irresponsibility to obligations. He fell in love with his stenographer (1931), demanded a divorce from his wife (1932), began to spend money lavishly and passed worthless checks (fall, 1932). At this time as a reaction to having an excellent position offered for the spring of 1933, he began to sleep poorly, was over-talkative, sang and shouted but always friendly and amenable. Admitted to the clinic (12/1/32) he showed a typically hypomanic picture without insight. He fitted moderately well into the activities of a quiet ward where patients received few privileges. His work in occupational therapy was inaccurate and group life presented difficulties because of his impulsiveness and a tendency to become easily excited and argumentative. Overstimulation was carefully avoided. He was therefore allowed no visitors. The patient soon saw that the physicians were unwilling to go beyond certain limits in the routine outlined and that some restrictions could not be changed. A brief personality analysis was made the basis for the psychotherapeutic approach, taking especially into consideration his proud, self-dependent make-up and his normal tendencies of becoming too enthusiastic and easily excited and getting overstimulation in athletic activities. In handling his tendency to spend money too freely, his present difficult financial situation and his personality feature to be generous (although as a careful business man well within his limits) were pointed out. Excessive smoking was curtailed according to the general rules of hygiene. Sufficient sleep was obtained by two-hour continuous baths before retiring and sedatives were unnecessary. He was advised to let the marriage problem drop for the present because his decision might be influenced by his elated mood in which he could not properly recognize obstacles and all the responsibilities involved with regard to his wife and children. It was pointed out that he might feel unduly obligated to the other girl as a result of his need for chivalry. His sex life illustrated to him his over-emphasis on sexual satisfaction which he was not always able to obtain with his partially frigid wife and attracted him to his passionate lover. He made attempts to smuggle letters out and was often untruthful. Such occurrences as well as the signing of worthless checks were merely stated as signs of his illness, in contrast to his previously very honest behavior. Arguments were carefully avoided. Because of occasional depressive features he had been put on suicidal observation from the beginning. After ten days, occasional brief depressive swings became more marked, for which he received psychotherapeutic help accordingly, but they did not last long enough to change the general treatment. He began to realize his tendency to moodiness and a readiness to react emotionally in life — at 18 he had a slight depression when he was unable to go to college, and life difficulties, strain, and success always produced corresponding mood swings. The previous manic excitement of his sister helped to characterize features of elation and overactivity.

His illness was formulated (after four weeks) as a reaction to business failure in 1930 after a previously very successful life and increasing marital maladjustment in which sexual life had become too much the center with neglect of the development of companionship and a healthy family formation. In several interviews the wife's attitude in general was modified and her outlook to sexual life, including the need for more affection, sympathy, and preliminary love play, changed. The girl's cooperation was gained by stressing that we were interested in the medical problem, which she was able to recognize, and would not force our conceptions on the patient's ultimate decision.

After four weeks the patient was quiet and cooperative and had gained insight into his illness but still insisted on his love for the other girl. At discharge (1/14/33), however, he was willing not to force an immediate decision and to live with his family till his business affairs were straightened out and he became successfully established in his new position. He planned to live a suitably adjusted general routine. When seen again in the spring of 1933, the patient was entirely well. He and his wife had developed a healthier family life, and the patient had spontaneously broken off with his girl, explaining his infatuation as part of his illness. In a review of the treatment before hospitalization, it became obvious that his physician had not recognized the hypomanic reaction until it had reached a marked intensity in the fall of 1932. By treating it correctly with restriction of activity and an analysis of all the features involved, and if necessary, a rest in a neutral environment, the increase most likely would have been prevented. From information obtained in 1947, the patient has remained in good health with a happy marital adjustment.

All the features which were discussed in the hypomanic conditon are much more marked in a manic excitement, and hospital care will almost always be necessary in order to protect the patient and to carry out adequate treatment. The treatment in the hospital is fundamentally the same. A brief physical examination at admission, which is absolutely necessary for diagnosis and treatment, is usually possible without too great difficulty. This examination also allows us to form rapport with the patient on the basis which he can best understand and accept, i.e., the study of his body. He will then usually be willing to accept hydrotherapy as a physical means of treatment. It is always advisable to administer a continuous bath as soon as possible and to formulate to the patient the treatment in general. He needs to understand the need for rest, not in the form of staying in bed but as a protection from stimulation and a means of diminishing activity. Separation in a private room is essential and the continuous bath treatment should be given in a single bathroom. Nurses and attendants must recognize the situations to which the patient is sensitive. Every occurrence of combativeness should be investigated and analyzed with the patient. In this way recurrences can usually be avoided. The patient's complaints about impolite or rough management should be taken seriously. Many manic patients have a great sense of pride and a need to protect their dignity, although their own behavior is not in accordance with it. It will always be wise for physicians and nurses to keep a professional distance between themselves and the patient. This does not mean a stiff or distant relationship, but should be the expression

of a healthy physician-patient relationship which avoids fraterniz-
ing. One should be willing to accept the patient's teasing, which may
frequently touch our own sensitive spots. If one feels irritated, it
is best to leave the patient. Furthermore, one should never try to
maintain professional dignity and authority by arguments or self-
assertion. One should also never permit anyone to tease the patient or to make fun of his delusions of wealth or strength.

The self-assertive manic patient clashes easily with self-assertive
persons around him. The desirable attitude of nurses and physicians
is one of patience and a willingness to overlook non-essential disturbances but to be firm along medically indicated lines. Every physician must be willing to assume full responsibility for his patient.
It is best to wait with discussions of clashes and outbursts of anger
until the angry mood has disappeared. If irritability or anger
appears during a subsequent discussion, the physician should formulate the reasons for it briefly to the patient.

Destructiveness, like combativeness, is usually the expression of
irritability and can often be reduced to a minimum by carefully individualized treatment in which the patient's personality is constantly considered. Both destructiveness and combativeness may,
however, be the outcome of a feeling of strength and the patient's
desire for outlet in activity. The room of an excited patient should
contain nothing of value which can be destroyed; the patient's
clothes and valuable belongings, such as jewelry and expensive
watches, should be removed. Such rooms, however, do not need to
be bare. It is possible in hospitals to have special furniture and
even attractive pictures, which can be inexpensive or protected in
some way. I have seen attractive wards for disturbed patients in
some of the English state hospitals, with pictures and flowers in the
halls. It is interesting to note how rarely manic patients destroy
flowers. One should offer reading and writing materials (pencil
and paper) to these patients. (It matters little whether the patient
tears up the daily paper after the other patients have read it. Every
hospital has old magazines for this purpose.) Many patients find a
good outlet in prolific writing. The physician should glance at the
content, which may offer valuable possibilities for an understanding
of the patient. One should keep these productions until the excitement has subsided, as many patients become considerably disturbed

if they hear that they were destroyed because they were considered nonsense.

It is frequently difficult to decide about the disposal of letters which these patients write. It is often possible to retain them and to secure the patient's consent in a quiet moment to have them destroyed. In persistent patients an arrangement should be achieved to have the letters sent for further disposal to a relative or friend on whom the physician and patient agree.

Manic patients often obtain great pleasure from decorating the windows and walls with pictures, papers, drawings, and writings. In a well-managed hospital with planned occupation these tendencies will be transient and should be accepted in order to prevent unnecessary irritation. In chronic manic patients a firmer hand is necessary for re-educational reasons.

Overtalkativeness, yelling, and singing are symptoms which can be overlooked at times, but the physician should not merely submit to this disturbance. Discussion, with careful formulation of the stimulating influence on the patient himself and the disturbance to the environment, helps greatly in correcting this tendency. The sound-proof rooms of modern hospitals have greatly simplified this problem.

It is wrong to believe that the overactive patient needs an outlet for his energy. Overactivity merely stimulates the patient. It should also be remembered that the manic patient is not aware of the normal sensation of fatigue and will exert himself even to the point of serious physical danger. Continuous bath treatment, which produces fatigue and relaxation, is the best means of relieving the desire for overactivity.

Even a highly excited patient should be invited to join in occupational activity. Although his work is usually poorly and superficially done, it depends on the patient to what extent this should be pointed out to him with encouragement to do more careful work. The hypomanic patient is usually more difficult than the manic in this respect because he has many plans with an inability to carry them out, and is unwilling to accept advice. The hypomanic patient should therefore be urged to finish his task and should not be allowed to begin something different except for definite therapeutic reasons. All these limitations help to decrease stimulation if correctly executed.

Content in the manic patient is formed by the elation, which expresses itself as delusions of strength, wealth, and self-aggrandizement, e.g., the belief that he is Christ or a great physician. The choice of the content is personality-determined and expresses the patient's strivings, interests, and fancies, and frequently underlying feelings of inadequacy. A careful recording of these expressions gives us a basis for a constructive analysis.

The main problems in the treatment of manic excitements are to diminish stimulation, to avoid reactions of anger and self-assertion by too much or wrongly executed interference, and to establish a plastic routine which will allow us to gain the patient's cooperation. Successful treatment is based on an understanding of the personality, especially the patient's sensitiveness and idiosyncrasies and his interests.

The hydrotherapeutic procedure, which has been outlined previously, is important to diminish overactivity and stimulation and to produce fatigue. It should be used freely, with necessary attention to somatic features and general hygiene. The value of psychotherapy in general and along specific lines cannot be too strongly emphasized. The final analysis of the dynamic factors is frequently neglected, partly because the physician does not recognize its importance in helping to achieve a more permanent stability and partly because so many patients leave the hospital during the hypomanic phase. It is considered advisable by some authors to keep such patients in the hospital, if necessary, for a few weeks after normal health has been regained. For many reasons, however, this is impossible from a practical point of view, and imposes an unnecessary hardship on the patient. Instead of assuming such an extreme attitude, better results can be obtained by prolonged consultation treatment after discharge, carrying out a well-planned constructive analysis. Rarely will it be indicated to resort to a thorough personality analysis as in the psychoneuroses.

In the following case the excitement was treated without great difficulty by the administration of continuous baths and the removal or diminution of stimuli, together with analysis of disturbing factors. The final synthetic analysis was carried out during the last two weeks before discharge and in two consultations afterwards.

Case 6:

A 25 year old garage owner suddenly developed a full-fledged manic excitement, characterized by marked elation, overtalkativeness with flight of ideas and rhyming, vulgar talk (sexual and swearing), and outbursts of anger when crossed or interfered with in his incessant drive of activity and planning. He broke small pieces of furniture and tore his clothes when angry. He became careless in his personal habits, often exposing himself and expectorating on the floor.

The illness developed about two weeks after it had become known that he was bankrupt. His failure came as a surprise even to his family, as he had concealed his business difficulties. The patient had always been a reserved man who hid his worries behind a cheerful face. He was sociable, jolly, and well liked, devoted to his family and supported them well. It had been his ambition to be independent, and he had bought his own garage business four years before his illness. Instability of mood had never been noticed, although there was a serious constitutional tendency in his family (his father committed suicide and his paternal grandmother made an unsuccessful suicidal attempt during a depression).

The patient came willingly to the hospital and presented no difficulties on the 40 mile trip. On admission he was exuberant, shook hands with everyone, and talked about his ability to make a great deal of money through bankruptcy. After brief psychiatric and physical examinations, the patient was advised that continuous baths would be helpful. He accepted this treatment readily. During the next two months he received bath treatments continuously every day from 10 A.M. to 9 P.M., occasionally starting at 8 or 9 A.M. He usually stayed in the tub, although he sometimes fretted about it. Occasionally he splashed the water or got out and walked around the tub-room. Attendants and nurses were told that he was a proud man who was easily angered by contradiction and interference and that he should not be treated in any way which might hurt his sense of dignity. He became combative with only one attendant, although he constantly called everyone vulgar names. The combativeness was due to the attendant's pushing him somewhat roughly. As the patient seemed irritated by that attendant during his whole stay, he was kept away from him as much as possible. When not in the tub, the patient was told to stay in his room, where reading and writing material were at his disposal. Regular occupational therapy was attempted. This, however, did not interest him for more than a few minutes at a time. Because of his high distractibility he was unable to stick to anything. As there was definite erotic behavior, nurses were advised to spend little time with him until he was less easily stimulated. He was usually careless about expectorating but took care of urination and bowel movements. Meals took a long time because he was so easily distracted. Visitors were not allowed to see him during the first six weeks of his excitement, but the patient's condition was always carefully formulated to them and their full co-operation obtained. The formulation to the patient was more difficult but it was successful as can be seen from his acquiescence to this advice and the absence of increased excitement or anger when other patients had visitors.

During the first two weeks the patient received 0.6 gm. (10 gr.) of barbital and 0.06 gm. (1 gr.) of phenobarbital between 8 and 9 P.M. He usually was sleepy when taken out of the tub at 10 P.M. and slept all night. Cathartics were not necessary.

After about six weeks the excitement began to subside. During the following two weeks of mild excitement the continuous baths were reduced to two hours in the morning and evening; i.e., at the time when the patient was still overactive and excitable. During the rest of the day he was quiet and was able to join in the routine of a disturbed ward. He slept without sedatives. Visitors, who after six weeks were allowed once a week, did not excite him. The physician urged him to remain on the disturbed ward, stressing that the greater activity on the other floors would still be too stimulating. At this time he became aware of sexual tension. High amounts of bromide did not produce a decrease and better results were obtained by directing the psychotherapeutic discussions, which were started at this time, to the problem of sexual hygiene, stimulating factors, and control of imagination. During this period psychotherapeutic discussions were not frequent. We endeavored to take care of all the problems which might come up, but did not push the patient too far in the analysis of the factors which were connected with his illness.

Their discussion was undertaken during the last two weeks of the hospital stay, when the patient showed normal behavior while carrying on a full day's schedule, including walks in the neighborhod of the hospital. He gained an understanding of his exaggerated need to be inde-dependent, his lack of plasticity, disinclination to share his worries with his intimates, and his need to become socialized on an easier and less restrained basis. The analysis of the sexual aspect did not lead far. It is quite likely that the erotic behavior was part of the elation in a passionate but sexually well-adjusted man and not of any special significance. From information obtained in 1947, the patient has remained in good health during the 20 years since discharge.

More difficult to treat are patients of a self-assertive make-up which does not allow them to yield and who are always inclined to project their difficulties onto others. Such a make-up resembles the paranoic, but paranoic features do not always appear clearly in the excitement. Some patients react to treatment with aversion, resentment, and frank antagonism, while others may even withdraw into a stupor. Such factors are well demonstrated in the following case in whom insulin treatment, together with individualized psychotherapy, alleviated resentment and manic excitement in a short time.

Case 7:

In the fall of 1943, when her father died and her husband insisted on sending her son to a boarding school, this 39 year old housewife became depressed. On March 28, 1944, after two months of increasing overactivity, overtalkativeness, and elation, the patient was admitted to the hospital. Her admission was precipitated by erotic behavior toward a casual acquaintance and toward her physician.

The patient had a mild depression with marked hypochondriasis during a five month period in 1940, followed by a mild elation of several weeks' duration. Otherwise she had always been in good health. She married a classmate in college, who since has become a successful business executive. She had a son of 13 years and a daughter of 8 years to whom she was greatly devoted and she resented being separated from them. Usually she was reserved and shy with strangers, sensitive to criticism, but concealing resentment, easily discouraged, and dependent on her domineering husband with whom she enjoyed a harmonious sexual life. A considerable overconcern to her health made her seek medical help readily.

In the clinic the patient was elated, talking incessantly about many plans, and constantly active with minor activities. She was erotic toward her physician and made frequent demands on medical and nursing attention. Resentment with regard to her husband was expressed freely. She became critical of the nurses and of the treatment. In April, she became suspicious and developed delusions that her utterances were recorded by some hidden dictaphones. Her sexual desires increased markedly. She became loud and intolerant of the other patients. She liked prolonged baths and relaxed in them. These were given daily two hours in the morning and evening, and she slept well with chloral hydrate 0.5 gm. (7½ gr.). Because of her increasing resentment and her paranoid projections, the patient became easily angered and less willing to accept the hospital routine. On May 15th, 20 units of insulin were administered, increased daily by ten units until on May 21st, 80 units were administered. Since the third day (May 17th), the patient reacted with mild drowsiness. She became less talkative but remained elated, resentful, and suspicious. To 80 units the patient reacted with sleep and myoclonic twitchings. Starting the next day the insulin dosage was decreased by 10 units and this decrease was continued till a dosage of 40 units was reached because the patient reacted with sleep to these smaller amounts. After ten days of treatment the excitement, resentment, suspiciousness, and erotic behavior subsided. Insulin administration was continued because the patient showed considerable underlying anxiety and mild depression. During the period from June 2nd to June 15th when the insulin treatment was terminated, psychotherapeutic discussion proceeded well. Anxiety and resentment, whenever they became stirred up, were alleviated easily by insulin. She discussed suspiciousness of her husband's infidelity and her own phantasies of promiscuity. For several years she had marked resentment to the responsibility with regard to her large house and social entertainment, whereas she was anxious to devote her time to intellectual pursuits. From June 15th to July 18th, when she left the hospital, she reviewed her husband's unsympathetic and aggressive attitude to her illness, and his accusing her of spoiling her son and therefore sending him to boarding school against her will. Much time was devoted to obtaining an understanding of a partial frigidity, of which her husband was unaware, of her choice of husband, and of her relationship to her father and mother in early childhood. The patient left in good health with a fair understanding of some of the important dynamic factors.

SCHIZOPHRENIC EXCITEMENTS

The most important factor in schizophrenic excitement (see Chapter X) is the tendency to withdrawal and autism. One is therefore not justified in segregating such a patient as in the manic cases, but should try to increase socialization, even during the excitement. It is best to keep the patient in his room for just a short time, i.e., until the excitement has somewhat subsided, and then urge him to mix with other patients and to take part in occupational therapy. During bath treatment, such patients should be distracted and not allowed to day-dream unless there are definite indications that the patient is falling asleep. There is always the possibility that nurses may become afraid of excited patients and therefore do not give them the attention which is needed.

The following case presents an excitement which is characterized by features of elation and withdrawal. The main problem therefore was to avoid stimulation and yet not to allow the patient to withdraw into her autistic preoccupations.

Case 8:

This 19 year old girl was anxious to leave her home town and to go to New York to study music. Her mother refused to allow this because of the sexual dangers in a large city. After a year's struggle, the patient finally forced permission from her. During the weeks of preparation she was quite "excited" and slept poorly. Arriving in New York on September 7th, she was invited to a party, at which she experienced her first flirtation with sexual implications. Within the next few days she developed a rapidly increasing excitement, characterized by elated mood, overtalkativeness and overactivity, irritability, and outbursts of anger when thwarted. At times she was terrified and tense, assuring others she was pure. At other times she delighted in marriage plans and spoke of being a famous movie actress. She refused food and had to be tube fed. On the 14th of September, when seen in consultation, admission to the hospital was urged. At this time she was staying with relatives in Baltimore whose means were moderate and who could not afford the expense of special nursing. They were advised to call the Health Department and not to inform the patient of the intended move until the ambulance was in front of the door. At that time the physician administered morphine 0.02 gm. ($\frac{1}{3}$ gr.) and scopolamine 0.001 gm. ($\frac{1}{60}$ gr.) hypodermically. The patient quieted after a few minutes. When informed of the need for hospital admission she protested but did not present any serious difficulty.

During the first six weeks in the hospital the patient was in a continuous excitement, playing the part of a movie actress, posing and greatly admiring herself, dancing and singing, usually very talkative, showing marked distractibility and flight. At times she was fearful of being murdered. She was careless in dressing, often tearing her dress, frequently urinating in the corner of her room, smearing feces on the wall, and masturbating frankly. It was soon noticed that she also had a tendency to expose herself freely to women. The nurses were instructed to avoid taking rectal temperatures and to keep in mind that any affectionate behavior of the patient was to be treated calmly and with reserve. There were times at which the patient was angry and combative when her desire to run around the ward was interfered with. By analyzing carefully the circumstances which increased her anger we were able to eliminate combativeness to a large extent. It was especially important not to contradict her or interfere with her acting. At times she was quiet for hours, complaining then of feeling homesick or lonely. These periods were utilized for establishing a better rapport and making her feel that she was with people who understood her and were anxious to participate in her preoccupations and worries. At other times she was puzzled, indecisive, and frequently showed definite ambivalency.

We therefore tried to make the routine as simple as possible, not producing any situations which would demand definite decisions. Her destructiveness, which had been a serious difficulty at home, was easily dealt with by removing anything valuable which could be destroyed. At times, the patient was quite suspicious, feeling that everyone made fun of her, that someone was spying on her, that there was a purpose in having the sunshine on the wall. These delusions never developed into anything systematized. Instead of contradicting her, we pointed out the possibilities of misinterpreting coincidences in a state of distress and insecurity. She heard her mother's and brother's voices calling for help and needed constant assurance that they were not here but were in good health at home. Occasional brief visits from her relatives helped to establish temporary confidence in the hospital. She made some attempts to explain her illness — she either felt that she was in prison because of sexual misdemeanors or that she was in a hospital studying nursing. These delusions changed according to her mood.

During this marked excitement hydrotherapy was used freely. The patient relaxed well in baths and cold wet packs. When she became too restless in the tub she was usually taken out and put in a cold wet pack, in which she then went to sleep. Sedatives were given only for the night. The patient ate when urged and we were able to keep her at a low but steady weight of around 100 pounds without having to resort to tube feeding. There was marked constipation, which was controlled by aromatic cascara.

From November to January, the patient showed phases of excitement which alternated with periods of marked preoccupation in which she stared and "day-dreamed" but was unwilling to share the content. There was little spontaneous talk during this period and answers were usually vague. Her mood changed frequently to anger or elation. She was troubled by the feeling that thoughts were snatched from her. This again was treated as a delusion by expressing doubt of the correctness of her observation. Periods of excitement were usually brief, characterized by irritability and resentment to being kept in the hospital. She felt she was treated as socially inferior and pictured herself as having developed into a lady of high social standing without showing corresponding behavior. This tendency was pointed out to her and she was urged to try to fit into the group on the basis of cooperation instead of futile imaginary compensation. She began to cooperate in dressing and could be allowed in the sitting-room with the other patients. As soon as signs of excitement appeared, she was taken to her room where newspapers and magazines as well as writing material were at her disposal. Separation from other patients was limited as much as possible. She was frightened occasionally, explaining that she was persecuted and that ghosts were after her. On several occasions she mentioned her flirtation in New York, stating that her dignity had been insulted. At another time she mentioned that at 10 she had had a sexual experience with a boy (apparently mutual masturbation) and that she had seen the boy when she came to Baltimore. She was worried about irregular menses and was afraid of pregnancy. Without minimizing her experience in New York, we showed her how she overemphasized it. She tried to find her own solution by believing that she was the Virgin Mary. Her frequent day-dreams about home and her homesickness received the necessary attention. During this period, we were still anxious to avoid any analysis and tried to keep the patient from becoming involved in too many fantasies and preoccupations. This danger was pointed out to her. It was stressed that we wished to discuss all this material later when she was more at ease and would not become so easily upset and excited.

She frequently complained that the nurses tried to dirty her room and that one had tried to cheat her. Her contact with the physician, however, was good during these three months and he therefore was able to clear up misunderstandings and establish a better rapport with the nurses.

Her behavior still presented many difficulties. She was not interested in her personal appearance, defecated frequently in her room, refused to mix with other patients, and did not cooperate well in routine. Occasionally there was definite negativism but most of the time she was on the defensive. She frequently expressed a need for more self-confidence. She believed that a general persecution of the Jews was going on in this country and therefore felt more at ease when with one of the Jewish nurses on her ward. This contact was not encouraged much, partly because it was a satisfaction on a delusional basis and partly because the patient showed definitely erotic behavior toward this woman. It was also noticed that she was attracted to another patient who showed latent homosexual tendencies. We tried to keep these two patients apart without making it obvious to either of them.

During this period, continuous baths were still frequently given, especially at night or at times when the patient showed signs of beginning excitement. Packs were omitted completely. The patient's appetite improved and her weight increased steadily. Her constipation improved. Another sign of her improvement was seen in the decrease of pulse rate, which now was never higher than 80 whereas before it was usually around 90.

The third phase (February and March) was primarily characterized by withdrawal with irritability, little talk, and depressive complaints. She felt homesick and was constantly preoccupied with her mistake in leaving home to go to New York. At other times she day-dreamed about good times and dancing. Occasionally she mentioned plans for taking a job as a stenographer after she was allowed to leave the hospital.

There was usually little actual understanding of being ill. She still did not feel well treated and reacted with temper tantrums when urged to join in the general routine with other patients. She insisted that she preferred to stay by herself. Her general apathy and lack of interest was one of the main obstacles. Occasionally she grimaced, laughed, and listened to voices, which she did not want to discuss. During these brief periods, she was kept at the usual occupation except when this tendency became too marked and indicated the possibility of an impending slight excitement. She then was put in a tub, where she always relaxed well. There was also periods when she was in good contact with physician and nurse and in which she discussed her worries about having left home. These brief periods of good contact were always utilized to solidify the rapport, to explain the need for routine and the desirability of acting instead of day-dreaming, the need to become part of the group and to be interested in others as well as oneself.

She began at this time to show increasing attention to her appearance. She was not allowed to use cosmetics because there were definite narcissistic tendencies which we did not want to foster. It was frequently difficult to stimulate attention to her personal appearance without encouraging her admiration of herself. Several times we allowed her to go out with her aunt. This was done primarily to increase her interest in life outside the hospital.

At the end of March and two weeks in April, the patient was cooperative but still showed little spontaneity. She had reached the point where she had some insight into her condition and a discussion of her personality features was started. During this period we were always watchful for signs of impending excitement or disorganization. Whenever the patient's pulse rate, which was now around 68, increased after a consultation or when there was any sleep disturbance, we took it as an indication that we had to go rather slowly and investigate whether the discussion of the previous day had really led to constructive assimilation. Hydrotherapy was no longer necessary. Her appetite was good and she did not have any constipation.

This last phase of treatment lasted about five weeks. It allowed us to discuss with her all the problems which had come to the foreground in the acute period of her illness in the form of delusions and hallucinations as well as general issues, preoccupations, and worries. We first discussed her leaving home, the breaking away from the small town where she had been brought up very carefully. This led to a brief discussion of her experience in New York, to which she became desensitized. She realized the danger of day-dreams and how she had anticipated great adventures in going to New York. In connection with this, general sexual hygiene was discussed. Her feeling of inadequacy and inferiority was not only linked to her being Jewish and living in a Catholic community but also to her lack of confidence in herself, partly because she had too high standards and partly because she had not given herself enough opportunity to test her abilities. She had always preferred to live in a world of dreams. She learned to understand the need of attention to personal appearance without giving in to self-admiration. Concrete plans for the future were made tentatively, outlining the possibilities of work, social contact in her own town, and possibilities for recreation.

The patient left the hospital at the end of April 1930. She has since made a good adjustment at home, working regularly in a physician's office, carrying a great deal of responsibility without apparent difficulty. Her social adjustment is much better. I do not feel, however, that this patient has a definitely good prognosis for life. She has not gained enough understanding of the various factors which played a role in her illness and of her many personality difficulties. Constructive treatment had to be limited because the patient was not willing to stay much longer and because of financial considerations. It would have been wrong to attempt a very far-reaching analysis. This would have stirred up many problems which the patient would not have been able to understand and which one would not have had enough time to analyze carefully. The last follow-up note was received in 1940 when the patient had finished training as a nurse. She had been in good health since discharge.

Many schizophrenic patients show manic admixtures which usually disappear after a few weeks. When they subside, the patient should be urged to participate in occupation and group activities. Sometimes, however, it is difficult to decide when such a patient can be urged into activity without stimulating him too much, as overstimulation may produce a recurrence of the excited phase. These considerations have led physicians to look for a treatment which would allow easier handling and more forceful adjustment to reality. The most outstanding procedures of this type are insulin and prolonged sleep treatment (see Chapter VII).

DELIRIOUS EXCITEMENTS

Delirious excitements of various origin are best treated with extensive hydrotherapy, which may be modified considerably in cardio-renal disorders. These patients are disoriented and have difficulties in grasp. All our procedures should therefore be simple and as few strange people introduced as possible. Because of marked fear the patient should be reassured whenever anything disturbs him — either real or hallucinatory experiences. The patient must be protected from suicidal attempts in an effort to escape from threatening dangers, and from incidental suicide caused by disorientation, e.g., mistaking a window for a door. Sedatives should only be given to secure rest at night. Constant attention must be paid to the physical condition and to etiological factors (see Chapter XII).

PANIC EXCITEMENTS

Panic excitements present a similar problem. One deals with extreme fear and insecurity, usually with paranoid projections, and often with marked difficulties of thinking. The acute excitement usually subsides quickly with insulin treatment. The main problem is to establish a rapport which will allow the patient to find some security in turning to somebody whom he can trust. He will then be willing to accept the hydrotherapeutic procedures which he may have rejected previously, because of distrust and fear. Topical discussions should be avoided entirely until the patient has found security and ease. We will have to formulate to such patients the reasons for all of our moves and to be prepared to offer formulations which will take care of their present needs. Their frequently dramatic behavior must be taken seriously, and reassurance offered. Such patients are always suicidal and should be carefully protected. In quiet moments the patients should participate in suitable occupations, with due attention to their thinking difficulties, overconscientiousness, and distrust. A more detailed discussion of the treatment of panic reactions is found in Chapters IX and XI.

OLIGOPHRENIC AND ORGANIC EXCITEMENTS

Distressing cases are oligophrenic and organic excitements (usually of the manic type but with much anger and suspiciousness). As a result of their congenital or acquired intellectual deficit, these patients have more difficulty in understanding our therapeutic approach. This is especially true of suspicious patients, who react easily with anger, impulsiveness, and combativeness. Patiently renewed attempts at establishing rapport, with careful utilization of the patient's previous interests and protection of their sensitiveness, will finally lead to good results, frequently before the excitement has subsided.

PSYCHOPATHIC PERSONALITIES

Excitement in psychopathic personalities presents similar problems. These patients, and also epileptics, are inclined to react easily with more or less brief outbursts of anger and combativeness even during quiet periods. When this happens they ought to be immediately transferred to a disturbed ward where correct treatment can be administered. They should not, however, be kept continuously on such a ward where there is not the same demand for control of one's behavior as in a quiet group. The patient therefore will not gain the necessary re-education. These patients are frequently dangerous in their outbursts of anger and any object with which they can injure others should be removed. Continuous bath treatment is most desirable. There is no danger involved with epileptic patients if they are under constant observation while in the tub.

The discussion of the various types of excitement emphasizes the need for the free use of a well-planned hydrotherapy which makes restraint unnecessary in a modern psychiatric hospital, the limitation of the use of sedatives for the night, individually modified psychotherapy, routine with occupation, and attempts at socialization. Separation from other patients may be necessary for various reasons and for varying periods of time, but old-fashioned isolation (in the sense of locked or padded cells) is no longer used.

BIBLIOGRAPHY

Pertinent literature is found listed under Chapter VII.

Chapter IX

DEPRESSIONS

IN DEPRESSIONS of any type the mood disturbance is generally accepted as the common feature. Kraepelin grouped them under the term, "manic-depressive psychosis," believing that both elation and depression are part of the same disease entity. This concept was founded on the observation that well-circumscribed depressions and elations (manic and hypomanic psychoses) seem to follow each other directly or with more or less normal intervals between. It is most doubtful that all depressions and elations show this cyclic character. The defenders of the manic-depressive disease entity have to bend clinical observations to force them into this clear-cut group. Many patients have recurrent depressions without elated phases. Other patients have only one depression which, for example, occurs at the time of the menopause or may be frankly situationally determined. The manic-depressive psychoses apparently form a large and well-defined group among the larger group of affective psychoses, but do not embrace all affective reactions.

Next to the mood disorder, the course of the illness is an outstanding characteristic of affective disorders. All these illnesses have a definite onset and end, terminating in recovery. Because of this and the frequent recurrence, the older writers spoke of cyclic and circular disorders. This feature is prognostically important and influences our therapeutic approach, but is not an exclusive fundamental principle. Other psychoses may occur in well-defined and recurrent attacks and some depressions end in rut formation and do not recover. In recent years the rhythmic character of mood disorders has been emphasized. There always seems to exist a definite diurnal rhythm which, however, may not be easily recognizable in deep depressions and marked elations. With improvement the rhythm may extend over several days.

Many authors stress the influence of heredity and therefore urge strongly against marriage and childbirth, or even demand sterilization. Although in many cases dominant heredity factors play an important role, one should not overlook the fact that dynamic factors enter and that their adjustment may prevent further illnesses. One should never assume a fatalistic attitude because of hereditary tendencies but try to determine what personality features can be utilized to counteract and overcome the hereditary danger. There are certainly few affective illnesses which occur automatically and without being considerably influenced by various dynamic factors. I have never seen one. Dynamic psychiatry has shown that there are always more or less strong dynamic factors.

Depressions are characterized by the depressed mood which is expressed by various individuals, with definite diurnal variations (usually more depressed in the morning), by the attack form of the illness, and by accompanying physical symptoms (loss of appetite and weight, constipation, sleep disturbance, decline of potency and libido, and menstrual disorders). These latter symptoms have led some authors to believe that we deal fundamentally with a metabolic disorder. Others point to specific endocrine factors. This claim is also supported by the frequent disturbance of mood in connection with menstruation, puberty, and menopause. Somatic investigations have not offered much, however, mostly because it is unclear how much is due to various secondary emotional reactions and what is really fundamental.

These introductory remarks are necessary because many treatments are based on the various theories mentioned. They will be discussed later whenever there seem to be facts in their support. For practical reasons this chapter deals entirely with the depressions. The hypomanic and manic reactions have been discussed in Chapter VIII. Depressions present a manifold group with various outstanding clinical pictures. This, as well as the varying importance of dynamic factors, has led to groupings which are therapeutically important. Some depressions are full-fledged, showing all the characteristics; others present less clear-cut pictures and should receive a different symptomatic approach.

The oldest distinction is between retarded and agitated depressions. In the latter group are usually included the anxiety depressions which frequently have a marked panic phase. Depressive stupors may be due to various dynamic factors, outstanding among them fear and aversion; they are only in a small number of cases the expression of depressive retardation. Aversion is frequently of fundamental importance and colors the whole picture, making acceptance of the illness and the help offered impossible. Such depressions may therefore end in depressive rut-formation with no recovery. Rut-formation may also be due to a fixation of mood on topical material, e.g., hypochondriasis or paranoid delusions. Not infrequent are catathymic depressions, i.e., reactions in which there is a harping on one set depressive topic, often without retardation of the pure affect of depression and tending to a more paranoid picture, with short stuporous phases, but without the features of the deterioration types (A. Meyer). In its original formulation "catathymic" meant the results of an affect-determined complex (H. W. Maier). Accepting this definition of catathymic, many authors, especially German authors, separate psychogenic and hysterical reactions. A large group of patients form the involutional depressions (for which the term "melancholia" is also used in foreign literature) with their characteristic picture of depressed mood with surliness and irritability, distorted hypochondriacal delusions, untidiness, and frequently incontinence of stool and urine. Careful psychopathologic studies have in recent years demonstrated the fallacy of the concept of involutional psychoses. These depressions in later life must be differentiated from organic, especially presenile, depressions. Seldom mentioned are menstrual psychoses. Puerperal psychoses are frequently depressions in which the puerperium is merely an important situational factor. It is therefore more correct to speak of a depression in the setting of puerperium. One also separates depressions according to their content, speaking especially of hypochondriacal and paranoid depressions. Depressions which occur with definite attacks of elation belong to the group of manic-depressive psychoses. In these depressions, catathymic features and content may play a less important role, and they are occasionally practically contentless. Mixed manic-depressive psychoses in the real sense of the meaning are merely phases, occurring when a depression (or elation) changes to the opposite mood. When a mixed picture persists, one should look for the explanation in the personality make-up (immature and psychopathic personalities), or in impure affects (fear, anxiety, and panic). It is of great practical importance to recognize depressions when there is affect fixation or outstanding content, e.g., hypochondriasis, anxiety, and obsessions. Whenever these complaints occur in definite attack form, one should look for a possible depression with its suicidal dangers. German psychiatrists referred to these depression equivalents. Also to this group belong some of the less marked tension depressions. For a well-planned treatment one should always determine first whether one deals with a depression alone, or whether the depression masks another underlying illness — e.g., structural changes in the brain, or a psychoneurosis. Many depressions have schizophrenic admixtures. It is then important to determine which of the features are dominant and whether schizophrenic features can be expected to subside with the clearing of the depression. A study of previous depressions in the same patient may be helpful in establishing the most likely prognosis. Depressions which are the direct reaction to circumscribed life situations (reactive depressions) are usually of shorter duration than the more constitutionally determined type and are more amenable to psychotherapy. The practitioner will frequently have to deal with recurrent mild depressive moods which do not reach the degree of an illness. They are primarily constitutionally determined (cyclothymic personalities) or dependent on situational factors. Depressed feelings at the beginning of the week, for example, are the expression of anticipation of possible unpleasantness, or actual dislike of one's work, or the dread of the impending work strain.

Offering a prognosis, one should be guided by the clinical picture, the personality setting, and the dynamic factors. The length of previous depressions may clarify the possibility of duration, but it is always hazardous to be too definite, and the patient should be advised to accept the final good outcome and not insist on a definite time promise. This is, however, important for the family and for necessary work and business arrangements. In some patients, recurrent depressions occur with photostatic similarity; in others each succeeding depression is longer (rarely shorter). The interval between each depression may become shorter or longer with progressing age, and allow a more or less definite life prognosis.

The first point in the treatment of a depression is the preservation of the patient's life, which is threatened by his suicidal urge and also by starvation. It is not always easy to detect the suicidal dangers, as many patients dissimulate either because they have a need to protect their private thoughts or are averse to any kind of interference, or because they want to make sure that they can succeed and definitely wish to deceive those who want to protect them. Whenever suicidal dangers exist, the patient should be put under strict observation with removal of all objects and drugs which could prove to be dangerous. Windows should be guarded, and the patient practically never left alone. To protect a cunning patient against a determination to commit suicide is extremely difficult, as the occurrence of suicides in psychiatric hospitals demonstrates. On the whole, however, one should realize that only under unusually favorable circumstances should a suicidal patient be treated outside a psychiatric hospital. Some physicians consider every depressed patient a suicidal risk and treat him as such. This conservative approach, however, cannot be shared by those who believe in an active and individualized treatment as I shall outline below. One will often have to take chances in order to help the patient, but one should only do this after careful evaluation of all the factors involved. It will always be wise to explain this carefully to the relatives and make them share the responsibility. Every hospital physician is familiar with depressed patients in rut-formations whom he was unwilling to push into outside activities because of suicidal dangers and who when taken out of the hospital against his advice, soon began to improve and to recover. There is, on the other hand, a deplorably high number of patients who commit suicide after being removed from the hospital against the physician's advice. To this group especially belong dissimulating patients, who suffer from tension and anxiety depressions, and panics.

In the evaluation of suicidal danger we are guided by the depth and character of the depression, the dynamic factors, and the patient's make-up. Complaints of hopelessness and the worthlessness of living signify serious dangers. Feelings of futility frequently indicate suicidal urges, especially in adolescence and in the late life period. Despair and fear drive to suicide not only in depressions but also in the various panic reactions, schizophrenic, and senile illnesses. In evaluating the content, all expressions of self-depreciation, and especially unreality feelings and depersonalization, should be considered suicidal indications. Most serious are catathymic suicidal urges as reactions to guilt feelings and a need for punishment. They also play an important role in schizophrenic illnesses, where they may take the form of sacrifice. One is frequently able to detect suicidal dangers from increasing brooding, casual remarks referring in some way to suicide, increased pulse rate, and sleep disturbance. After the patient has decided on suicide, he may show temporary and superficial improvement which deceives the persons in the environment and causes them to relax. Suicidal attempts occur in acute and chronic stages of depressions and are frequent when improvement has started. Suicides in the family history are often an attraction to similar attempts or even impress themselves with such strength on the patient that he develops the conviction that it his unavoidable fate. Attempts in a previous depression should always warn the physician against renewed attempts in the recurring illness. Incidental suicides occur frequently in a delirium and occasionally as the unintended result of a pretended suicide for dramatization in an hysterical or psychopathic setting. It is never wise to take dramatizations lightly. If suicidal attempts recur, the patient ought to be sent to a psychiatric hospital for observation. Spite suicidal attempts, which the patient regrets immediately and following which he tries to secure help, are frequent in feebleminded and psychopathic persons, adolescents, and alcoholics. Not infrequently the latter make suicidal attempts and have to be especially guarded when they develop full-fledged depressions. Suicides on a philosophic basis, in persons who are not depressed, are rare. More frequently they occur as the expression of resentment to life. The choice of the method varies greatly. It may be premeditated, frequently carefully hidden behind dissimulation, or impulsive (often occurring in one of the brief periods of more marked hopelessness during the period of improvement when an opportunity presents itself), or violent (especially in panics). Many patients are attracted by the methods of friends and relatives. There are definite fashions, poison and shooting at present predominating. From this discussion it is clear that any physician who treats a depressed or otherwise suicidal patient assumes a great obligation in which the responsible relatives must share. Nobody can guarantee absolute protection. Nurses should not be kept too long on a suicidal case because their vigilance is bound to relax after continued strenuous observation.

As a result of poor appetite, markedly depressed moods, and distorted hypochondriacal delusions referring to the gastrointestinal system many patients present a marked feeding problem. Spoon feeding and occasionally tube feeding is necessary. Tube feeding may stir up the patient's antagonism and increase an attitude of aversion. Yet, if the feeding aspect is neglected, the patient may become greatly undernourished and show signs of starvation. Because of this and faulty feeding, with the neglect of sufficient vitamins, the patient may die from central neuritis (A. Meyer). With improved institutional care, these cases are now rare. The two patients whom I saw die from central neuritis suffered from serious involutional depression with unwillingness to live and marked aversion to treatment, vomiting all the food after tube feeding. With all the modern means of institutional treatment, we were only able to postpone the fatal outcome, but not prevent it.

In every depressed patient the need for a high caloric diet must be considered. In obese patients, one's attempt at reduction of weight should be carried out cautiously or delayed until the patients have practically recovered from their depressive illness. In all instances of weight reduction, sufficient protein should be given. In general, the daily diet should contain about 1 gm. of protein for every kilogram of normal body weight. Food should be offered at frequent intervals. This and activity will be more helpful than medication to stimulate the appetite. It is, for example, wise to request the patient to take some milk and crackers at 10 A.M., a sandwich, malted milk, or eggnog at 4 P.M., and a glass of warm milk or chocolate before retiring. In summer time ice cream is easily taken. Such a routine can be carried out even if a patient is living his full routine outside the hospital. It is wrong to assume that such measures are not very important because the patient begins to gain weight with improvement. It is essential that we increase the patient's resistance by keeping him in as fit condition physically as possible. One should take care of minor gastrointestinal complaints, including the frequent complaint of distention, in a general hygienic adjustment through activity and a well-balanced diet.

Constipation is a complaint which should never be neglected. Otherwise, marked discomfort and, in undernourished, dehydrated, and elderly patients, impaction may occur. In the latter, the removal of impacted feces manually or by instrument may present a serious problem. Impaction should not occur if a physician watches a patient closely and does not depend on his vague description of bowel movements. The treatment of constipation depends on the type and on the setting in which it occurs. I shall not go into a thorough discussion, which should be part of one's medical training, but merely stress a few essential and practical points. One should determine whether one deals with spastic or atonic constipation. Spastic constipation is frequent in an anxiety picture, occurring in psychoneuroses and various types of psychotic pictures. A low residue diet is of great benefit in spastic constipation, by allaying the added irritative features that roughage would cause. Rectal instillations of oil (cotton seed, olive, or corn) each night, seem to have a soothing effect on a spastic colon and are often very helpful. As a rule, however, rectal administrations, especially enemas, should be avoided as much as possible. Their liberal use cannot be recommended from a psychobiologic point of view. There is considerable controversy as to the effectiveness of the administration of belladonna. If used at all, it should be used up to the point of individual tolerance. The best way to determine this point of tolerance is to begin with a small dose, increase one drop per dose daily until the patient begins to notice either visual changes or dryness of the mouth; then stop for a day and continue with a slightly smaller dosage than had caused symptoms. In most depressions and in many organic psychoses, one deals with atonic constipation. It is essential that a patient receive bulky foods such as vegetables, sufficient fluids, and salt. This is not easily achieved in non-cooperative patients. Cathartics need to be tried out on the individual case and the dosage varied according to needs. Mineral oil is helpful in mild degrees of constipation. In the more marked type one needs to resort to aromatic cascara 0.3 to 0.6 gm. (5 to 10 gr.) and Epsom Salts (1 to 2 oz.). In many patients, a pint to a quart of isotonic salt solution before breakfast is very effective. Others react well to senna tea. In older patients, attention should be paid to mild hypothyroidism. Thyroid administration 0.2 gm. (3 gr.) relieves such constipation promptly. Many physicians combat constipation by physical exercise, postural training, abdominal massage, and the use of Scotch douches which are directed to the abdomen. Attention also needs to be directed to healthy toilet habits. A regular time of the day for bowel movement should be cultivated, preferably immediately after breakfast, and this habit should be maintained regardless of whether or not movement occurs. In psychoneurotic constipation, attention to all these factors is essential and helpful in many cases, especially if the physician utilizes the strong suggestive influences which are inherent in well-formulated hygienic advice.

Whenever a depressed patient presents a definite suicidal danger, when the feeding problem cannot be taken care of sufficiently, when undesirable outside influence increases the depression or prevents improvement, when the danger of rut-formation threatens, hospitalization in a psychiatric hospital is indicated to secure protection of the patient, remove him from disturbing influences, and keep him occupied in a carefully adjusted routine.

The affective rhythm is utilized psychotherapeutically and in working out the most helpful routine. When more depressed in the morning for example, the patient suffers from increased thinking disorders; difficulties in spontaneity, decision, and activity; fatigue; restlessness, and varying degrees of irritability. During his morning visits, the physician should encourage the patient, urging him to look forward to the lifting of some or all of these symptoms in the afternoon or evening. When he feels better, however, the patient should remember that there will again be an increase of his symptoms. He should develop a philosophy of acceptance, with a willingness to make use of the better periods and not give in to discouragement at times of more marked depression. This attitude is similar to that which one has to pain in a physical illness. No physical or mental distress can last incessantly with the same intensity.

The routine prescribed for the patient should utilize the individual mood rhythm. At periods of more marked depression, occupation which requires little spontaneity, decision, and concentration is advised. More strenuous activity, physically and mentally, and social contacts are postponed to the time when the patient feels less depressed. Routine in home and hospital treatment is fundamentally the same. Handicraft, walks, reading the newspapers are the means of occupation for more depressed periods; reading, intellectual work, visitors, modified social activities, and athletic outlets for the less depressed time. A routine should not become monotonous and occupation therefore should be changed after about an hour. Individual interests, assets, and handicaps are duly considered. With the improvement or increase of the depression the routine should be adjusted accordingly. It is of utmost importance to realize that a depressed patient is usually inclined to undertake too much, then becoming worse when faced with his incapacity to live up to his own expectations. The physician who knows the patient well should be able to foresee and forestall this. Occupation should encourage the patient and help to distract him from his problems and dissecting self-observation. In some patients, inborn conscientiousness and rigid standards demand repeated formulations for greater plasticity and for being satisfied with what one is able to do at the time; in others the life-long attitude of inadequacy needs to be counteracted; the averse patient must be led gradually to accept occupation as a well established and helpful kind of treatment; the apathetic patient needs to be investigated for the possibility of certain interests which can be utilized. As a result of the incessant search of his physician, many patients have learned to recognize interests and capacities in themselves of which they had not been aware or which they had forgotten. An analysis of the patient's youth frequently reveals such interests.

Modern treatment demands an active routine under which the patient will gain more weight and improve faster than under any of the various kinds of rest cures. Bed treatment, which has been especially advised for agitated depressions, has been given up by most physicians. In some patients modification seems wise, e.g., bed rest for one to two hours after the noon meal. I personally doubt the wisdom of this except when there are definite physical indications among which, however, I would not count fatigue and undernourishment. The fatigue is mood determined and therefore shows the corresponding daily rhythm. This type of fatigue does not react well to physical rest but to varied activity, including recreation. General mild hydrotherapeutic procedures may prove to be helpful. Treatment in hospitals shows clearly that the average depression improves most quickly under a routine which extends from 7:30 A.M. to 9 or 10 P.M.

Visitors and mail should be evaluated individually. It is always best to have as few visitors as possible and to prevent the carrying on of disturbing business activities. In patients with deep depressions all these transactions must be handled by someone else. Excessive smoking, which is due to restlessness has to be curbed. Alcohol should be omitted entirely. There is always grave danger that a patient will develop chronic alcoholism because of a depressed mood and that he will resort to alcohol during minor mood disturbances later in life if he has become aware of its stimulating and ease-producing influence in a depression. Sexual activities should be strictly prohibited. They are usually attempts by the patient to reassure himself that he is still potent or that he is still devoted to his partner. The diminished potency and libido, which in women leads to frigidity, causes failure, increased inadequacy, and self-accusatory reaction — the more so if the patient has even lost the normal feeling of affection for his partner. Careful explanations are usually received with relief. The recurrence of libido and potency shows itself in the return of morning erections, sexual thoughts and dreams, and later, dreams with discharge. These signs should be explained as a return of normal vitality. Sexual relations should not be resumed until the patient has practically recovered. In women, menstrual disorders need to be discussed and explained as part of the depression, if no specific factors can be found. With improvement, regularity of menses returns.

If operations of any kind are necessary, they should be performed as soon as convenient. Their psychotherapeutic value lies in the fact that they may help by distracting the patient from his mood fixation or eliminate some definite body concern. In patients who are averse to accepting treatment for their personality disorders or who reiterate topical hypochondriacal complaints, the physical treatment may offer an opening for psychotherapy. Unfortunate news, such as deaths in the family, loss of position, financial reverses, should be told to the patient as soon as possible, either by the physician or by responsible relatives in cooperation with him. These may bring the patient closer again to the problems of real life and can often be used to the patient's advantage. Any resulting increase in the depressed mood is usually of only short duration.

The content of a depression should be carefully studied. The frequent hypochondriacal overconcern and delusions need to be treated by reassurance and explanations ("persuasion" of Dubois), according to the patient's intelligence, offered in strongly suggestive form and based on a careful physical study. No complaint should be minimized without a thorough investigation. I remember the case of a man of fifty-six who suffered from a severe depression and whose stomach complaints were never thoroughly investigated during a six-month hospital stay. When transferred to our hospital, a gastric ulcer was found. Unreality feelings and depersonalization are distressing and persistent symptoms which yield only slowly to continued distraction and stimulating routine. A thorough analysis for possible dynamic factors should be delayed until the depression has cleared up. Delusions of sin, especially in the sexual field, and guilt to actual past misdemeanors are treated similarly. One should, however, always offer an opportunity for discussions which are terminated by constructive formulation. In religious scruples, the aid of a minister may be required, but one must keep in mind that the minister is a helper and not a healer and that he should work in cooperation with the physician and under his supervision. Too many visits by a minister will tend to cause the patient to consider his illness a religious problem. Delusions of poverty should be met with the actual statements but not by financial arguments. The treatment of the content is that of the treatment of delusions, i.e., tolerant listening with the injecting of doubt through suitable formulations and only frank contraindications when necessary and when the physician is in complete command of all the facts. The physician should make use of the affective rhythm and utilize the more or less marked insight which the patient has been able to acquire during less depressed periods. Obsessions and compulsions are treated similarly, their final analysis postponed until after recovery from the depression.

When transferring an improved depressed patient to a quiet ward, one should always consider carefully whether the patient will be put under too much responsibility. His degree of conscientiousness, thinking difficulties, and whether he will fit well into new surroundings should be evaluated. There is greater danger that such a patient will be transferred too soon, and will have a relapse than that improvement will be delayed by keeping him longer on a ward with simple demands. The same factors must be considered with regard to discharge to his home and return to work. It is certainly most desirable that such patients be sent home repeatedly on brief furloughs and start work on a part-time basis. This, unfortunately, is only possible when the psychiatric hospital is in the patient's community.

This entire discussion should demonstrate that active and individualized treatment is necessary in depressions and that the claim that little can be done beyond preserving the patient's life and letting nature take its course cannot be maintained any longer. The following case will illustrate this.

Case 9:

A 42 year old clerk developed increasing irritability and restlessness in June 1933. In August, after a visit to the World's Fair in order to distract himself, he became more preoccupied and lost interest in his daily activities. He now developed a definite depression, with increase of depressed mood and thinking difficulties in the morning, a feeling of futility, suicidal preoccupations, and fear of insanity. In October, he began to lose weight, developed marked constipation, had difficulty in falling asleep, his sleep became broken, and there was a marked decline in sexual desires. Self-depreciation increased; he became restless and developed anxiety symptoms. Admitted to the clinic on November 2nd, he presented a definitely depressed picture, especially in the morning, but with a marked tendency to dissimulation. He was resentful of hospitalization, feeling that he did not need a physician. We learned from him that he had had a depression lasting several weeks when 24, when he had to leave home, and that his father had suffered from three marked depressions. He had always been cheerful but inclined to be moody and easily worried by his work — a man who had a definite inadequacy feelings, who was highly conscientious, and had high standards. He had always been sociable but rather reserved, somewhat shy and sensitive to the opinion of others about him. He had carried responsibility well in his work.

The first four weeks of treatment were used to develop a better attitude to his illness and to medical help. His averse attitude gradually changed to one of trust and seeking help. With this, his depression became more obvious. He was restless, smoked incessantly, and felt he was unable to participate in routine. We urged him to limit his smoking considerably, learning to take it as recreation and not as an outlet for restlessness, and to participate in the full ward routine, including playing games and talking with other patients. He resented most the locked doors and limitation of his personal freedom. Using his own statement of suicidal preoccupations, the restrictions were explained to him carefully. Noticing that he was usually worse after visiting day, we tried to discuss this but the patient was unwilling to do so. Finally, after four weeks' treatment, he discussed part of his preoccupations, stating that he was worried over a sodomitic experience with a sheep at the age of 15, when he was a butcher's helper to his uncle. He felt guilty about this act and upset by the killing of the animal. Since then he had had an aversion to killing animals and frequently refused to eat meat. During his visit to the World's Fair he visited the Chicago stock yards, again saw slaughtering, and his old preoccupations returned and increased greatly. When asked to discuss his sex life, he mentioned his masturbation during adolescence and promiscuity after the age of 22, and finally a sexual relation with a married woman. After discussion the patient felt relieved. It was pointed out to him that he was not in a condition to do justice to himself during a depression; that it was best to try to push these thoughts away through active routine and to limit thinking about them to the consultation with the physician. In other words, he was not told merely to forget these thoughts, but to avoid self-analysis and self-accusation.

This married woman, being a relative, was one of his few visitors. He was advised to accept a limitation of visitors to one friend who did not stir up any special preoccupations. No personal topics were to be mentioned during these visits. After these topical discussions, there was a brief improvement of a few days which was due to relief from the discussion. Then, however, he again became more depressed, developing a depressive rut attitude with reiteration of self-depreciatory statements because of his past sexual misdemeanors and with marked hypochondriacal concern about his body sensations and poor sleep. The physician formulated to him the need to control his imaginations, urging him to discuss them freely. However, the patient was unable to do this. His body sensations were explained as symptoms of tension, and it was stressed that careful watching of the body makes us aware of, and intensifies normal body sensations. Sleep hygiene was carefully formulated — the need for relaxation, achieved by accepting a passive attitude with regard to sleep and imaginations; the sleep-destroying factor of the efforts to fall asleep and of worrying over the inability to sleep; and the relief obtained by a full discussion of imaginations. It was pointed out to him that sleep had become the central problem of his hypochondriacal attitude. After the first few discussions there was improvement in sleep (about six hours), but then again a drop to only two to three hours a night. The physician tried to produce sleep by hydrotherapy and by the administration of various sedatives in high amounts without, however, more than temporary results with each new drug. During this period, he received continuous warm baths from 7:30 to 8:30 P.M. and barbital 0.6 gm. (10 gr.) Later cold wet packs and barbital which at other

times was combined with alurate were administered. Trional and sulpho-
nal did not help either.

The patient remained in this depressive hypochondriacal rut with
considerable anxiety from January to April. During this period he was
allowed more visitors and urged to accept rides with two friends who
could be trusted to protect him against possible suicidal impulses. Unfortunately, he saw his woman friend twice on such trips before he informed us, denying that it had stirred up any undesirable preoccupations. The daily routine helped him considerably during the daytime but
in the evenings he was left too much to himself because there was no
congenial group on his ward.

At the end of April, the patient was transferred to another ward,
and his new physician was advised to depend primarily on psychotherapy
and to omit medication entirely. During the previous month his physician had been urged unsuccessfully to carry out the same procedure.
It had been pointed out that medication would destroy any suggestive
influence of his sleep therapy. The sleep problem was presented briefly,
using direct suggestion strongly. The need for a control of imaginations
with a willingness to accept fleeting sexual preoccupations on a physiologic basis, indicating in itself improvement, was re-emphasized. Interviews were offered freely but were always brief because repetition was
not permitted. Each discussion had to lead to something new and constructive or was terminated. The changes in occupational activities and
in social setting with wider recreational possibilities on this quiet ward
were utilized freely. All advice was offered in a marked suggestive way.
The patient's sleep improved rapidly (six to seven hours), hypochondriasis and apprehension decreased and self-confidence began to increase.
When urged to begin part-time work at the office (middle of May) he
agreed but became panicky the day before, afraid to face his colleagues.
He was advised to tell them frankly that he was a patient at the clinic
if asked about it, but not to volunteer information as it was entirely
his private affair. His attitude to his illness was again formulated.
The next day the patient went to work and adjusted well. His self-
confidence increased, and he was discharged, working full time, at the
end of May.

Discussion during the last week dealt constructively with outstanding personality features and their modifiability. Sexual hygiene was
treated as one among many other problems. Much attention was paid
to better possibilities for socialization and recreation. After discharge,
he came for further psychotherapeutic discussions, first twice a week,
later once a month. The outlook for the future is good and little likeli-
hood for further depressions is seen, if he is willing to turn to his
physician when he is confronted with more than he can deal with or
when he notices signs of depression.

It is quite possible that the "confession" at the end of December relieved this patient considerably for a short time but was followed by resentment at having been urged into it and therefore an inability to develop a healthy permanent rapport with his physician occurred. The change of physician created a more suitable basis for psychotherapy. Catathymic factors played a considerable role but only became active, expressed in guilt feelings, after the depression had started. It is therefore not an essentially catathymic depression. The case illustrates the need for an individualizing treatment of depressions and the possibilities of modification by psychotherapy. (There was no follow-up note obtainable on this patient in 1947.)

Many patients with marked anxiety develop panic reactions which may be brief or extended over weeks or months, characterized by intense fear and insecurity with suspiciousness, projections, misinterpretations, ideas of reference, and delusions of persecutions which are usually, but not always, self-depreciatory. During acute panic outbursts the patient is more or less inaccessible. In the intervals between these outbursts he may be in good rapport or suspicious and on guard. Insecurity demands self-assertion which leads to paranoid projections and impulsive acts. In milder degrees, or when fear is subsiding, the patients are arrogant, sarcastic, uncooperative, or evasive, especially when pushed with questions. This seems an important self-protection as patients react frequently with severe panic when a zealous physician pushes through his defense and forces the patient into a realization of the leading threatening factors.

Whenever one deals with a panic reaction the patient must be considered dangerously suicidal, and hospitalization is indicated. The suicidal attempts may be impulsive and violent as a result of fear and insecurity, or carefully planned. The adjustment to the hospital is a difficult task because of the patient's suspiciousness and insecurity. A frank attitude on the part of the physician and of those who come in contact with the patient is necessary. Admission and every step of routine must be carefully explained and considered, with modifications as may be necessary. Hydrotherapy and repeated doses of barbital 0.15 gm. (2½ grs.) three to four times a day decrease tension and permit a basis to be established for cooperation and confidence. In prolonged intense panic reaction, insulin therapy may be very effective. One ought not to expect more from a patient than seems wise according to his make-up. His conscientiousness and feeling of inadequacy ought to warn against giving him tasks that are difficult for him at a time of fear and thinking difficulties. There is usually a tendency to push such patients too fast when they begin to feel at ease. Premature transfer to a more active ward, sudden withdrawal of sedatives, or an attempt at analysis of underlying factors may precipitate an increase in insecurity and cause a panic outburst. Spontaneous discussions should be terminated with a constructive formulation which takes care of the patient's need but is not to be utilized for an investigation of the factors involved. A discussion of the more fundamental factors must be delayed until the patient is able to face his shortcomings and can also give his assets due appreciation. The prognosis is good if dealt with correctly but many of these depressions may last from one to two years. Many patients end in suicide, either in the hospital, or when discharged too soon or when taken out against advice. Insulin therapy frequently has a prompt effect in panic reactions. I have found its use especially indicated when a patient is brought to the hospital in a full-fledged panic and does not react within 48 hours to the barbiturates, hydrotherapy, and psychotherapy.

Case 10:

A 56 year old principal of a large preparatory school developed a depression in February which gradually increased with thinking difficulties in the morning, loss of appetite and weight, indigestion, poor sleep, and accusing himself of not having carried out his work well and of being a failure. He became indecisive. All the symptoms increased a great deal during the summer vacation. He became convinced he had contracted syphilis while swimming in a public pool and that he was a danger of infection to everyone, that he mismanaged the school's business, and was to be punished for it. He often refused food because he thought it was poisoned and began to refer remarks to himself. He became silent and usually declined to discuss his illness. During this period, the physician treated him with reassurance and advised recreation but did not outline a definite routine. On July 28th the patient suddenly seemed better and laughed about his ideas. That night, however, he became panicky, begged his wife to lock the door and to call the police for protection. In despair he tried to jump out of the window. The next day he was admitted to the hospital, entering willingly. He was restless and agitated, felt hopeless, and said the only out would be by suicide. The need for hospitalization and hospital life was carefully formulated to him and he accepted continuous warm bath treatment, food, and medication with urging.

The history from the family revealed that we dealt with a proud, very conscientious man who had always depended on himself and confided in nobody but his wife; he was sociable and well liked. He always preferred reading and research in modern languages to social and athletic recreation. There had always been a marked tendency to pay careful attention to his health although no frank hypochondriasis was present. His standards had always been high in ethics and work, and he was a rigid, stubborn man who was never able to yield. His life had been successful, and he had held his present position for four years. His father and two brothers were prone to slight depressions.

During the first two and a half weeks the patient talked little, usually sitting around motionless or pacing the floor restlessly. He looked sad and tense, often apprehensive, and was resistant to help offered. We realized that it was of utmost importance to gain the patient's confidence but that we could not expect good rapport in a short time in this patient. The physician saw the patient several times a day when passing through the ward, inquiring with a few words into his general condition, explaining minor steps of treatment, encouraging him to help the nurses, and to join in occupation which would help him to forget his preoccupations. No inquiry was made into the content, but the patient stated spontaneously during the brief period of a few minutes, after two days, that he was depressed because of having made a failure of his life, that he was unable to earn enough money, and that he had been dissatisfied with his present work. At night he was apprehensive and needed reassurance with regard to his health and personal safety. He was afraid that someone was trying to compromise him by making it appear that a woman was with him. During the physician's visits he usually did not talk, but when the former was leaving, the patient grabbed for him. This behavior induced us to increase a feeling of security by our formulations. To decrease his marked tension he received barbital 0.15 gm. (2½ gr.), three times a day, and two hours' continuous bath before retiring. Every other night barbital 0.3 gm. (5 gr.) was offered in addition because his sleep remained poor and he was afraid of the nights. On a few occasions cold wet packs were administered. These the patient was able to accept for one hour, following which, upon his request, it was necessary to remove him. Although he ate sufficiently with constant urging, he still lost weight (10 lbs.). The marked constipation was treated alternately with magnesium sulphate (30 cc.) and milk of magnesia (40 cc.) in the morning, or aromatic cascara (30 cc.) in the evening, and the bowels were well controlled. The second day he was advised to get up and join in carefully modified manual activity. This type of occupation was selected because one

expects thinking difficulties to be present in depressions. The patient
denied this difficulty at admission but complained of it a week later.
He was advised to read the daily papers, especially in the late afternoon, but not to try books yet. His wife visited him twice a week and
encouraged him to cooperate. The physician usually dropped in on these
occasions to discuss the various therapeutic procedures and hospital
occurrences with the wife. This was used as an indirect approach to the
patient and also considered especially important to prevent an undue
dependence on his wife, which would have interfered with establishing a healthy medical rapport. The pulse was a good indicator of the
patient's tension and fear. The first three days it ranged around 100,
afterwards between 80 and 90, and with the slight improvement (decrease of restlessness, apprehension, and resistance, and more spontaneous activity) it dropped to around 70. The definite improvement was
substantiated by gain of weight after two weeks and satisfactory sleep.
No attempts at getting more of the content were made. When he mentioned that he had been greatly upset by a spontaneous discharge during his wife's visit, the opportunity was utilized for a brief formulation of sexual physiology.

A second phase of treatment started at the time of this definite
improvement with the accompanying feeling of more security and some
confidence in the hospital. During the following three months, the
patient was still tense and more frankly depressed, crying occasionally,
describing his mood as hopeless, and complaining of marked thinking
difficulties. He occasionally mentioned some of the content. The physician always attempted to take care of whatever came up without pushing further, although offering encouraging opportunities for discussion. On such occasions the patient was advised to accept his depressive
difficulties in making decisions and to depend on others for the time
being. His "feeling ashamed" was related to his high standards, his
"despair" and "fear of consequences of mistakes" of the past to his
marked conscientiousness and exactness, and the exaggerated difficulty
in approaching tasks to his depression. He was urged not to chafe
against his illness and to accept the necessary observation by the nurses,
which he resented, as help and protection against impulses to harm
himself in despair and hopelessness. In all formulations the patient's
own expressions and what he had mentioned were used constructively.
The delusions of syphilis and persecution for his imagined failure were
undermined by repeated statements of his health and reference to his
depressed self-depreciation and to related personality features. Arguments were carefully avoided. He began to appreciate the help gained
through occupation which allowed him to forget his worries and accept
better socialization. Walks on the hospital grounds distracted him but
were limited because of the still persisting tendency to depressive ideas

of reference. Conversation on impersonal topics was cultivated. The increasingly more obvious daily mood variations were pointed out and utilized. The physical improvement was offered as a sign of general progress with stress on the relative value of minor changes. He was urged to be patient with himself and not to insist on his transfer to a quiet ward because that step involved more spontaneous activity and responsibility and should always be considered carefully in an over-conscientious person. Every opportunity was utilized to lead him to an acceptance of his illness and medical help and advice. When he insisted that he could not talk with a young physician, a consultation with an older member of the staff (of his choosing) was arranged. (The consultation took place in the presence of his ward physician.) Nothing essentially new was obtained, but the consultation, during which the above-outlined procedure was followed by the consultant, made it easier for the patient to form better rapport. A short set-back was caused when he had to endorse a check because it made him think of the treasurer of his school who had defaulted, and of his own neglect of supervision. This situation was utilized for a brief constructive rediscussion of these factors, stressing that he should allow our judgment to predominate for the present.

On November 11th he was transferred to a quiet ward. He reacted with slight increase of restlessness and apprehension which subsided after a few days. It was, however, taken as an indication that the treatment should not be changed yet. When the patient was again feeling at ease, medication was decreased gradually. First the noon dose was omitted; a week later the morning dose; and after another week sedatives were entirely discontinued. He joined in full activity and tried to fit in with the group of patients. The value of socialization was discussed and the need to develop various kinds of recreation. He was permitted to read more in the evening and could choose books suited to his own interest because the thinking difficulties cleared up entirely in the afternoon. His behavior was now normal except for decreased spontaneity. He still felt depressed and hopeless in the morning. The patient tried to forget his depressed mood and disturbing preoccupations by constantly keeping occupied. It was therefore necessary to point out to him that he should learn to do things with ease and to find forgetfulness also through recreation and group activities. Only after he had improved considerably (at the beginning of December) was he allowed to take up his research interests to which he then devoted most of the time which was reserved for occupation. Outdoor activities were increased (walks).

In December he went home every Sunday. This was advised to increase his confidence in himself and to help him overcome his uneasiness in meeting acquaintances, to re-establish broken connections, and to overcome his doubts that he would be able to find a way back to an

active life. His wife was aware of the still persistent suicidal potentialities but was anxious for him to attempt trial visits because she felt
that he was unwilling to stay in the hospital much longer. Therapeutic
interviews occurred every three to four days. In the intervals the physician watched carefully for signs of increased depressive tendencies.
which might have indicated the need for shorter or less frequent discussions. They dealt first with his school difficulties, his interest in research,
and lack of interest in administrative duties which were a burden.
Aggravating factors were his need for exactness and orderliness and
unwillingness to make quick decisions. There had always been marked
difficulty in carrying responsibility, and he had therefore never wanted
to have children. He then discussed personality features which made
it difficult for him to exert leadership, and later his ambition for research
and the need to earn money in a school. This was followed by a general discussion of interests and possibilities for a broader and also less
self-centered life. After a discussion of socialization, and especially of
the features of reserve, rigidity, and pride, the patient volunteered the
question as to whether he should conceal the psychiatric nature of his
illness. After a study of all the factors which were involved in this
problem, the patient decided to offer the correct explanation if asked,
as he otherwise could not establish the necessary social ease. He discussed his professional future again but felt unable as yet to arrive at
a definite decision. In this connection he tried to gain a better understanding of what life was able to offer him and whether his religious
and philosophic views were broad and plastic enough. A brief study
of his sexual life, especially of an increase of desires and preoccupations
in the last few years which had caused him to resort to masturbation at
the time of the onset of his depression, led to a constructive understanding of sex control and hygiene. When he left the hospital on January
2nd he was still undecided about his future, feeling unable to resign
because it would indicate failure and financial restrictions.

During January and February he was treated in regular consultations
in which his illness and the factors involved were discussed, but special
attention was paid to a study of his assets and interests and their cultivation, and his need for success along lines which were not of fundamental importance for his personality. The patient was active in a well-
balanced routine which included physical and social recreation. At the
end of this period of treatment he decided to resign from his position
and to accept an opportunity for teaching and research in a near-by college. Since then he has been in good health, satisfied in his work and
better adjusted to the group and to life in general. The patient has remained in good health (1947).

Depression around the age of fifty and later is frequent. One is
inclined to connect it with endocrinologic changes but attempts at

verification by careful somatic study and at modification by glandular therapy have not led far. It is quite possible that the general, although slight, decline in physical and mental strength and endurance is of importance. However, one should also consider the phase of personality development and situations which are likely to occur, i.e., loss of general plasticity, the feeling that one has spent one's most active years, curtailment of ambition and resignation, difficulties in reorientation, and fewer possibilities for new positions. The change of living conditions frequently proves to be too much. We therefore find depressive reactions to moving into a new environment.

In depressions occurring during the menopausal and postmenopausal periods, the vasomotor symptoms seem to be beneficially affected by estrogenic hormones. This improvement may be helpful in patients with hypochondriacal concern and should therefore be utilized psychotherapeutically. No evidence has been presented in literature that the depressive illness and its course can be influenced by endocrinologic treatment. In male patients, androgenic hormone may increase sexual desires. These urges may lead to psychodynamic difficulties if suppressed or repressed unacceptable sexual desires become provoked.

The treatment of depressions in the fifth and sixth decade has become much more efficient since the introduction of convulsive therapy. On the other hand, in a considerable number of these patients, the depressive illness may be influenced temporarily only, or to a limited extent and followed by a prolonged course of convalescence. It is important that each patient be studied carefully for several weeks before convulsive therapy is started if one wishes to use individualized psychotherapy and strive for more than merely symptomatic improvement.

Case 11:

A 50 year old banker was admitted on September 6, 1946 in a deeply depressed state with marked slowness of movements, self-accusation, and expressions of worthlessness. His depression had developed over the preceding eight months and had become much worse in the last four weeks. Four days before admission he had a brief paranoid panic and made a suicidal attempt.

The patient was an intelligent man who despite success never developed full self-confidence. He had been moody and obviously overly concerned about his physical health during the last 10 years. Greatly impressed by childhood poverty he had a strong need for financial security. He appeared to be well adjusted sexually, was devoted to his family, and well liked by his friends.

In the hospital the patient remained depressed, appeared suspicious of being watched, and had the delusion that his eating well was depriving other patients of their food. He continuously spoke of his feeling of unworthiness. His agitation subsided under the administration of barbital .15 gm ($2\frac{1}{2}$ gr.), three times a day, and three hours of warm bath, and he slept adequately. There was a persistent marked resentment to the hospital and to his being sick, but he cooperated well in occupational therapy. On October 2nd conclusive therapy was started. Two convulsions a week were administered. After his fifth convulsion (October 19th), he showed fast improvement. He felt depressed but the delusions had subsided; he felt at ease with the other patients, and was less concerned about his bowel movements. There was fear, however, that the convulsions might have harmed him because he had headaches. Sedation which had been reduced gradually, was discontinued. During the period between October 16th and 25th, he received three additional convulsions. This period was used to review his family life and social adjustment and he was urged to participate in group activities. At the end of October he made plans for leaving because he wanted to be with his family and to assume his obligations in his bank. He again became more depressed and suspiciousness returned. After a review of his present status he accepted the physician's advice to stay in the hospital. He was transferred to a floor where the social requirements were less. On November 11th, convulsions were readministered and he completed his second series of eight convulsions on December 2nd. He again improved fast. Psychotherapy played a major role. In November, his sexual life and his attitude to his body were reviewed and later his work and lack of recreation. Resentment to his socially ambitious wife began to be expressed. Financial insecurity and lack of confidence in his work, the type and amount of responsibility he had to carry, and his relationship to his superior officer were studied. In December, his illness was reviewed as well as the factors which played a role, his aversion to hospital treatment, his sensitivity to others, his ambitions, his high sense of obligation to his family, and his body insecurity. His self-confidence returned and he began to work January 2nd but remained a patient in the clinic till January 31st because the social contact with other patients and recreation in the evening permitted him to feel at ease. Since his discharge the patient has remained in good health.

In patients in whom convulsive and insulin therapy do not bring about the desired improvement, one should consider the various phases of the illness and plan treatment which may last from one to two years. Otherwise one loses sight of what has been achieved and what the present demands. The outstanding problems are the correct dealing with anxiety and panic phases, persistent and far-reaching delusions, rut-formation, and an attitude of aversion and resentment to the illness, to medical help, and frequently to life and family. Feelings of futility and unreality are distressing problems which can only be modified by painstaking treatment in which one attempts to create situations that may stimulate the patient's interests. One should be careful not to push the patient and cause undesirable reactions by exposing him to situations which make him painfully aware of his inability to appreciate things the way he did previously. A ride in the country in the spring time is usually pleasant and distracting, but what was beautiful before may appear unreal to a depressed patient and distress him greatly. The psychologic interpretations of unreality and resentment, and of what is interpreted as sadistic strivings and repression to narcissism, cannot be used therapeutically. In rut-formation one is inclined to urge the family to try an outside adjustment. This is rarely advisable because of suicidal danger. Transfer to another hospital or to a different ward or building in the same hospital is preferable. It is also never wise to keep the same nurses over a long period of time on such a case.

In later as well as early life, the emotion of tension may take the place of the depressive mood. In such patients, the dynamic factors are marked conscientiousness, a need for self-reliance coupled with inadequacy, habits of anticipation, and developmental short-comings (insufficient emancipation and immature habits), together with specific life situations (increased responsibility and insecurity). These patients react frequently with an attitude of aversion to their illness and to the help which physicians and nurses offer. Repeated small amounts of barbital and hydrotherapy relieve the tension. If sleep difficulties persist, the psychotherapeutic approach is essential. To prevent the increase of tension which may lead to serious panic reactions, the same therapeutic principles which were discussed under panic need to be considered. In many cases, the main goal for a considerable time is the prevention of panic and rut-formation, and the influencing of the aversion and hypochondriacal attitudes. The analysis of the underlying factors has to be postponed. On the other hand, the psychotherapeutic discussions are frequently postponed too long. The physician must evaluate all the factors and choose the most suitable phase for more aggressive psychotherapy. As a rule patients are amenable to this when tension and depression have subsided, as seen by the general subjective and objective improvement and the decrease of the pulse rate. The beginning of rut-formation is usually an indication for more active psychotherapy. In patients with slight tension depression, a distributive analysis is indicated early. One should always consider these patients suicidal and advise hospital treatment if the symptoms reach marked intensity. Many cases of slight tension depression are mistaken for hypochondriasis, neurasthenia, or anxiety neurosis and may be lost by suicide.

Catathymic factors play a certain role in tension depressions. In the catathymic depression more specific factors are usually at work and produce guilt reactions. In these depressions, marked need for atonement may cause the patient to resort to suicide or self-mutilation. It is very difficult to guard against such acts. Protection of the patient is important as these patients usually recover with a good life prognosis. During the deep depressive phase the guilt reaction needs to be treated by injecting doubt into the justification of such a rigid philosophy which is unable to accept reconstructive possibilities. The physician should avoid forcing his own views on the patient and participating in argumentative discussions. As these attitudes have the strength of delusional beliefs, the attempt at modification through religious means proves to be futile. A constructive analysis is not possible until the depression has largely cleared up and even then, many patients are averse to a thorough discussion. The recovery may, nevertheless, be lasting because the patient has satisfied his ethical needs by atonement through his illness. In others, repression may be strong enough for life if no new dangers stir up the same conflicts.

Obsessions and compulsions, which occur frequently in depressions, are usually the manifestation of a general personality reaction rather than the result of specific factors, as in obsessive-compulsive neurosis. An analysis of the personality is therefore essential after the patient has recovered from the depression. During the depression the patient should be distracted from his preoccupations and compulsions, and should try to find relief from the accumulating tension resulting from this suppression in discussions and activity. The physician should lead the patient from mere repetition, complaints, and self-accusation to a constructive discussion. It will be best to offer the patient a few minutes for spontaneous expression of his complaints but then urge him to seek possibilities of connection. In occupational therapy the marked conscientiousness, together with inadequacy, has to be kept in mind. These patients have to learn to accept a task as finished, even if there is a need to make it perfect. In some cases, there is an increase of compulsions during the depressive illness which must be treated before dealing with the underlying neurosis.

Case 12:

A 39 year old successful business man became worried after a revival meeting in September 1927, thinking that he was not saved and that he had not been quite correct in business transactions. After a few days, he developed more depressive features — increases of life-long constipation, decrease of sexual potency and desires, and poor sleep, waking after three or four o'clock in the morning. He became increasingly restless and hesitant in his actions, feeling an urge to repeat them. He was greatly distressed by obsessive thoughts of lewd content and of cursing the Lord, and by increasing compulsions. During two months' vacation in Florida he became definitely worse. He then took a rest cure with very modified activity in a nursing home, but showed no improvement. In August 1928, he was transferred to our clinic, showing about the same picture as has been mentioned above.

A brief orientation with regard to the patient's past life and personality make-up revealed that he had always been a timid rather shy person who had many friends but few intimates. There had always been a definite tendency to moodiness, especially when feeling that he had made a mistake. His conscientiousness had been marked since childhood. Since adolescence he had shown definite tendency to compulsive acts — for instance, to look repeatedly to see whether he had closed a door or locked the safe. He had always been very religious, taking an active part in church activities, but was also active in sports of all kinds. Shortly after his marriage in the spring of 1917, he developed a slight depression which increased markedly after the draft legislation had been passed. He was greatly afraid that he was avoiding the draft, heard voices saying that he would be killed, and accusing him of not doing his duty. At that time the depression lasted several months. He was entirely well until 1924, when he developed a depression after a revival meeting. This illness, with content similar to the present attack, lasted about six months. There was a definite depressive strain on the paternal side.

Obtaining this history from the patient offered a basis for a preliminary formulation which stressed his personality make-up and the need to consider his present condition as an illness. He was urged to enter into full ward activity and to force himself to stop compulsive activity. We tried to utilize his interests and advised him to play golf and to take walks to points of interest in the city. It frequently took half an hour to get him through his morning bath and many of the activities were constantly interrupted by his compulsive repetitions and rituals. The nurse urged and encouraged him patiently but persistently. From the beginning there was a definite improvement noticeable in the afternoon. That was the time of day when he was asked to enter into more activities. In occupational therapy, he was encouraged by telling him that his work was done satisfactorily; he was not pushed because this too conscientious man tried to do more than he was capable of doing. Cathartics were necessary. His sleep was well managed with a cold wet pack from 8 to 10 o'clock and barbital 0.3 gm. (5 gr.) at 9:30. He slept six to seven hours every night.

After four weeks there was a definite improvement in his depression. At this time we were informed of financial strain which would cause termination of the hospital stay. This was frankly discussed with the patient and it was stressed to him at the same time that he was improving. Under this financial strain the patient definitely showed more improvement. He was able to control his compulsive activities better, the depression diminished, sleep improved, and sedatives and packs were entirely left off at the beginning of October. The last four weeks in the hospital (discharged November 2nd) were utilized for establishing a better understanding of his personality and of the development of his compulsive and obsessive tendencies. He was urged to give up the fatalistic point of view which had been instilled into him by the psychiatrist who treated him in 1917, and who had tried to prepare him for recurrences of his depression. Instead of such an acceptance, we analyzed with him the situations which had brought on the various depressions, pointing out the assets and interests which could be utilized to counterbalance strain. He decided that it would be best for him to restrict his active interest in church affairs and to recognize his sensitiveness to revival meetings. He also learned to understand that he was too much aware of himself, unable to throw off his thoughts, as well as being constantly concerned about his body welfare. In the last few discussions, his wife was included in the hope of making her more plastic and making them both aware of depressive mood reactions and their management. Since discharge in 1928 the patient has been doing well.

The treatment of a depression with much catathymic material was outlined briefly to illustrate what can be done in any well-managed hospital. We were not able to adjust the underlying causes because the patient was unable to undergo treatment for a sufficient length of time. It was, however, an active and carefully planned treatment. Previously, when treated merely for depression according to the general rule of treatment, he showed little improvement. When routine and psychotherapy were adjusted to his personal needs he improved rather rapidly.

Psychoneurotic features and impure affects are especially marked in depressions in psychopathic individuals and adolescents. These personality make-ups may also show a tendency to recurrence of depression on slight provocation. Hate, suspiciousness, resentment, and aversion to treatment are frequently observed. A prolonged depressive stupor may be caused by aversion. One of my patients, a thirty-five-year-old unmarried woman, developed her depression in the setting of unsatisfactory attempts at sexual gratification. When unable to manage the treatment in her own way, she became stuporous for over two years and then recovered completely from her illness, fostering since then, however, marked resentment to the treatment. In depressive stupors many factors play a role and have to be considered therapeutically during the stupor and in the final adjustment. A thirty-five-year-old man developed a depression with one and a half years' stupor (catalepsy, drooling, and complete immobility) when suspicious of his wife's fidelity. During the stupor we used the wife's regular visit for an indirect psychotherapeutic approach. The stupor cleared suddenly and within a week he developed a manic excitement of one and a half years' duration and then recovered. This proud, unbending person was, however, never able to discuss the jealousy reaction. In others, the need for atonement may be dominant. Stupor occurs frequently in the setting of apathy. Relatively few cases present this reaction as the expression of maximal retardation.

Hallucinatory experiences and paranoid trends are frequent in psychopathic depressions. The problem of re-education is more important and handling more difficult than in the average depression. These patients may disturb a wholesome ward atmosphere greatly through their resentful and criticizing attitude. It is therefore necessary to keep them longer on a disturbed ward. In large hospitals it should always be possible to offer possibilities for adjustment in a quiet group but with brief transfers to the disturbed ward if the behavior becomes disturbing to the other patients or when the patient becomes uncooperative. The general principles of the treatment of psychopathic personality should guide us. Disciplinary routine is undesirable and provokes reactions of aversion to the physician and the treatment. In adolescents, similar considerations with due attention to the tendencies and reactions of adolescence should guide us.

In primarily constitutionally-determined recurrent depressions, situational and personality factors need to be investigated. When such affective reactions develop with great frequency in a person who has been in good health until the age of 30 or longer, one should look for catathymic factors. A thorough analysis is then indicated after the patient has recovered from one of the attacks. Many recurrent depressions occur in poorly organized psychopathic personalities. Although the leading factors may be clear to the patient he is unable to do much about it and personality re-education needs to be carried out in regular well-spaced consultation treatment over years. Recurrent affective disorders in adolescence do not necessarily offer a poor life prognosis. In many patients these attacks subside when a better stability of the personality has been reached with maturity. The treatment should therefore be directed towards increasing the natural tendencies toward stability and towards preventing life situations which are too much for such an adolescent.

Many depressions terminate with a brief hypomanic elation. Others, belonging to the manic-depressive cycle, are preceded or followed by manic excitement. It is important to recognize these changes early so that the patient is not pushed too far and an excitement can thereby be prevented. Mixed conditions, i.e., brief periods of elation and depression interchanging readily in the course of the day, necessitate a curtailment of activity. The patient needs to be made aware of the undesirability of undertaking too much in his elated mood and to recognize these reactions as part of the illness and not to mistake them as normal push. Suicidal danger can be considerable during the brief depressive moods. The older conception that the elation is a normal reaction of relief to having recovered has often led physicians to accept increased stimulation, thus precipitating an excitement.

In the declining years of life, depressions of a persistent type occur with a tendency to apathy and rut-formation, mood fixation on delusions, and hypochondriacal concerns. In presenile and arteriosclerotic settings these features are also predominant. The treatment attempts to create situations and a routine which are stimulating to the patient and also to reconcile him to his illness. Irritability and rigid, often unmodifiable delusions, especially of a hypochondriacal type, demand special psychotherapeutic attention. It is frequently possible to reach an improvement in which an outside adjustment can be achieved although delusions persist. In other cases permanent hospitalization is necessary. Even then therapy should be active, utilizing the patient's previous interests, and stressing the need for socialization and healthy routine with regular occupation and recreation. Treatment should never become a mere taking care of the patient.

BIBLIOGRAPHY

1. HINSIE, L. E., and KATZ, S. E.: Treatment of Manic-Depressive Psychosis; a Survey of the Literature. *American Journal of Psychiatry,* 11, 1931.
2. JAMEISON, G. R.: Suicide and Mental Disease — a Clinical Analysis of One Hundred Cases. *Archives of Neurology and Psychiatry,* 36, 1936.
3. BENDER, L., and SCHILDER, P.: Suicidal Preoccupations and Attempts in Children. *American Journal of Orthopsychiatry,* 7, 1937.
4. RIPLEY, H. S.; SHORR, E., and PAPANICOLAOU, G. N.: The Effect of Treatment of Depression in the Menopause with Estrogenic Hormone. *American Journal of Psychiatry,* 96, 1940.

Chapter X

SCHIZOPHRENIC REACTIONS

UNDER this heading are discussed those illnesses which are characterized by "twists and fundamental or fancy-born incongruities more or less foreign to average mature waking life." (A. Meyer.) Developing largely in shut-in and tense persons, these reactions lead to indulgence in unfulfilled and vague autistic fancy, day-dreaming and withdrawal from reality, automatic and dissociated thought processes frequently expressed in the form of projection (delusions of reference and hallucinations). Outstanding in the content are projections with passivity (being under an outside influence), dramatic, mystical, and religious experiences, and often fantastic episodes and grotesque incongruities of judgment. Other psychopathologic symptoms are strange actions and oddities of behavior, disorders of thinking in the realm of discrimination with vagueness and use of generalities, unaccountable interruptions (blocking) which may lead to disconnected and scattered stream of talk, condensations and misplacement of affect, ambivalence, and indifference, often interrupted by impulsive episodes.

In his genetic-dynamic conception of schizophrenia, A. Meyer stressed the importance of the personality make-up which predisposes to this reaction and of the life factors which cause them. These patients are poorly socialized with a marked tendency to withdraw into preoccupations and day-dreams. They lack healthy aggressiveness and constructive goals. Conflict results from empty ambitions and inadequacy of performance. These patients have many unsatisfied longings and frequently strong feelings of inadequacy. A poorly directed instinctive life and the untimely stirring up of instincts and longings result in conflicts which affect the balance of the total personality. In some cases, the habit disorders preponderate in the side-tracking and curbing of leading interests and the creation of disastrous substitutions. In others, definite life experiences play a special role. This concept of schizophrenia takes into consideration the wide range of possibilities for psychobiologic habit-formation and the possibility of the development of a cleavage along distinctly psychobiologic lines, incompatible with reintegration. This may result in permanent disorganization of the personality and possibly far-reaching deterioration.

The therapeutic procedure depends much on one's conception of the illness. Dementia praecox stresses the terminal dementia as the essential feature. Fortunately most schizophrenic patients do not end in dementia, and a fatalistic attitude is therefore unjustified. One should realize that the term, "dementia," has been extended by some psychiatrists to such a point that any persistence of schizophrenic symptoms is used as a proof of its existence. This leads to academic discussions which are rarely of practical value and frequently interfere with constructive treatment. Let us accept the fact that we still know little about "normal thinking" and its many variations. It is well known that erratic and somewhat vague thinking need not make an adjustment impossible in every field of life and that some exceptional persons with this type of thinking have even achieved high success. Each case has to be studied and treated individually. In the expectancy of our therapeutic results we should not be influenced by too narrow a concept of normality. It is also essential that one recognize that patients who suffer from schizophrenic illnesses may recover and that the life prognosis may be good. The prognosis for the present illness and for the future depends on the type of schizophrenic reaction, the personality setting in which it occurs, and the personality and other resources which are available for treatment. Nothing definite is known about structural changes in the brain or possible etiological somatic factors. The treatment must therefore deal primarily with personality functions. This brief discussion demonstrates why the term, "schizophrenia," as introduced by Bleuler, does not correspond to Meyer's concept which is used in this book. These introductory remarks should eliminate any misunderstanding.

In treatment, one should consider all the modifiable factors, and be guided by the facts obtained from the patient's life history and from direct observation. One makes use of all the opportunities for correcting endocrinologic involvements and toxic factors without, however, considering them the causal factors as do some investigators. The importance of a narcissistic reaction and the factors of regression in general have to be kept in mind, without making them the only guiding principles in the therapeutic approach. The treatment tries to modify fundamental factors as well as disturbing symptoms. As a rule, a constructive analysis as the immediate treatment is possible in the incipient schizophrenic illness, while in the full-fledged illness a symptomatic treatment must be carried out. This should be based on an understanding of the patient's personality with attention to autistic withdrawal, and to behavior and content disorders. The psychotherapeutic efforts deal with all these features and make full use of opportunities for socialization, occupation, and re-education. With increasing reintegration, a more or less far-reaching constructive analysis becomes possible. In many cases, one has to be satisfied with a life adjustment on a less satisfactory level, and in a relatively high number of patients, permanent hospitalization is necessary. The latter, however, should not mean mere care but a constant creating of opportunities for helpful activities and contacts and the utilization of new situations which, occasionally in apparently hopeless cases of years' standing, may lead to surprising improvement.

From a clinical point of view, four types of schizophrenic reactions are usually distinguished: catatonic, hebephrenic, paranoid, and the simple type. The catatonic reaction is characterized by motility involvement and frequently by the attempt at a mystical submissive solution of the difficulty. The illness is often phasic, with stupor or excitement, or with intermissions of short or long duration. The hebephrenic reaction is of the vague, scattered type. It may present a wealth of psychopathologic material or take a more psychopathic form which allows the patient to live in society for a considerable length of time. When the content is definitely of systematized delusion-formation with hallucinations, automatism, and behavior involvement, one speaks of a paranoid schizophrenic illness. This type will be discussed in Chapter XI (paranoic and paranoid reactions) because the treatment of delusional illnesses is fundamentally the same whenever they occur. Simple schizophrenia or early schizophrenic symptoms will not be treated separately as they primarily present problems of withdrawal and habit-deterioration. The rules which should be followed in the other schizophrenic reactions should also be applied to this rather ill-defined group.

The treatment is always based on the understanding of the individual who has reacted with a more or less marked autistic withdrawal, i.e., an indulgence in phantasy without the test of reality. Such phantasy leads to an increasing loss of group contact and interest in reality. Fancies offer compensation for cravings and inadequacy, real or imagined. The first, and frequently most difficult, therapeutic task is to establish a rapport which utilizes the patient's interests. Socialization is most important. Isolation should therefore be avoided as much as possible. The patients should not even be allowed to stay in their own rooms except for definite therapeutic reasons. By living in a group and by means of accordingly planned psychotherapy, the patients learn to depend more on the consensus of opinion than on their own isolated evaluation of experiences or desires. They gradually become interested in other individuals. In wealthy patients, special nurses are frequently the only means of socialization. This is less helpful than being with a small group of patients which keeps changing and contains a variety of different persons. A carefully planned routine should stimulate their interests, allowing them to be cultivated. However, an increasing ability and need to share pleasures and disappointments with others should be fostered. This should prevent them from indulging in autistic creations except for definite therapeutic reasons, i.e., when these creations reveal personality strivings which one wishes to analyze. Through routine, undue preoccupations are forestalled. They do not occupy the center of attention and importance while the patient is busy, and many problems are allowed to subside or even be forgotten. On the basis of therapeutic considerations the physician must decide whether these problems should be left undisturbed or used for a helpful analysis at the opportune time.

The content is of utmost importance. It is frequently most difficult to obtain in a concrete form. Life experiences also are often not well given, or the accurate time of their actual occurrence is only generally indicated. If one wishes to use life experiences of any kind constructively, one should find out when they happened in order to be able to recognize what factors played a role at the time. To obtain an understanding of the underlying strivings, one must analyze the meaning of experiences, fancies, and projections, but this cannot be done indiscriminately. Although the psychiatrist may clearly understand the underlying factors which form the symptoms, he should not interpret them to the patient but use this knowledge as a guide in his approach and treatment. A schizophrenic illness disorganizes the personality. Therapy should help to regain a sufficiently secure personality organization. The analysis of symptoms as well as personality features should be stopped whenever new signs of disorganization appear. Disorganization is indicated by the appearance of contradictory strivings and behavior without the attempt to adjust them to each other, by concentration and specific thinking disorders, motility disturbances, and mystical features. Temporary interruptions of varying length of the analysis is necessary, especially when more material than the physician can handle securely has been stirred up. The above-discussed routine will allow this material to settle down. Analysis of the sensitive topics should not be resumed until the physician is sure that the patient has definitely improved. This, however, does not imply an aloof attitude or a refusal for discussion when the patient has need of relief. Active therapy is possible even in disintegrated states if the physician can create more ease and thus achieve reintegration by offering constructive advice based on an understanding which has been gained in a brief analysis of the topic. Much depends, however, on the physician's grasp of the whole illness and of the special problems under consideration, and on his therapeutic imagination which allows him to foresee and prevent dangers which could be stirred up. It is essential that discussions do not merely bring within the patient's field of grasp the underlying disturbing factors and that rediscussion of sensitive topics does not reopen wounds and interfere with the healing process. When using analysis in schizophrenic illnesses, the physician must assume an active role and know when he should stop the exploration. The free association method can therefore be used only in patients who have no signs of serious disorganization, and even then should be interrupted if such signs appear. Through a distributive analysis by question and answer (see Chapter VI) the physician is much more apt to avoid dangerous situations and to remain in command of the therapeutic procedure. The goal is the analysis of the content, the personality, and the life setting, so that the patient can recognize faulty conclusions and the factors which played a role in his withdrawal reaction as well as personality features which he can use constructively for an adjustment.

The use of insulin treatment to alleviate anxiety now permits a more active analysis than previously. Signs of disorganization in the form of incoherent thinking, transient delusions, or hallucinations may subside with decreased anxiety and analytic therapy can progress constructively if the patient receives insulin every day (see Chapter VII).

Symptomatic treatment is necessary in any content disorder. It is essential, for instance, that one deal correctly with hallucinations and delusions. The physician must listen willingly without contradiction yet without accepting them as correct. Instead, he will close the discussion with a formulation which does justice to the patient's sensitiveness and beliefs but at the same time injects doubt in their validity. The patient is urged to consider the possibility of fallacious conclusions when one depends entirely on one's self. The wisdom of discussion with others is pointed out, and therefore the desirability of the continuance of interviews with the physician.

In re-education, which plays such an important role in this reaction type, symptomatic treatment is important but should not lead to a neglect of the whole personality. Re-education has long been considered important in patients with schizophrenic illnesses because these patients react with definite habit-deterioration. This term is broad and refers to the development of poor habits in personality functions. It does not refer merely to the general behavior but involves habits of thinking, decision and action, emotional control, and attitude to life and its problems. The need for re-education along the lines of group adjustment and socialization has already been stressed. It is important that one keep the patient's personality in mind and not expect a self-conscious or shy person to utilize the opportunities offered without being constantly encouraged and urged. A brief analysis of these recurrent difficulties is the basis for success. It requires a tactful and firm attitude to correct table manners, general appearance, and poor habits in general hygiene. This is especially difficult in patients who have a great need to protect their dignity and a lack of insight into their difficulties. Such poor habits may have developed gradually and become part of the personality. Re-education is a slow and tedious procedure. It is wise to keep this in mind and not to become discouraged by the slow progress. One will then also be willing not to expect a perfect adjustment in every patient.

Difficulties in social adjustment, lack of interest and therefore of persistence, or catathymic factors (influence of life experiences, frequently dissociated) often cause the patients to give up their work and to become shiftless. This problem offers good possibilities for re-education in many cases. Difficulties in decision and action can also be gradually corrected. To re-education also belongs the development of a healthy attitude to life and its manifold problems. Such re-education cannot be accomplished without an analysis of the person's desires and needs, his assets, and shortcomings.

The re-education of patients suffering from schizophrenic thinking disorders has probably received least attention, although considerable improvement can be achieved. One has to know the type of thinking disorder, i.e., whether one deals with vagueness or illogical thinking, use of generalities (especially in mystical and philosophic concepts), condensations, scattering, or lack of concentration. A more secondary type of thinking disorder is due to affective and catathymic influences and should be adjusted by means of analysis. In re-education, one should point out to the patient his lack of concreteness and his fallacious conclusions, his lack of sharp discrimination leading to faulty fusion, and the need to stick to problems until they are solved. One should suggest a selection of problems for work which the patient is able to do at the time. By advising a patient to read a brief article and to discuss it with others one tries to re-educate the patient's thinking, increase his socialization, and correct his withdrawal tendencies. With some, translations are helpful. Abstract discussions and reading ought to be avoided. The main difficulties are usually to lead the patient into a willingness to make these efforts which frequently seem unimportant or not interesting enough to him, and to urge the patient persistently without becoming irksome.

Modern psychiatry stresses the need for well-planned occupation but frequently considers only work and neglects well-planned recreation. This is the main criticism of Simon's active therapy, which revolutionized European psychiatric hospitals twenty years ago. His criticism is, on the other hand, justified — that most American hospitals have a relatively small and expensive occupational therapy department which cannot offer enough work to all patients for the whole day and neglects to utilize the simpler possibilities of work which can be done by patients for the hospital. The fear that in such a place valuable workers will be kept when they should be ready for discharge can hardly be considered a valid excuse for not putting the patients to useful tasks. One should be able to trust the physicians in charge of the hospital and the supervising authorities. If this is not possible in any state, the whole hospital system needs a thorough reorganization. Simon and others have demonstrated for years that a medium-sized state hospital can be organized accordingly, so that regular work is done on all the wards, with nurses carrying out the tasks of specialized occupational teachers. Our teaching of nurses is at present inadequate from this point of view. Relatives' complaints, based on prejudices with regard to the simple work to which a deteriorated schizophrenic patient can be assigned, usually subside after a while if the physicians take care to reformulate the value of occupation to prevent habit-deterioration and withdrawal into an autistic world. The relatives will also be aware of the more cheerful and active atmosphere in such a hospital.

Any kind of occupation should be well planned according to the patient's original interests and include sufficient changes during the day to prevent monotony. The goal is to teach the patient to obtain satisfaction from his task. This can best be done if the patient is required to finish the whole task so that he can see the end result. Most schizophrenic patients become easily bored and wish to change to something else. Correct occupational therapy will teach the patient the need to stick to his task and not allow the fostering of the patient's shiftless attitude. It will also emphasize the need for balanced work and modify exclusive preference along any special line. Handicraft, physical labor, intellectual work, outdoor recreation, reading, music and shows, cultivation of special talents and group activities and games all form part of occupational therapy. Athletic games should stress primarily the socializing aspect rather than the competitive one.

The most serious mistakes in the treatment of schizophrenic illnesses are ruthless analysis leading to disorganization and the utilization of destructive features. To this latter group belongs the mistaking a homosexual or heterosexual attachment for having established good rapport. This error is mentioned first because it happens easily and may have disastrous results. Nurses and physicians both should be aware of it without becoming sensitive to the problem so that it does not disturb their ease in dealing with the patient. Less frequent is the mistake of trying to utilize recognized homo- and heterosexual erotic behavior as the basis for rapport. Some physicians feel that they can use such tendencies for producing a therapeutic transference which seems to them necessary to correct the narcissistic withdrawal. I would hesitate to call this psychoanalytic treatment although these proponents consider it such. It is really merely the application of psychoanalytic principles but without working them into an individualized treatment of schizophrenic illnesses. It is possible that the principles of transference in the above-mentioned sense as well as narcissism can be made the therapeutic issue in some cases, but they are no doubt rare and would have to be carefully selected. I do not know by what indications one would have to be guided in such instances.

Narcissistic tendencies are occasionally utilized therapeutically. This is a fundamental mistake in an illness where narcissism is such a destructive tendency that the psychoanalytic school coined the term, "narcissistic neurosis," for it. Nevertheless, I have seen psychiatrists who believed they were establishing the basis for treatment by trying to utilize the patients' interest in themselves — rouge, perfume, expensive clothes, etc. Bargaining on such a narcissistic basis cannot be defended. To this group also belong patients who have the desire to help other patients. If this is done on a narcissistic or autistic basis it is not constructive to the patients themselves. It increases their conviction of having to find their own solution. These remarks do not refer to that degree of helpfulness and interest in others which is part of socialization.

Case 13:

At 18 this patient had a brief period of discouragement during which he felt that nobody liked him, and therefore showed definite resentment to his teachers and fellow-students. At 20 he had a similar episode during which he noticed difficulties especially in concentration and the inability to attend to his work with the same persistence. At that time he was appointed a fellow at a large university. He became preoccupied with the fear that there was something wrong with him but could not figure out what. Under the stress of examinations (at 22) he experienced automatic writing — he wrote a brief letter to his successful brother stating that the brother was doing what the patient was meant to do. He wrote another letter to his step-mother stating that no woman was to give him advice, and a third one to his teacher accusing him of being aristocratic. He had to write these letters as if he were forced by some strange power and could not explain this occurrence to himself. A few days later he began to have a feeling that things which he had imagined previously began to happen. He felt a strange compulsion to walk around a train on the railroad track and to jump aside at the last minute. He stopped his work entirely, usually lying preoccupied with his imaginations. He felt people were reading his letters and began to hear voices which constantly asked him questions. It seemed to him that he was thinking other people's thoughts and he felt there was a magical relation between himself and others. He became disturbed and puzzled by the observation that things which he had predicted to himself happened (they were the banal occurrences of daily life). Delusions of reference increased and automatic actions developed — he had to smoke and type like his teacher and to act like his successful brother. After a week of this marked disturbance the patient was admitted to our hospital. He was very untidy, dirty, and mumbled to himself, never finishing any sentence, preoccupied with trying to find a system of philosophy. Voices asked him questions and he felt compelled to answer them. His mood was described as indifferent, his concentration was poor, and he was unable to pay attention to anything for any length of time. He felt under a strange power and thought he had to do what his teacher thought. His stream of talk was disconnected and his actions were few and impulsive.

This patient was an intelligent, quiet, seclusive, reserved person, who did very well in high school and in a small college but was unable to adjust to the other students, feeling easily slighted, mildly sensitive about the impression he made on others, irritable when contradicted, and unable to adjust to school discipline. His interests were primarily in psychology and biology, only moderately in athletics. On the whole he was a day-dreamer who tried to find his own solutions. With girls he was shy; little was known about his sex life. The patient had been unable to adjust to his stepmother (at 12), who was a somewhat overbearing and oversolicitious woman. His father was a queer and seclusive person. His mother, who died when the patient was an infant, had suffered from two psychiatric illnesses characterized by day-dreaming and depressive mood. A maternal uncle had committed suicide. His brother had an illness of a year's duration of a vague type characterized primarily by withdrawal. He had since made an adjustment and was a college teacher.

During the first week the patient improved little. He was immediately put on full routine. In the therapeutic discussions the physician tried primarily to establish rapport and point out to the patient the need for taking care of himself in order to fit into the group. He was urged to participate somewhat in conversations and the nurses were advised to try to discuss topics which were of interest to him, such as biology. It was frequently necessary to remind him of personal hygiene, but as this was done in a tactful way it did not upset him. After a week he was definitely improved. The simple routine was now increased by urging him to begin to read magazines and newspapers, but to avoid any lengthy stories. The physician began to inject more doubt into the reality of his experiences and urged him to depend more on the fact as to whether or not others could hear the voices too. Doubts were also injected into the reality of his past experiences. He gradually developed a more objective point of view and after a few more days the voices subsided, but he still showed marked indecision and a tendency to get panicky when urged to go outside. In the hospital he felt easily "shaken" by conversations with the patients. When he mentioned plans for the future his voice again became mumbling and his talk incoherent. He also complained that there were still "forces drawing me — a dynamical power," and that he still had the vague feeling that he had to act like others. All of these complaints which he mentioned were immediately discussed with him thoroughly. The issue was always to produce doubt of the correctness of his interpretation. After four weeks in the hospital the patient's behavior became more normal. During the next two weeks he was urged to add to his routine; that is, to read more and to discuss what he read with the nurses and patients, to develop more interest in other people's ideas, and to make suggestions with regard to change of routine in his special case.

During the last two months in the hospital, (the entire hospital stay was three and a half months), the patient frequently showed a tendency to untidiness and preoccupations especially when disturbing life problems were discussed, but on the whole he improved steadily. The discussions turned first to the automatic actions, which he analyzed as relief from tension and anger resulting from minor interferences from his family, teacher, or students. In connection with these considerations, he discussed freely his need for independence and marked reaction to dictation from anyone. A more thorough discussion of the beginning of his illness two years previously was started. He described having felt suspicious and that there was a barrier around him which prevented him from feeling close to other people. In this connection, we went into a discussion of his attitude to the group in general, his anxiousness to make a good impression and be admired by others, but his unwillingness to adjust to others and find out what they actually thought about him. He became aware of the fact that he had never had any close friends and that he probably had definitely kept people away from himself. We then discussed the reaction a year ago when he began to develop definite untidiness and the feeling that he "was breaking." This occurred when first entering the university. He felt especially inferior to a teacher who was a well-known scientist and whom he began to admire and idolize. This teacher hurt his feelings several times by somewhat abrupt criticism and the patient's emotions toward him became mixed with hate. The discussion led to an understanding of his need for hero worship and the formation of ideals and his unwillingness to accept shortcomings in his heroes. Instead of this, he had usually reacted with an ambivalent attitude of admiration and resentment and hate. The same attitude was expressed toward his brother and a former college teacher. To all these people he had written automatic letters. There had been a marked resentment to the molding of his personality by others in his environment since early childhood. It developed especially towards his stepmother, whom he otherwise liked quite well. (These factors caused the automatic letter to her.)

During the last two weeks he discussed primarily his attitude to the future. He had found out that he had an interest in, and a talent for, carpentry and was willing to accept our advice to spend the rest of the academic year with a relative who was a carpenter. Later he might consider teaching in a small school with possibilities for various kinds of interests, instead of planning for a research career. The patient understood that this did not mean an adjustment on a lower level but on a different level, which was more suited to his personality. The discussion of his sex life led to an understanding of considerable sexual desires which he had pushed aside and which had caused frequent emissions. He had been concerned about them, feeling they would harm his body. For the same reason he had given up masturbation, which he had practiced from 14 to 16. He began to see now that the adjustment to girls is not necessarily sexual, but to a large extent one of friendship and companionship. He began to be able to control his imaginations better and to feel more at ease with the nurses and girls he later met socially. The attitude to his father was clearly seen after his father's visit two weeks before discharge. The visit was apparently pleasant but the next day the patient was angry and irritable. This situation was utilized for an analysis of the father-son and stepmother-son relationships.

During this illness few sedatives were used. For the first six weeks he received 0.3 gm. (5 gr.) of barbital at night. When he improved generally and felt more at ease the barbital was omitted completely. The underlying tension was usually well recognized from a high pulse rate, which subsided after four weeks in the hospital but increased again slightly when the question of discharge came up.

Since his discharge in the spring of 1927, the patient has made a good adjustment. Since 1930, he has been teaching in a private school and is well liked by his superiors and the students. He is satisfied with his type of work. His social adjustment is good and his ease with women was established within a year after discharge. Although his standards are still high, he is willing to adjust them to the requirements of his life. He married in 1931 and has a child. The new responsibilities as well as financial struggles did not affect him unduly. There is, however, still an underlying tension noticeable when the patient has been working under strain for several weeks. It is especially obvious at the end of the teaching year and leads to brief irritability and a tendency to anger. The patient takes these as indications that he is carrying as heavy a load as he can afford and that he has to be satisfied with his present achievements in life from which he is able to get full satisfaction. (These notes were written in 1936.)

In the spring of 1942 (37 years old) the patient felt sexually stirred by a woman acquaintance, and struggling unsuccessfully against his desires, he felt guilty. In January 1943 he was admitted to the Payne Whitney Clinic in a mild schizophrenic confusional condition. With an organized routine and the reassurance that he need not fear a recurrence of his previous illness, his anxiety and with it the confusion subsided. The psychotherapeutic discussion led to a brief constructive analysis of his rigid and high standards, of his perfectionism as a defense against insecurity, of his recent dissatisfaction with teaching and accompanying ambitious day-dreams, and of his antagonism to his driving headmasters whom he admired. The patient recognized patterns similar to those discussed 15 years ago. His sexual life was reviewed and practical advice was offered with regard to the adjustment and control of sexual drives. The patient left the hospital after two weeks and has been in good health during the last five years.

Many schizophrenic illnesses contain affective features which give the illness a more or less frank depressive or manic coloring. Although these affective features are of secondary importance, they may demand considerable therapeutic attention. There may occur prolonged phases of depression or excitement during which the treatment corresponds to that of affective disorders. Even so, it is wise to keep in mind the possibility of withdrawal and autistic tendencies and try to prevent these dangers by carefully adjusted routine and planned psychotherapy. In contrast to the pure manic excitement, segregation of the patient is undesirable and should be used as little as possible. Constant attempts at socialization should be resumed. Separation from other patients may be necessary for a few minutes, a few hours, or even several days, depending on the patient's behavior, the stimulating factors, and the phase of the illness.

Fearful excitements and incidental panics must be dealt with carefully. The treatment of the acute condition is the same as in panics of the depressive and paranoid types — protection against suicide and establishing confidence in the hospital environment, avoidance of any procedure to which the patient is sensitive and of tasks which are difficult for him at times of fear and insecurity. Sedatives in small amounts during the day and hydrotherapy are useful. A discussion of the more fundamental factors should be postponed until the patient has reached a level of security. Interviews ought to be short and end with a reassuring formulation. In schizophrenic excitement, including panic reaction, excellent results are usually obtained with insulin treatment (Chapter VII). Convulsive therapy may also be helpful. In my own experience I prefer insulin therapy but, if not effective, follow it with convulsive therapy.

Temper tantrums are treated mostly by re-education, but should always be briefly analyzed. They are an indication of underlying tension which should be relieved through personality adjustment. Anger outbursts are similar problems. It is always desirable to study these behavior reactions closely and not to deal with them merely by general re-education. Less frequent are sudden outbursts of brief excitement for which the term "raptus" is used. They are seldom purely automatic and their analysis is frequently helpful. If this is not possible, the physician should be able to deal with them correctly by means of hydrotherapy (especially cold wet packs), or chemical procedures (scopolamine-morphine or amytal intramuscularly — see Chapter VII), or by repeated convulsions. These outbursts should be discussed with the patient later and the treatment carefully explained to him.

In catatonic reactions, one should consider that one deals with submissive patients who are inclined to give up the struggle with reality. There results an attitude of diminished motility, spontaneous and reactive, which may lead to a deep stupor. It is therefore essential that one avoid anything which might increase the tendency to submission. With kind and untiring patience, nurses succeed in having a patient feed himself and attend to his personal hygiene. In more advanced stages of submission, the nurses may still be able to spoon feed the patient and to regulate his defecation and urination, i.e., the patient is willing to make an effort although not spontaneously. These same patients are driven into a deep stupor by domineering and abrupt physicians and nurses. Ambivalency and ambitendency are symptoms which require tactful help, wisely offered when necessary. However, decisions should not be made readily for the patient. Mannerisms can frequently be prevented or corrected by direct advice, often after an analysis of their meaning. Posturing, cataleptic phenomena, stereotypies are frequently hospital products — signs of a domineering or too appreciative environment, lack of individualized occupation and socialization.

It is important to have a clear understanding of the treatment of patients with diminished activity, which can reach the state of stupor of varying degree. The main principle is to recognize these conditions as reactions of submission. The therapeutic task is to avoid any increase of submission by tactful and encouraging help. It is incorrect to assume that the treatment of a stupor is a mere nursing problem. The nurses will have to carry the main burden but they need careful instruction from the physician, who formulates the nursing approach on an individualistic basis. The nurses must know the factors to which the patient is sensitive and what might stimulate his interest. The physicians and nurses who succeed in creating situations which appeal to the patient and stir up spontaneous activity will be successful in the treatment of stuporous patients. It requires a great deal of a certain type of imagination and a willingness to look for new opportunities which will bring the patient out of his stupor step by step. A careful knowledge of the patient's personality and interests is essential.

The second therapeutic point is correct nursing care. Attention to general hygiene is an individual problem. Care should be given to general appearance, toilet habits, teeth, and skin condition. In deep stupors, washing of the eyes with boric acid solution is indicated because of the danger of developing corneal ulcers as a result of immobility of the eyeballs. The joints should be mobilized to prevent contractures. Passive movements and massage are frequently necessary even in stupors of only a few weeks' duration. Self-feeding by encouragement should be kept up as long as possible. The next step resorted to is skilled spoon feeding. If the patient still masticates, a soft diet can be offered. Otherwise, food in the form of fluids becomes necessary when the patient refuses to open his mouth or to swallow, but tube feeding should be delayed until acetone appears in the urine or general malnutrition is serious enough to demand such a step. Nasal feeding, which can be learned easily, is the choice of procedure because it can be done with less struggle than tube feeding by mouth. Before each tube feeding the nurses and doctor ought to encourage the patient to eat, and psychotherapeutic remarks should always be made. Tube feeding should never become mere routine.

If a patient is not fully cooperative, it will be best to have him put in a dry pack for the few minutes of feeding instead of struggling with him. After insertion, the free end of the tube should be placed in water to see whether it has safely reached the stomach. Bubbles in respiratory rhythm would indicate that the tube is in the trachea or even in a large bronchus. After the feeding, some water should be added to be sure that the tube is washed free from the feeding. In removing the tube, the physician should press the end closely with his fingers so that no food drops escape during the fast withdrawal. Some patients develop a habit of catching the tube with the tongue and keeping it in the mouth. It is usually easy to prevent this by careful observation of the patient during the insertion. If one is unsuccessful, it will be wise to insert the tube by mouth. The latter may also be best if a patient vomits the feeding while the thin nasal tube is still in the stomach. A wide mouth tube will readily prevent this, especially if the tube is inserted no further than through the cardiac opening of the stomach.

The feeding has to be in fluid form. The following mixtures, used at the Payne Whitney Clinic, contain well-balanced feedings which can be given over a long period of time and satisfy varying physical needs. The regular tube feeding contains 3,000 calories per day, consisting of 88 gm. of protein, 198 gm. of fat, and 234 gm. of carbohydrate. It is adequate in calcium, phosphorous, iron, and Vitamins A, B, C, and Riboflavin (B_2 and G), but slightly low in Vitamin D, depending on the kind of oil used. Usually two feedings a day are necessary, each feeding containing 1,500 calories, consisting of: Milk — 480 cc., Lactose — 15 gm. (2 tsp.), Sugar — 30 gm. (4 tsp.), Eggs — 3, Malted Milk — 60 gm. (8 tsp.), Tomato Juice — 240 cc., Oil (olive or vegetable) — 60 cc., Salt — 5 gm. (½ tsp.), Water — 240 cc. If a patient is unable to tolerate this large amount of fluid, it might be necessary to divide the day's nourishment into three feedings, offering each time 1,000 calories. These feedings would consist of: Milk — 320 cc., Lactose — 10 gm., (1 large tsp.), Sugar — 15 gm. (2 tsp.), Eggs — 2, Malted Milk — 33 gm. (4 large tsp.), Tomato Juice — 160 cc., Oil (olive and vegetable) — 40 cc., Salt — 3 gm. (⅓ tsp.) Water — 160 cc. When high protein feeding is indicated, the 3,000 calories per day contain 102 gm. of protein, 184 gm. of fat, and 230 gm. of carbohydrate. If offered in two feedings of 1,500 calories, each feeding contains: Milk — 600 cc., Lactose — 15 gm. (2 tsp.), Sugar — 25 gm. (3 large tsp.), Eggs — 4, Malted Milk — 46 gm. (6 tsp.), Tomato Juice — 240 cc., Oil (olive or vegetable) — 42 cc., Salt — 5 gm. (½ tsp.). If given in three parts a day of 1,000 calories, the feedings would consist of: Milk — 360 cc., Lactose — 15 gm. (2 tsp.), Sugar — 18 gm. (2 large tsp.), Eggs — 3, Malted Milk — 28 gm. (4 tsp.), Tomato Juice — 160 cc., Oil (olive or vegetable) — 27 cc., Salt — 3 gm. (⅓ tsp.). If a high vitamin intake is necessary, vitamin supplements may be added or the following procedures used: In feedings offered twice a day, 20 cc. of cod liver oil and one yeast cake should be added, the oil in the feeding being decreased to 40 cc.; in feedings offered three times a day, 15 cc. of cod liver oil and one-half a yeast cake should be added, the oil being decreased to 30 cc. Medication (sedatives, cathartics) should be given at the beginning of the feeding. Usually two feedings a day are necessary. If sedatives are given to secure sleep, the evening feeding should be administered between 8 and 9 p.m.

Negativism often makes the therapeutic approach difficult. Studying the patient's personality may offer us a lead in overcoming it — the utilization of special interests and the careful avoidance of anything to which the patient is sensitive (to this belong also therapeutic discussions by too zealous physicians). Indirect remarks, directed to other physicians, nurses or relatives, frequently penetrate and exert a strong helpful influence. This indirect treatment should be used constantly in negativistic schizophrenic patients (and aversion depressions, see Chapter IX). The indirect approach also tries to create opportunities which appear merely casual to the patient and which he may therefore utilize. In contrast to this, the same patient will resist developing an interest in anything which he recognizes as being offered by persons in the environment. The choice of situations depends on the patient's original interests

— a certain magazine or book, other patients, animals, outdoor or athletic possibilities.

Insulin therapy is helpful in catatonic patients and often leads to fast symptomatic improvement. Intravenous administration of sodium amytal may offer the patient an opportunity to express himself and the physician a possibility to establish rapport. To have a dynamic discussion followed by sleep is probably desirable in any disorganized patient. The results depend to a considerable extent on the physician's ability to utilize this therapeutic situation. If one wishes to use such aids, one must know the patient and his illness in detail and have definite plans as to the actual procedure and after-treatment. In some patients a combination of insulin therapy with occasional sodium amytal interviews in the afternoon may be indicated.

The dysplastic make-up of many schizophrenic patients and certain features of the deteriorated cases, especially their general sluggishness and marked gain of weight, have directed attention to possible endocrinologic factors. Clinical tests and postmortem examinations do not substantiate such a claim. Endocrinologic therapy should be administered only when there are definite clinical indications. Some authors argue for autointoxication, referring to the gastrointestinal tract or the liver as the source of the disturbance. These are theories which deserve the attention of further research but are by no means ready for therapeutic utilization. After the success of non-specific treatment of general paresis, the previously dropped attempts at non-specific treatment of schizophrenic reactions have been revived. Tuberculin, nucleic acid, and chemicals have been used to produce therapeutic fever. Incidental infections, and minor as well as major illnesses, such as pneumonia, have always been observed to produce temporary improvement in autistic and negativistic patients. Interests and established rapport, however, subside frequently with physical improvement. It apparently depends largely on whether the physicians are able to utilize the opportunity therapeutically.

The value of indicated surgical procedures is well presented in the following case. A young woman in an acute catatonic excitement showed symptoms of definite hyperthyroidism and marked improvement after partial lobectomy. The brief analysis at the end allowed a correction of the dynamic factors involved.

Case 14:

In July 1928, this 28 year old married woman began to complain of weakness and fatigue and was concerned about her scanty menses. When moving to a new town on August 1st her complaints increased. With the onset of her menses on August 11th she suddenly became excited, stated that she had given birth to twins which were kept from her by her husband and her physician. She showed marked mood changes from cheerfulness to crying, and was afraid that colored men were trying to break into the house. At other times she exposed herself and threw her wedding ring away. On August 30th she believed her house was on fire and was in great fear. Her husband had been away during the whole month. On his return he arranged immediately for admission (September 1st). In the hospital the patient was excited, irritable, easily angered, resistant and combative to interference, tearing clothes and bed linen, suspicious and fearful. Then again she would suddenly change to cheerful or sad behavior, listening constantly to voices of various people and of her husband, who corrected what she said. She was preoccupied with the delusion of being pregnant and the fear of being shot, but talked little, usually staying by herself and staring into space with queer posturing. Her general physical condition was good but she had a symmetrically enlarged pulsatile thyroid gland. There was a diffuse regular hyperemia over her neck and the upper third of her chest, and a slight cyanosis of the hands. Her face was flushed and the pupils dilated. The pulse rate varied between 120 and 160. The skin was warm and moist; no exophthalmos was present. Her teeth were carious and she had infected tonsils. She had an infantile uterus.

We felt that we dealt with an acute catatonic excitement in which the exophthalmic goiter played an incidental, but definitely aggravating, role which had to be considered seriously in the whole treatment. Her thyroid had apparently been enlarged since 1918 (at 18) and the swelling had been especially marked during menses and when the patient was under emotional strain. At 15 she had to leave high school for one year because of "nervousness" and chorea-like movements. She graduated as a nurse in 1920 (at 20) and did private duty, which she continued after a sudden marriage in 1925 (at 25) until a year previously. Her family informed us that she had been engaged from 20 to 24 but then broke the engagement for unknown reasons and a few months later married a widower of 40 with two children. Her family objected because of his age and because he was not Catholic like the patient. Her husband was a sea captain and was frequently away from home for weeks at a time. After her marriage she had often felt lonesome and had wished for children, often teasing her husband for his inability to impregnate her.

The patient grew up in a large family and little was known about her early youth. She was considered a cheerful and sociable person but sensitive about a squint, rather retiring and reserved, home-loving and industrious and efficient as a nurse. Her father was a chronic alcoholic.

The treatment was that of an excitement but in which considerable attention had to be paid to her physical condition. It was impossible to keep the patient in bed, and continuous baths usually had to be stopped after one or two hours because of her fear and unwillingness to stay in the tub. On such occasions her pulse rate increased to 160. She reacted well to cold wet packs of one to two hours' duration, especially in the evening. She usually slept about six hours. Spoon feeding was satisfactory. Rapport was difficult to establish. The patient was usually negativistic and did not answer but seemed to relax somewhat to reassurance and repeated explanation of every therapeutic move. From the time of admission she had been digitalized and small amounts of barbital were given because of her cardiac condition.

The third day after admission, with the onset of menstruation, the patient's excitement increased. She began to masturbate openly and marked motility disturbance developed — posturing and queer movements, catalepsy, and frequent mutism. She was in a dreamlike state, believing she was in a general hospital being delivered of a baby. Her talk became disconnected and was of the baby-talk type. Tube feeding had to be administered twice daily. With the night tube feeding (9 P.M.) she received paraldehyde 4 cc. (1 dram.) This period of marked excitement lasted ten days. She then became less excited, mostly standing or lying around in queer postures, negativistic, and mute. She voided and defecated on the floor. The latter could usually be prevented through thoughtful nursing care. Oral hygiene also demanded much attention. On September 23rd treatment with Lugol's solution (5 min. three times a day with feeding) was started. As bed treatment, which was indicated for the protection of her heart, was impossible because of her overactivity, the patient stayed in the tub from 7 A.M. to 6 P.M. She usually moved about in slow rhythm, often assuming grotesque postures, alert, but negativistic. After her husband's visit catalepsy increased. He was therefore advised to remain away. The reasons were carefully formulated to the patient. During this whole negativistic phase much use was made of indirect remarks, either of an explanatory or suggestive nature. After October 13th the patient was in better rapport and her illness was now repeatedly formulated to her in a way which took care of the present needs of treatment and considered her own understanding of the various factors involved.

During the treatment with Lugol's solution, the pulse rate had dropped to below 110 but increased again around this time and the thyroid gland became more swollen. After repeated careful explanation to the mute patient, a double lobectomy was performed on October 17th, followed by an uneventful postoperative course during which the patient became increasingly more cooperative, although still maintaining cataleptic postures. She complained spontaneously with regard to her throat symptoms and was greatly puzzled by her physical condition. She expressed fear that her teeth would fall out if she opened her mouth and that her legs would break if she bent them. Her throat symptoms too were "uncanny." The psychotherapeutic issue therefore was to give her an increasing understanding of the meaning of her complaints through well-planned explanations which took care of the minutest observations and were frequently offered daily. It proved to be more effectual to offer them as casual remarks, often directed to by-standers (e.g., the nurses) than to try to clarify the puzzling observations directly. This latter approach was naturally used when the patient made complaints or asked for an explanation. On this basis a medical rapport dealing with her physical health was established. Topical discussions were purposely avoided.

At the end of October the patient began to swallow food which was offered in spoon feeding and to sleep without paraldehyde. In the first week of November she was up all day, and began to take interest in occupational therapy but was still inclined to void on the floor. She spoke little spontaneously but answered questions. Obsessive swear words worried her but she learned to ignore them when occupied. As she was frequently playfully overactive in the evenings, we were careful not to push her into too many interests and administered baths and some small amounts of sedatives (barbital 0.3 gm. — 5 gr.) at night.

During December her rigidity in posture and gait gradually disappeared but whenever questions regarding topical material were asked, her motor negativism increased. As the same reaction was observed after her husband's visit he was advised to see her only once a week for a few minutes. The therapeutic value of occupation and socialization had to be frequently re-formulated. To solidify our rapport we allowed her to sleep in a private room for three weeks but only with the understanding that she would spend the day with the other patients in the day-room. According to increasing improvement minor privileges on the ward were given. We stressed at the same time that more privileges, such as wearing her own clothes and walks outside of the hospital grounds, could only be granted when she was ready and willing to be transferred to a quiet ward. With the renewal of her religious interests, a visit from a neighborhood priest was arranged. The patient did not discuss much with him.

In December several carious teeth and later tonsils and adenoids were removed. Various uneventful postoperative treatments were used psychotherapeutically to intensify the rapport and to increase the patient's willingness to turn to the physician for help in all her puzzling

complaints. At the end of December the patient explained that the
rigidity of her body and especially of her arms after her husband's
visit and before menses was an effort to overcome sexual desires and
corresponding physical sensations. We urged her to learn to use relaxation instead and successfully reduced the sexual tension through
daily sitz baths. She also talked now of her sexual tension during her
husband's absence, especially shortly before the onset of her present
illness when she frequently had had sexual dreams, awakening with
orgasm. She often had examined her body to find the cause for a general burning feeling. Anxiety attacks had developed and made her
afraid of death. These facts were mentioned spontaneously in several
of the interviews which were offered freely. The physician was careful
not to urge her too far in such discussions because of her general vagueness of thinking and marked difficulties of concentration. Each brief
discussion was terminated with a formulation which took care of all
the present needs.

Slow progress was made in January and February, the patient still
showing lack of interest, vagueness of thinking, slight incoherence, and
occasional posturing. When on various occasions she discussed spontaneously the delusions of the delivery of twins, her desire for children
and the brutal treatment which she had received as a child from her
alcoholic father, she showed an increase of her symptoms for several
days. These warning signals were heeded and not too much opportunity
for analysis of her past was offered. A psychogalvanic test taken at this
time revealed marked reactions to topics of religion and sin, masturbation, and her desire for a child.

The last three weeks in the hospital (discharged March 9th), the
patient showed normal behavior although still with a tendency to day-
dreaming and definite vagueness of thinking. She was able to fit fairly
well into the group on a quiet ward and showed a normal reaction to
visitors. This time was utilized for constructive personality discussions
in which we avoided going beyond what the patient was clearly able
to grasp. Her social adjustment had always presented difficulties because of her overconcern for her personal appearance and anxiousness
to please others. She realized the need to have interests in common with
others and not merely to join social activities for the sake of having
a good time. To please her husband she had tried unsuccessfully to
change her church affiliations. Usually cheerful, she became easily discouraged and had a definite tendency to moodiness. Although she stated
that she loved her husband, there had been a constant tendency to com-
pare him to her previous fiancé. Her great desire for children and family
formation had not been fulfilled. She became resigned to the fact that
pregnancy was unlikely (infantile uterus). Previously she had blamed
this on her husband. There had been marked jealousy of her step-
children and even the deceased wife. Intercourse had been taken as a

means for procreation only and she had always made efforts not to let herself relax into orgasm. During the prolonged absence of her husband she had given in to masturbation, of which she was ashamed afterwards. The content was always sexual relations with her husband. These discussions led to an understanding of the essential principles of sexual hygiene and to a broader outlook on married life. The general hygiene of living, with special attention to regular eating habits and suitable recreation, was stressed. She became desensitized to unpleasant memories of her father. Her illness was accepted by her as a personality reaction, although she still overemphasized the importance of her thyroid condition.

Since discharge the patient has made a good adjustment. Resigned to her inability to have children, she has succeeded in creating a home and family life for her husband and step-children. Her sexual life is apparently satisfactory and intercourse usually ends with orgasm. Her social adjustment is probably least satisfactory. The prognosis for the future is certainly not definitely good but, if the patient is willing to return promptly for an interview if difficulties arise, probably better than we had originally anticipated. The thyroid factor was not fundamental but important enough to demand special treatment. Its correction removed a disturbing factor and permitted us to establish rapport on a basis which was easiest for this patient to accept, i.e., the treatment of a physical ailment.

The patient has remained in good health (1947).

This catatonic reaction illustrates modern hospital treatment of submissive and autistic cases. Until thirty years ago hospitals were filled with stuporous patients, or patients standing or sitting around with odd posturing, catalepsy, and stereotypies. These symptoms are rarely seen in modern hospitals where sympathetic and patient understanding prevails instead of brusque and domineering behavior. Occupational therapy prevents autistic elaboration and causes these hospital-produced symptoms to disappear.

European authors have placed special emphasis on early discharge, forcing the patient into a stimulating outside adjustment as soon as a reasonable improvement has been reached. This is done in order to prevent a relapse and a getting accustomed to a protected hospital environment. This danger no doubt exists in many cases but is less great since planned occupation and routine has become part of a well-managed hospital and since an analysis of the dynamic factors is considered essential for any kind of adjustment. There is, however, a great deal to be said for the early discharge of patients who show few available assets and small chance of modifiability. In such cases, a careful analysis of the home environment will permit the physician to decide whether the patient can be discharged to his previous living conditions, whether these can be modified if necessary, or whether a more neutral and more favorable place can be found. The parole system of some Swiss hospitals has proved to be most efficient. These hospitals have made contacts with farmers and small business men with whom the patients can be placed, with a well-regulated and supervised routine and family life. One of the physicians follows the cases carefully, calling in person, and through social workers, at their new homes regularly, straightening out minor difficulties, and proposing increasing responsibilities according to the patient's improvement. Other hospitals have tried to create small colonies of patients in suitable communities. These attempts are of utmost importance because they allow many chronic patients a modified life outside the hospital and greatly relieve the heavy expense to the state. There is always a danger, however, that the psychotherapeutic approach may suffer and the possibility for better adjustment may be overlooked when early discharge is considered of predominant importance.

In chronic cases, the same rules of treatment should be applied but with more attention to symptomatic adjustments. One should avoid neglecting individual needs in general management and try to utilize the hospital opportunities for stimulating interest and working possibilities. Deterioration of behavior can be prevented in most patients if psychotherapeutic planning is the basis for hospital routine. Many symptoms formerly attributed to regression are now rare in a hospital which creates an environment that cultivates normal social demands. Transfers within the hospital or to other hospitals can frequently be used advantageously. Even in apparently hopeless cases, the physician should never develop a nihilistic attitude but carry out a planned and individually adjusted treatment. The treatment which has been outlined in general in Chapter II (utilization of occupational therapy and hydrotherapy and attempts at re-education) is of importance.

In suitable cases, constructive analysis may lead to permanent adjustment. The main principle in any analytic approach is to establish a certain stability of the personality before allowing the patient to be confronted with experiences to which he is sensitive, desires and strivings which are against his standards, and the need to modify his expectations of future life. Overaggressive psychotherapy will interfere with the natural healing tendencies which exist in every case and which it is our task to recognize and support as early as possible.

Psychoanalytic treatment with adjustment in technique according to the individual patient is successful in cases of schizophrenic illnesses which do not have any signs of disorganization. To repeat — one should always watch for the appearance of symptoms of disorganization and then either stop the analysis temporarily or shift to a less disturbing topic. It is also important to space the treatment and inject periods of analytic rest. Analysis should be active and include an adjustment of the patient's routine.

The following case demonstrates the therapeutic possibilities of constructive analysis in a serious schizophrenic illness. Less far-reaching psychotherapy, but fundamentally along the same lines, was carried out in the previously discussed cases.

Case 15:

A 27 year old student in biology, who did research work, began to show irritability and vague thinking in the spring of 1927. In January 1928, she complained of marked difficulties of concentration ("muddled thinking"), increasing self-consciousness, and feelings of inadequacy. All these symptoms increased during the summer of 1928 and were then accompanied by poor sleep and headaches. Her family physician urged her to take a rest cure (June 1928). On June 17th, the day before menstruation, she suddenly expressed the fact that she had a marked need for sexual relations. That night she developed a sudden excitement with combativeness, felt as if she were "going crazy," and suffered abdominal pains and headache. She was erotic toward the physician and spoke of having sexual relations with him. At times she masturbated openly and exhibited motions of intercourse. There were quiet periods lasting several hours during which she denied all this. Then again she had ecstatic periods, believed she was in heaven with angels and heard beautiful music. She felt that the nurses were against her and that she was under their influence. At another time she tried to jump out of the window. This phase lasted one week and was followed by three days' stupor. In July she again became excited and made an attempt to stab and hang herself because people were after her and wanted to injure her eyes. She exposed herself at the open window. The following four weeks she was quieter, showing childish behavior, not wanting to see people, often impulsively angry and combative. During the excitement, her family physician had a special nurse constantly in the room, gave her high amounts of sedatives for the night and bath treatments and cold wet packs. During the quieter period, the four weeks before admission, he tried the patient out in a more active routine including walking, playing games, and riding in her car.

In August she was admitted to the hospital. During the first four weeks the patient was restless, resistant, and occasionally destructive in outbursts of anger. To a large extent, all these features were an expression of fear and apprehension. She showed little spontaneous activity, was usually disinterested and merely mumbled to herself. She masturbated freely and exposed herself to nurses and male physicians. She refused to feed herself but swallowed food when spoon fed. At times she spoke of being "hypnotized" and of "ultra-violet lights being after" her. She was occasionally uncooperative and listless, doing very little in occupational therapy. At other times she whined and giggled, then again showed sudden outbursts of restless agitation.

In order to deal intelligently with such a patient, the physician must understand the personality involved and what factors might play a role. The patient was an only child, highly intelligent, always ambitious, successful in her studies, quiet, reserved and well liked, deliberate and slow in her judgment, self-reliant but not self-assertive, self-conscious and ill at ease with strangers, tactful and sensitive in her own feelings, and easily stimulated by pleasures. She had a strong family attachment but had occasionally resented her mother's urging her constantly to make more money. The mother was a suspicious and excitable person. Otherwise, there were no definite heredity features known. Menstruation had been normal since 15 but scanty for a year before the onset of the present illness. There had been definite warning signals which the family had overlooked, i.e., a prolonged vomiting attack before examinations at the age of 20, and anxiety attacks when visiting Niagara Falls at 23.

During this excited period, the patient was put on full routine from the beginning but she was allowed to retire to her own room whenever she became too disturbed. It was considered important to prevent autistic withdrawal and to recognize the need for definite stimulation. Conversation with the physicians and nurses was planned accordingly and the patient was invited to join in games with others. She received continuous baths daily and cold wet packs, to which she reacted with marked relaxation. At night sedatives were given. Her father was allowed to visit her once or twice a week, while her mother was advised not to come more than once in two weeks. To both was explained the importance of not discussing her illness but rather topics which would have interested her when she was well. The ward physician frequently joined in these visits and in this way began to be accepted by the patient.

After the middle of September, the patient showed definite improvement. She now ate well and slept better and showed some interest in occupational therapy, but there was still considerable masturbation in the morning. She still stared erotically at the male physicians. Her main complaints were that she was afraid that something was going to happen to her, that she was going crazy, and going to be killed. She now began to read books which we had sent for and discussed them with the physician afterwards (books dealing with animals — the patient liked to talk of her own dog). She was encouraged to start sketching, which she had not done for years. By reassurance, her fears were overcome. When visitors seemed to depress instead of cheer her in the beginning of October, the physician explained to her the desirability of discontinuing them for two weeks, which advice she accepted willingly. He formulated to her the need for sedatives in order to obtain sleep and rest from disturbing thoughts. She was sensitive to receiving baths and to exposure of her body. Brief discussions helped her to change her attitude and to obtain an understanding of her general feelings of inadequacy.

In October, she reacted well to formal social behavior when going out for walks. Menses occurred for the first time since June. In this connection she mentioned her fear of pregnancy, which we were able to destroy. She began to appreciate occupation as an aid in breaking her continuous day-dreaming and keeping away troubling thoughts.

In November, therapeutic efforts were especially directed at her complaints of difficulties in thinking. Purposely, difficult books had not been given to her. She now saw how she was able to read much more difficult books than previously. Her occupation and general routine were adjusted according to her improvement. She was allowed to retire to her room and read there when she felt irritated. Long walks were utilized not only for recreation but also to increase her confidence in seeing strangers. The need for remaining in the hospital had to be constantly reformulated because of her reiteration, "I wish to go home." The same need for constant reformulation over a period of weeks existed with regard to the value of ward routine in breaking her day-dreaming habit.

It is quite likely that the patient heard voices during most of this period, but she was unable to discuss them or to explain her feeling afraid. The change in behavior was very slow. She seemed to feel gradually more at ease with the physician, less restless, and less disinterested. There was less of a tendency to pouting and it was less necessary to help her in getting dressed. With increasing interest in routine there was an increasing interest in her personal appearance. During interviews, however, she mumbled and turned away, giving only short answers. There were times when she was more uncooperative. Most distressing was her lack of plans, her desire to talk but her inability to offer much, and her desire not to be bothered by physicians.

There was again definite improvement in January. She stated that she felt scared when she looked at certain people. We noticed that it occurred more with certain nurses when they leaned over her, and instructed the nurses to avoid doing this. She voided in bed because she refused to get out of bed when no bathrobe was readily available. This again was apparently self-consciousness in the presence of nurses. There was marked sensitiveness in discussing any sexual preoccupations and she asked for a woman physician. This, however, was not granted, but one of the women physicians saw her a few times to gain an opportunity for discussion, which the patient was not able to use. Her letters became less vague and she was able to write longer sentences. In this period we started to give her thyroid extract 0.06 gm. (1 gr.) four times daily, and kept this up until March. The indication was a slight degree of hypothyroidism. Because of her amenorrhea and the suspicion of some deficiency of ovarian secretion, agomensin had also been given for several weeks without any definite result.

In February the patient was more alert and cheerful, showed some spontaneous interest, and reacted better to being urged into activity. She was able to enjoy walks in the city, feeling at ease, although there was still an underlying fear that she might not feel at ease on meeting old acquaintances. There were preoccupations with regard to her work and the sense of failure. In this period, personality features were discussed in daily interviews and the patient began to develop an understanding of her sensitiveness to people's reaction to her, especially nurses and physicians, and to criticism. (This tendency had increased considerably in the last few years.) She was also aware of her defense whenever she felt that someone might break through her reserve. She was able to socialize better by meeting patients on a quiet ward, joining in group activities and general discussions. Her interest in music helped in socialization. She discussed her work, obtaining considerable pleasure from achievement and gradually overcoming her marked feelings of inadequacy. Complimentary and encouraging remarks about her work helped her greatly.

During this period her father informed us of heavy financial losses which would mean premature termination of her hospital stay. The patient was told by her physician immediately. The occasion was utilized to stir up a healthy desire to leave the hospital and find work. In reviewing the illness, minor hospital annoyances were explained and the situation utilized to point out to the patient the need to resign herself to life obstacles. Week-ends at home increased self-confidence and ease and gave us also an opportunity to discuss her sensitive reaction to her mother's grumbling and complaining behavior, which she had concealed from us previously. The final discussions dealt with the parental adjustment, the problem of emancipation, and the need to be able to share responsibility without getting panicky.

After her discharge on March 10th, the patient was seen regularly once or twice a week. No further personality analysis was attempted and no special study of the factors which had caused her illness. It was felt best to give the patient a chance to settle down in outside life with as much normal activity as possible. The discussions dealt with practical issues, leading to stabilization through increasing self-confidence, self-reliance, and desensitization. In May and June consultations were increased to three times a week. The patient now worked on a study of her personality. As she was more at ease in writing than in free discussion, after every consultation a number of questions were given to her and she wrote out the answers. Her physician was anxious, however, to point out to her the need to do this writing at definite times of the day and not to indulge in self-analysis at any other time. This constructive analysis was along the following lines:

The basic principle for this analysis was to establish general stability before going into detailed analysis, and to delay the study of the more sensitive or fundamental factors. The first discussions dealt with her body functions and her attitude to them, leading to an understanding of her need for a considerable amount of sleep and her disturbing tendency to plan the next day's work or to try to solve the difficulties of the day before falling asleep. At such times, recurring dreams with marked anxiety helped to illustrate this sleep disturbance. Another indication of apprehension and anticipation was indigestion. Her eating habits needed some correction. Her sexual life was merely superficially discussed, the physician offering her a brief biologic and psychobiologic formulation, thus laying the foundation for later discussions and establishing temporary security.

The next topic dealt with her concept of God and eternity, the value of reality, and the danger of overemphasis on mystical interests. (These factors had never played an important role.) A preliminary understanding of her mood reactions emphasized her serious attitude to life and her lack of obtaining full satisfaction from achievement because of too high expectations. It also clarified her tendency to indulge in day-dreams in which she would shape the world to suit herself. Her excessive need for self-reliance made the modification of attitudes and expectations most difficult. There was a constant drive to succeed without sufficient time for leisure and well-selected recreation.

The first important difficulty discussed was her poor group adjustment, passive in type, although connected with a marked need for contact with others. Again too high expectations and the need to feel close to others without being willing to give up her own reserve came clearly to the foreground. The same tendencies prevented a close relationship with father and mother, both being the ideals for her standards and giving her a feeling of security. The set attitudes of all of them and the inability to communicate freely, however, made family life difficult.

Instead of analyzing these important factors in detail, we changed the approach to a detailed study of her life history in order to give her an understanding of her general development and of special traits, to study their plasticity, and to find concrete proofs for reaction tendencies. The patient now remembered her tendency to loneliness and slight depression in adolescence and her trying to find security in group adjustment by developing crushes on some girls and teachers, and also her marked unhappiness when they became estranged later. Unrecognized sexual sensations when riding on a bicycle between 14 and 16 were not discussed. Greater attention was paid instead to her reaction to tasks and responsibilities, her feeling panicky in anticipation and marked elation to success, and her attempt to escape in research, for which she was not fitted, from work and home difficulties. The relationship to her parents was again reviewed and she learned to understand them not as ideals but as they really were. Summarizing the factors which had been elicited and her specific life reactions, the patient was able to accept and appreciate certain reactions previous to the acute onset of her illness as definite danger signals which, if recurring and heeded, should allow a correction of difficulties.

A more thorough analysis of her mood and reaction to responsibility covered her marked excitability, the tendency to exhilaration, worry, anxiety and apprehension, to depression with feeling lonely and not understood, to anger, jealousy, and hate. She recognized her self-consciousness as being due to unreachable, fixed standards and to a lack of mutual interests with others, expecting too much response from them without being willing to offer enough herself. All these features were increased by her need for self-importance and to be admired by others. The actual possibilities for a needed outlet in creative work were stressed. The concepts of freedom and individuality, of self-reliance and being part of a group were formulated.

It was then considered wise to go fully into the development and actual difficulties, fancies and preoccupations of her sexual life. Early childhood masturbation from 4 to 6, sensations and unrecognized desires at puberty, adolescent attractions and the sexual upheaval at the onset of her illness, fancies relating to married life and sexual preoccupations, the return of masturbation and uncontrollable desires and homosexual sensitiveness during the excitement were viewed in their totality and not as mere incidents. The patient had previously claimed she was unable to remember her behavior in the hospital. Realizing the wisdom of not breaking through a wholesome reticence at a time when the patient was not stable enough to face her past upheaval, this point had not been stressed. However, it was important at this time to desensitize her to her experiences and to utilize them for a final constructive analysis. This was possible with little distress to the patient and was a good indicator of her present degree of stability.

During the whole treatment, analysis was considered the means to synthesis, the goal being a well-integrated personality in which the various features and tendencies were adjusted to each other. Some were stressed more by her than previously, some (e.g., her overestimation of intellectual features and achievements) reduced as far as their unique importance went. Some interests were decentralized, and certain topics and desires were tested with regard to their desirability and practicability. Her attitude to real and fancied experiences and desires was desensitized, and contradictory strivings were adjusted through culitvation of the acceptable and suppression of the unacceptable. The result was not a perfectly harmonious personality but a person who was able to maintain sufficient balance and unity to allow her to lead a healthy life but one in which she still needed occasional guidance from her physician.

Three months after discharge, the patient obtained regular work as a technician and has been doing well since (seven years). A few times, when under pressure of work, some feelings of inadequacy reappeared, but one or two consultations were usually sufficient to give the patient the necessary ease and self-reliance. She is socially well adjusted, has been able to modify her ambitions without developing a sense of failure, and has learned to deal with life problems in a less conscientious and set way. Although not married, she has no difficulties with sexual desires and is not upset when she is aware of them at times. Physical activity and planned recreation help her to deal with them. There is less tendency to preoccupation with herself, to concern about her body, and to withdrawal in day-dreaming. She has reached an emancipation from her family which allows her to be devoted to both parents without losing her independence and without shrinking from seeing their shortcomings. Even with this improvement, one cannot help feeling that there is danger of another illness if the patient gets involved in any situation to which she is especially sensitive. However, one also has the impression that by seeing a psychiatrist once or twice a year, catastrophes can be averted.

Information from her psychiatrist in 1947 revealed that the patient has been able to work steadily. Since the spring of 1945, delusions of reference have been present, accompanied by increased day-dreaming and decreased efficiency in work.

In both Case 14 and Case 15 problems which have not become thoroughly clear to the patient remain. I refer, for example, to the probable desires for promiscuity in Case 14 and the homosexual factors in Case 15. It is quite likely that the patients were correct in denying that such factors had been of importance in their lives. Desires and strivings which are ineffectual in the well-integrated personality may become obvious and disturbing in the disintegrated phase of the illness, and again become ineffective with re-integration. One should keep in mind that a perfect solution of all problems is practically impossible. The possibility of gaining a more or less thorough understanding depends on the individual patient and the illness. Such a clarification of all the factors involved is of theoretical value and highly interesting to the physician, but frequently detrimental to the patient. Only in a few carefully selected cases is this possible. On the other hand, these cases are not as rare as was believed by the older therapeutic schools, which were not based on a genetic-dynamic approach. Complete and lasting recoveries are possible, either through an understanding of the factors involved or through the dissociation of disturbing factors. The latter result, which is primarily brought about by the healing tendencies of the personality, is not desirable as it always presents an uncertainty in the future life.

Cases which have not led to an ideal solution have been selected purposely. Such cases are more frequent and show more clearly the therapeutic approach. Nothing fundamentally different is necessary where a more thorough analysis is possible. This part of the treatment should always be undertaken as the last phase of treatment, lasting over a short or prolonged period of time. The technical procedure will depend on the physician's interests and training. The treatment of chronic conditions is guided by the same principles. Hospital routine and management should offer opportunities for well-planned occupation and recreation. Along these lines, active treatment is always possible and mere custodial care prevented.

BIBLIOGRAPHY

1. HAMILTON, S. W.: The Treatment of Schizophrenia. *Association for Research in Nervous and Mental Disease,* 5, 1928. P. Hoeber, New York. (Discussion of literature.)
2. THOMPSON, C. E.: Family Care of the Insane. *American Journal of Psychiatry,* 91, 1934.
3. WERTHAM, F.: The Active Work Therapy of Dr. Simon. *Archives of Neurology and Psychiatry,* 24, 1930. (Discussion of German occupational therapy.)
4. DUNTON, W. R.: *Prescribing Occupational Therapy,* 2nd ed. Charles C Thomas • Publisher • Springfield, 1947. (Presentation of methods and crafts.)

Chapter XI

PARANOID AND PARANOIC REACTIONS

THE CHARACTERISTIC features of these reactions is systematized delusion-formation with formally correct conduct and grasp but the inability to adapt to reality the beliefs, convictions, and inferences concerning others or personal topics. We speak of "paranoic" when there is no evidence of disorganization of reasoning and behavior as such, beyond logical short-circuiting, and of "paranoid" when dissociation (hallucinations, passivity reactions) and behavior disorders occur. These reactions are an expression of personality assertion on false premises, with all the rigid short-circuited reasoning and inability to sense the need of correction. Although such reactions when merely part of an affective illness do not belong to this group from a therapeutic point of view, they deserve similar but considerably modified attention.

A. Meyer's psychodynamic formulation stresses the constitutional make-up, the disturbances of the balance of instincts taken in a broad sense, and various grades of development of the illness. It recognizes that the course is usually chronic but not necessarily progressive and that it may be influenced considerably by therapeutic interference. A paranoic development may come to a standstill at any of the various grades. Episodic course is relatively infrequent. It is recognized that incidental paranoid episodes may be superimposed on other reaction-sets, and that conflicts of a fundamental nature are favored by hereditary predisposition as well as discrepancies of endowment and ambition or deteriorative processes of the brain. A. Meyer formulates the therapeutic task clearly by stating that our only hope today is to discover and correct all the modifiable factors in the discrepancies between endowment and ambition. These factors may be physical, psychologic, or environmental. In this way a readjustment of the foundation of the convictions may be possible.

The characteristic features of the paranoic personality are its set organization, which does not allow submitting to insurmountable obstacles and handicaps; a sensitiveness about the attitude and behavior of others and concern about his impression on others; a tendency to brooding and rumination along the line of set suspicions and fancies with the inability to make concessions, and constant anticipation of possible future developments. This leads to uneasiness and suspense, and in many cases to resentment and anger reactions, loneliness, and often more definite moods of unhappiness, and slight depression. When these characteristics are so pronounced that they lead to obvious maladjustment in life we speak of paranoic psychopathic attitudes and reactions. In the development of a definite paranoic reaction the first step is characterized by the appearance of dominant notions and suspicions, or ill-balanced and frequently frustrated ambitions (inventions, claims of other parentage, or more mystical explanations), or projections in the form of jealousy, interpretation, and persecution with the more or less marked need for vindication. Hypochondriacal concern, which is frequently present, is the expression of inadequacy in the realm of body interest. These features have an irresistible tendency to systematization by false interpretations with self-reference (second stage), with or without retrospective, and often hallucinatory, falsification which is no longer controlled or verified (third stage). In the fourth stage, intercurrent acute episodes, megalomanic development, or deterioration occur. To the latter belong paranoid schizophrenic and paraphrenic developments. At any period antisocial and dangerous reactions may result from the lack of adaptability and excessive assertion of the sidetracked personality, and the prevalence of hate and suspicion.

In literature, the classification of these various reactions is still disputed. Paranoia is distinguished more or less definitely from the paraphrenic and paranoid schizophrenic illnesses. The minor and abortive reactions which are therapeutically very important have not attracted attention till relatively recently and are most frequently allocated to the psychopathic personalities. Kretschmer's "sensitive delusion-formation" also belongs to this group. The querulous paranoic reaction has been considered similar to hysterical reactions. Jealousy is usually taken separately. The frequent observations of paranoic reactions in the setting of brain injury and tumor, arteriosclerotic, and senile or involutional changes, and in toxic and thyroid disturbances, (which have been described as independent reactions) should be understood as personality reactions and treated accordingly with due attention to all the factors involved.

Bleuler's conception that the important feature is the fixation of the results of dominant experiences which were charged with much affect, as well as his observation that ideas of grandeur are a compensation reaction and not of an explanatory type have helped us greatly in understanding these reactions better. They occur in personalities in which strong affective forces, together with high aspirations, are in contrast to inadequate ability. The claim that there is always an affective root, e.g., distrust, is still held by many. The therapeutic question, however, is what causes the distrust and what can be done about it. Freud's investigations directed our attention to the importance of homosexual factors. He formulates paranoid reactions as a defense against homosexuality. The most loved person of his own sex becomes the persecutor. Ambivalence of feelings, the intrinsic connection of love and hate, is the source for the reversal of affects. When the patient feels persecuted by persons of the opposite sex, the person originally involved was of the same sex, and the delusional projection has been transferred to the other sex. Grandiose delusions are the expression of an increasing narcissistic regression. With his unconsciously increased homosexuality, a conflict leading to repression and projection develops. (In persecutory paranoid reactions we deal with the dynamic development of "I do not love him — I hate him — He hates me — He persecutes me." In erotomania the projection develops from "I do not love him, I love her — The fact is: she loves me.") Freud's dynamic interpretation is of therapeutic value if it is utilized as a guide for procedure and if a definite attack can be deferred until the patient has reached a stage in treatment at which he is able to deal constructively with such factors. In recent years, the theory has been proposed that in some patients the illness is caused by his fixation in the period of maximal sadism or by a masochistic identification. The modern German psychiatric approach (Kehrer) points to the importance of precipitating and situational factors. The treatment which is outlined takes all these factors into consideration, evaluating their relative importance and seeking possibilities for modification. It is a causal therapy but with frank realization that in many cases we must be contented with achieving a practical life adjustment which also includes a satisfactory hospital life if necessary. A thorough analytic correction is only possible in the minor paranoic reactions or in unusually fortunate cases. Bleuler's hopeless attitude is in no way justified, and even Freud's pessimistic view deserves correction if one wishes to be practical rather than perfectionistic. Modern psychodynamic formulation and treatment can be contrasted with the older psychiatric attitude which considered paranoia a disorder of the intellect or of degeneracy, stressing its chronicity and incurability, and planning at best merely symptomatic treatment.

Hypnosis is contraindicated in paranoic states. The patient frequently involves the hypnotizing physician in his system of delusions and may become dangerous to him. The dynamic forces behind these projections and transformations seem to be of homosexual or heterosexual nature. This is not surprising when we consider our observations in the hypnosis of normal persons. Suggestive therapy in its frank form influences the paranoic constitution very little, but suggestions in general play a considerable role in the reassurance offered and in environmental changes.

Treatment must be adjusted to the varying course of the illness if one wants to utilize the best possibilities for attack and to consider how much and what kind of aggression is involved and its direction expressed in content and underlying strivings. In some cases the delusions form a full-fledged wish fulfillment (prison manic psychoses) with or without explanatory, or persecutory, delusions which may finally dominate the whole picture. In others, megalomanic features of varying degree and extent prevail. Strong ambitions and a need to be appreciated or admired, or in some, inadequacy feelings (Kretschmer's sensitive reaction), or depressive affect (delusions with persecutory features) may be of importance (Lange). The role of resentment in delusion formation and in paranoic fixation is not well understood. Little is known about heredity and racial predisposition.

With the first contact the basis for treatment has been laid. A physician should be prepared to listen sympathetically, without disagreeing yet without committing himself to acceptance. It is the same attitude which we assume in daily life, when listening to somebody's strange creed. Deception and "humoring" should never be resorted to. The patient receives considerable relief from being able to present his problem and will be able to form some rapport. In patients who are on the defensive and unwilling to see any features which deserve discussion, the physician should ask the patient about physical complaints which are usually present. Interest in one's body, and thus an overevaluation of bodily symptoms, which may be on an organic basis or the expression of emotional tension, is part of the paranoic picture. Having obtained a history from relatives previously the physician will be able to recognize the best possible points for an opening discussion. It is essential that he determine the extent of the delusion, the direction and strength of the dynamic factors in the whole setting, with special attention to dominant affective features, toxic and organic factors, situational influences, and the personality background. A thorough psychiatric and physical examination is therefore necessary and can be utilized for establishing a medical rapport.

In this first consultation the decision with regard to further treatment must be made. Danger to others, suicidal possibilities, and refusal to attend to the necessary needs of physical hygiene are absolute indications for hospitalization. Many paranoic and paranoid patients are willing to accept temporary hospitalization if the physician presents it as a possibility for a thorough study of the whole situation. In others, commitment is necessary because the patient is unable to agree that a review with a neutral person in a neutral environment is desirable. Some are afraid of being "put away" permanently on the basis that they are considered insane or because their persecutors have the power to incarcerate them in a hospital. Incipient or minor paranoic reactions can frequently be treated outside of hospitals. It is then essential that a relationship of dependable cooperation with the physician be established. This may be possible without any deep or disturbing change in the patient's life. In others, it is advisable to have the patient leave his environment for a more neutral or directly helpful atmosphere, accompanied by proper medical care. Patients may have friends or relatives in other cities where they can be referred to a psychiatrist, staying there in a hotel. Even then, it is important that a regular routine of work and recreation be established. Traveling with a suitable companion is occasionally helpful as a distraction, but on the whole is merely a postponement of treatment. The patient should realize that he cannot get away from his own sensitiveness and will probably soon notice disturbing situations somewhere else.

When entering a hospital voluntarily, the patient usually has at first a feeling of safety and confidence. He frequently adjusts surprisingly well to the group. It is then important not to transfer the patient too soon to a new group. After a few days or weeks, however, he may begin to make disturbing observations, and projections which do not necessarily involve the physician develop. He will then begin to consider new plans and ask for discharge, which can be postponed for a while only. It then depends on how much has been accomplished as to whether the patient can be tried on the outside or has to be committed. In some cases transfer to another hospital may offer the possibility of an individually more attractive therapeutic setting. Occasionally a change of physicians is desirable. Another physician may succeed because of his personality where one equally well-trained failed. All these considerations are important in the treatment of a committed patient. The patient's life should be shaped so that constructive improvement is possible and even in permanent hospitalization, the patient can lead as satisfactory a life as possible. In formulating to a paranoic patient his impression, the physician should point out the unusualness of the whole problem and that therefore further discussion would be desirable; that there is a possibility that the patient's sensitiveness, which he is willing to accept for his life in general but not for specific situations, may cause him to overemphasize certain observations, and that he should learn to develop a need to consider the opinions of others.

The next step in treatment is to determine the patient's delusions. It is wrong to argue about delusions and misinterpretations. One deals with convictions (i.e., akin to belief) and not with errors which can be clarified by explanation. The physician agrees that the patient's interpretation may be correct but points to other possibilities which would be more likely acceptable to the average person. It will be best to do this in detail in observations in which the physician knows all the factors, practicing it more warily in less clear situations. The physician should guard against putting the patient on defense by constantly pointing out misinterpretations. He must stress the need to depend on a consensus of opinion, encouraging the patient to turn especially to those he can trust. The danger of bias and preconceived attitudes, of dominant moods, and of not being able to throw off impressions and experiences is discussed, as well as the dangers of forming conclusions without definite proof. This leads to a discussion of outstanding personality features which predispose to such reactions. In many patients one is not able to go beyond this stage which, however, may be sufficient to secure a temporary adjustment.

An analysis of the most outstanding past experiences which promise to be most modifiable can be attempted after a foundation of some tendency to doubt has been laid. One should try to lead the patient to study not only the motives of others but also their personalities and reactions. With a broader understanding of others, the patient will become more plastic and more tolerant of himself. The tendencies of misinterpretation, which have been previously studied, are constantly reviewed in this connection. It depends on the physician's tact whether he can do this without irritating or antagonizing the patient. He may then turn to a more thorough analysis of the personality features which cause misinterpretations and projections and study the patient's type of self-assertion. An analysis of group integration is essential and may clarify the dynamic factors which cause a feeling of loneliness in these patients.

An analysis of the paranoic system can be attempted if one has been successful in undermining the patient's convictions and attitudes and in producing some constructive understanding of his personality. At this stage, the patient frequently has begun to doubt that the physician shares his belief and will confront him with it. It is therefore important that the physician be prepared with a formulation which expresses his views in an acceptable form. Many patients break off treatment at this point. In others, a sufficiently strong rapport or sufficient undermining of misinterpretations has been achieved so that the patient can accept the need for further investigation. If the patient does not ask for a definite statement of the physician's attitude, I urge an analysis of the delusional system on the basis that it might be wrong (the previous attitude was always as if it were right). This now leads to an investigation into underlying factors. Here again patience and caution are indicated.

Through a distributive procedure, one analyzes first what is least important and correlates it constructively with the whole personality setting. Gradually this leads to the more important factors to which the patient has been so sensitive that he has not been able to accept them but had to project them. Finally a constructive solution is achieved.

Only a few cases of full-fledged paranoic reactions reach this point. The reason may be, as Freud believes, the inability to reach a complete transference because of marked narcissism or rigidity of the personality. One should, however, consider that these illnesses have an insidious onset and development and the patients do not come to the physician before an advanced state has been reached. It is quite possible that the treatment of paranoic personalities can prevent an otherwise progressive paranoic development. There is no proof at present that these developments have an unmodifiable course. Many minor paranoid reactions yield successfully to this treatment. In the more symptomatic paranoid reaction the same treatment must be applied, but the final distributive analysis usually has to be delayed till the more fundamental illness has cleared up.

Case 16:

A 46 year old unmarried man had been complaining to his brother for two years that he was persecuted by the Ku Klux Klan, which at that time was very active in his state. He confided in his minister, who, however, did not discuss it with the family, but tried to reassure him. Because of increasing delusions and irritability, a brother took him to the family physician, who advised him to seek treatment at the Johns Hopkins Hospital for brain tumor. Although this was an unfortunate way of sending the patient to us and prevented him later from trusting that physician, the patient was cooperative and talked freely in the first consultation, accepting our advice to enter the hospital for rest and a more thorough discussion of the whole problem. Within the first few days the following history was obtained:

At about 32, when working as bookkeeper in a bank, a vice-president was particularly kind to him because he knew that the patient partly supported his family. One day the vice-president dictated a letter to an uncle whose name was the same as that of a boy who had founded a boys' society at the school which the patient had attended. The boys of this society had not liked to play with him. The patient found some similarity in the employer's face to that of this particular boy. This made him think that his employer was of the same family as the boy. A few days later he saw that his employer, who had been away for two days, looked "mischievously" at him and the patient thought the man had seen that boy. He became sure that his employer no longer liked him. The patient stated, however, that these observations became clear to him only when he realized this man's persecution (at 40).

A few weeks later it happened that his sister was sent away from school for having stolen a corset from another girl. He and his family were sure that it was a wrong accusation, but it was never cleared up. The following day his mother became paralyzed. The patient brought all these events into connection. "The banker who had some money in that school is the cause of the misfortune of the family." This idea became slowly fixed in the next few years. Two weeks later he left, trying his luck in another state. A few days later he came back again to the city, asking his former employer for a new engagement, which was refused.

The patient was never able to forget these incidents. He opened a store in a small town and was fairly successful. After six years (at 37) his business began to fail, and two years later he had to sell out. He then tried unsuccessfully to build up a dairy farm, changed two years later to another farm, borrowing money for these enterprises. In the last three years he has been working as a salesman for his brother, his work becoming increasingly less satisfactory because he is too preoccupied with himself.

Shortly after the failure of his store, the patient (at 40) conceived the idea that the banker might be the founder of the Ku Klux Klan and that his suspicions were true — "That man knows that he caused all the misfortunes of the family and persecutes it, for fear the sons would later take revenge upon him." He felt that the man had persecuted him for many years and had caused the failure of his store. From that time (1920), the patient increasingly developed ideas of reference and misinterpretations of remote and recent events, and in October 1922 (42) he had the feeling of poison gas blowing in through the window (not a hallucination). From 1920-22 he often had a burning sensation in the stomach and believed it was some poison in the milk he had had for breakfast.

Since then, the delusion that the banker was the founder and leader of the Ku Klux Klan and was using this organization against him has become fixed. He also used the Germans against him, whose leader he was in this country, because his family was of German origin. Jews and Catholics, being persecuted by the Ku Klux Klan, helped the patient. The leader of the Ku Klux Klan in his home town, his birthplace, was the physician who gave him a book about masturbation when he was a young man. He noticed many indications for this constant persecution, became increasingly more suspicious and seclusive, and felt lonely and unhappy. He tried to establish himself in three different localities but was not able to make a success with any of these stores and farms.

The patient readily related this story, which was not changed later although important additions were given, and obtained relief from telling it. He asked for our opinion, which, however, was deferred until we had a chance to go more into detail. He expressed his gratitude for having found physicians who were willing to listen and were sympathetic. The physical examination, and a preliminary formulation of palpitation caused by anxiety and indigestion caused by strain, reassured him.

The psychiatric examination revealed no other involvements and there was therefore no doubt from the start that we dealt with a paranoic reaction (the observation of the case since, which has extended over ten years, has further substantiated this diagnosis). A brief personality review revealed the patient as an intelligent man of high ethical standards, who had worked since the age of 16 to support his family and secure an education for his brothers and sisters. He was always unbending in what he considered right; he was self-reliant and domineering, wishing to be appreciated for what he called his self-sacrifice. Even in his family he was proud and reserved but more so to outsiders, always feeling a need to protect his own and his family's pride and dignity. He was easily inclined to see slights and held dislikes and grudges. He had no friends but was friendly to people. Financial needs were the excuse for not being able to join in social life or to marry. An increasing slight hearing difficulty in the last few years had made him more sensitive and suspicious. Otherwise he had always been in good health, but was always considerably disturbed by minor ailments. At 11, he was infected with gonorrhea and had not had intercourse since, resorting to masturbation until the age of 20. After reading a book about the dangers of masturbation, he tried to stop and reproached himself for this practice. After one year he finally succeeded, finding aid in ardent religion. He ate practically no meat until he entered the clinic because he had read that it produces sexual desires. At 19, he fell in love with a cousin, but did not wish to consider marriage because he felt it was his duty to help his brothers. He was never able to forget his first love. A shy approach to a young teacher at 29 was rebuffed, hurting the patient's pride greatly. The same happened again at 34. He wondered at that time whether the girl's father had not been told that he might have syphilis and had therefore interfered. Since the age of about 37 he had noticed frequently that girls and women made advances to him, interpreting a look or a greeting as such, and became convinced that with regard to some girls it indicated their desire to marry him, whereas others were employed by the Ku Klux Klan to compromise him.

The latter delusion developed shortly after he realized the origin of the persecutions at 40. Of interest was the family picture which the patient and his brothers described alike. The father was still living (70), a proud man of aristocratic bearing who, like the mother who died at 60 (when the patient was 37) after seven years' invalidism after an apoplectic stroke, impressed the children with family pride and ancestry. The father was unsuccessful and the mother had impressed it upon the patient as a boy that she expected him to bring the family back to its social standing before the Civil War. The patient was greatly attached to her and also to his sisters. They represented the ideal of womanhood, deserving great respect from everybody.

In the beginning the patient felt secure in the hospital, but after a few days began to observe in the newspapers and then also in the hospital things which indicated that the Ku Klux Klan was using its power even in the hospital. These observations referred to outsiders and not to the physicians and nurses. Doubt as to their correctness was injected and a few misinterpretations were analyzed in greater detail. There was no doubt that the history of his present illness contained definite falsifications. The fallacies of an ordinary person's memory were pointed out to him and further review was urged with an attempt to correlate events to definite years (above-given history is the story as we were able to correct it within the first few days). These discrepancies were used to inject doubt and to provoke a more critical attitude.

For two months this treatment was pursued. It served to collect material and to inject doubts in acute misinterpretations and led to an increasing study of the personality setting. Every morning the patient discussed disturbing observations, frequently obtaining a more or less clear understanding of his tendency to connect facts and to read meanings into them without using any criticism. He became more willing to consider impressions and opinions of others. The improvement which occurred, however, could be explained more by the relief from ventilation and the feeling of security in the hospital (and was probably also due to a certain amount of pride in the attention he was receiving for the first time in his life) than to actual symptomatic insight. In further discussions of his life and personality reactions he mentioned his lonely life and his inability to form friendships, although he had a marked longing for it. He expressed marked resentment to his brothers and sisters, whom he considered ungrateful. This need for appreciation was expressed with regard to his present situation as: "I suffered so much. It never happened in the history of the U. S. that a low man had to suffer so much. It is not the same for a man in a prominent position, he becomes a hero — I am only an old bachelor." He believed that the banker had the power to have him killed at any time but enjoyed seeing him suffer. This heroism of suffering and the duty to fight persisted with little change. There was also only temporary confidence established in the normal functioning of his heart. At times he related how many leaders in political and business life had died from cardiac failure, which might indicate that they were poisoned. His own fear of poison gas being blown through the window was connected with this. On the whole, however, he had a resigned attitude and formed no plans for the future. This made us feel that he was not dangerous to others but, on the other hand, also indicated that there were not sufficient strivings to be utilized for a constructive readjustment. At the end of this phase of treatment, the desire to leave could be recognized in his projections — signs and remarks in the newspaper ridiculed him for his unwillingness to leave this secure place and do his duty. He felt that a remark of one of the nurses indicated that he wished to be with bad women and that she and one of the physicians were directed by his enemy. Through a critical review of all the facts a more definite delusional formation was prevented, but the whole trend of the development urged us to try to get closer to the fundamental factors.

In my own formulation of the dynamic factors involved, I considered the patient's personality make-up and the whole family situation which forced the patient into an ill-adjusted attitude, a struggle of high ambition, and inability to succeed. The business failures seemed to be merely a precipitating factor. His hypochondriacal attitude seemed to be more circumscribed and was probably related to definite, rather than general, factors. It also seemed important to gain a better understanding of his relationship to the vice-president and to test Freud's formulation of erotomania. It was not felt, however, that further study would even help the patient to gain such an understanding, but that we should be guided by this formulation to secure a better understanding of the personality development. It was also unclear why this paitent should develop a heroism of suffering.

On our advice the patient, while staying in the hospital, went to work every day in a candy factory. He was interested in the work and we hoped that he might be able to use the acquired knowledge in connection with his brother's dairies. The patient felt encouraged and recognized that distraction would be helpful, and that one's need for inquiry is valuable if done critically, and does not lead to paying too much attention to what is going on around us. He also recognized that the anticipation of work caused indigestion and that anticipation in the past had produced similiar disturbances. A discussion of the relation to the vice-president revealed that on one of the first days in his office his employer asked him to stay and help him with his work one night. This man invited him to have dinner in his home because his family were on their vacation and let him sleep in his daughter's bedroom. During the following days (he had not made definite arrangements for his lodging yet), the patient stayed at this house at the invitation of the banker who went to join his family. In the weeks that followed he often had dinner with the vice-president in his home. Often other young fellows of the bank teased him because of his friendship with his employer and told him that other boys of the bank had received similar favors. The patient was convinced, however, that this was untrue and that they were envious. After having left the bank he often thought of the banker as a kind friend. Five years later (at 36) he wrote him at Christmas (previously he had sent the customary greeting), telling him that he could never forget him and his kindness. He received a brief but kind answer. A year later (at 37) he went to see him and asked for re-employment. The banker was unable to offer him a place. At this time his business had begun to fail. A few months later he wrote the banker that he did not want to earn much money but only wanted to be near him, if necessary as "his chauffeur or to blacken his shoes." Two years later (39) the patient wrote again, telling him about his failure in business. "I want to be close to you as I was the time when I worked at night for you in your office." He never received any answer to these two letters. When he went to see his former employer a year later (at 40) the man was rather cold to him, inviting him to dinner but not at his home. Shortly afterwards his store failed. At this time the patient suddenly saw clearly that the vice president persecuted him through the Ku Klux Klan.

In adolescence, the patient had formed a similar, but not so intense, attachment to his first employer, who was to him the ideal gentleman. Asked about earlier attachments, he stated that at about 9 he had been greatly under the influence of a boy of 11 who mistreated him in every way but from whom he was never able to free himself till late adolescence. This boy urged him into sexual relations with the colored prostitute who infected him with gonorrhea and teased him about it publicly. He then advised him to take up masturbation. This boy was the founder of the school society which ostracized him, and the resemblance which he thought he detected between him and the vice-president made him suddenly realize his persecutions (at 40).

In a discussion of his sexual life he mentioned that he had dreams with discharge but could never remember the content of these or other dreams. He was frequently afraid that his enemies might misinterpret the proof of his sexual desires. He had often been astonished to notice his lack of sexual desires, but explained it by the education of his character, and weakness from adolescent masturbation. He was relieved, but also ashamed that he no longer had sexual desires. He reviewed in greater detail his love for his cousin, and the school teacher who had rejected him, and the "advances" of other girls because he was attractive to them. He had been unhappy about his failure to marry and felt that it soon would be too late. The spontaneous statement, "My heel of Achilles is my sex life. If I could settle these things I would be better" was, however, not indicative of his gaining insight, as I had hoped. In the last six years he had been greatly concerned about the possibility of his favorite sister's indulging in sexual misdemeanors and although she never gave any cause, misinterpreted observations along this line.

These discussions were spread over four weeks. The patient became increasingly more suspicious and restless. After some discussions he slept poorly. He began to fear that there might be a way for his enemies to infect him with syphilis. (This and an increase in his erotomanic misinterpretations occurred after the sexual discussions.) After the discussion of his boyhood friend, he developed the delusion that dictaphones were installed in the office and persisted in this belief until discharge. Suspiciousness increased after a rediscussion of the banker. An awareness of odors which might indicate poison also increased. At this time he mentioned that his father's colored cook had tried to poison him four years previously. He felt discouraged and unhappy and wanted to leave. One evening he suddenly asked whether the physicians believed that his persecutions were real or imaginary. It was formulated to him that we had never been able to find a proof for their real existence and that he himself never had. He had repeatedly stated that he would go to court as soon as he had proof. On the other hand, we pointed out that there were many occurrences which he, under our observation, misinterpreted. We wanted him to stay in the hospital hoping that we could make him look more critically at daily happenings and take them more easily so that he would be able to avoid misinterpretations, which made him unhappy. The need to have friends like his physicians who understood him was stressed. The patient was unhappy about this formulation and left a few days later, asking for a statement from us with regard to his sanity. He accepted the following letter as satisfactory:

"Mr. X left our clinic with our knowledge and consent. During his stay here he has been very cooperative. It is difficult for him to understand a number of experiences of the past as we see them, and he still shows sensitiveness and interpretations along lines of his former impressions. His ability to cooperate makes us feel that he should be able to work under reasonably convenient circumstances."

Feeling reasonably certain that there was at present, and probably in the future, no serious danger to others, we let him return home where he worked for his brothers for two and a half years. His family physician kept us informed and we had to agree with him that permanent hospitalization was necessary when his family no longer felt able to stand the strain of his suspicions and the talk of people in the community. We hoped, however, that after a few months' hospitalization he might again try to make an adjustment on the outside. This has not been possible largely because his family is unwilling to make another attempt. In the hospital (16 years) the patient is pleasant, quiet, and cooperative, keeping busy in regular occupation. He never discusses his persistent delusions except when something arouses him, e.g., when somebody mentions Negroes, a term which in his mind refers to his intercourse experience. The commitment he blames on his enemy, who forced his family to this step.

The case is interesting because some of the fundamental factors are demonstrated rather definitely; i.e., the homosexual fixation to the man who persecuted him and the projection of his heterosexual desires into erotomania; the ethical conflict and the inability to adjust fundamental strivings in his personality to the possibilities of real satisfaction, his personality development and the destructive influence of unfortunate life situations. His precocious sexuality is striking. It is possible that a definite masochistic tendency forces this patient into the attitude of the heroic sufferer and prevents aggression toward the environment. There are also, however, personality features which may determine this course independent of specific sexual factors. The frequent observations that paranoics are not interested in having children also applies to this case. Whether this is due primarily to sexual factors and in connection with the sexualization of his social tendencies through erotomania, or to other personality features and fixation on his brothers and sisters, whom he had brought up like his children, cannot be decided.

The treatment had been successful in destroying secondary delusional developments, elaborations, and misinterpretations, but failed to modify his personality and to shake the center of the delusional system. Even after our own attitude had become clear to the patient, he was able to maintain confidence in our personal integrity and returned twice for advice about future positions. In other patients this contact has permitted us to keep them outside of hospitals for many years. Even in this case, the two and a half years outside of a hospital is gratifying to a physician who does not always expect perfect results. In treating a paranoic reaction, the physician is bound by his duty to society and to the patient. The need for hospitalization must be evaluated individually and never be considered permanent in the sense that no further attempts should be made to create situations to allow the patient to live at his best in or out of the hospital. Dangers in discharge always have to be evaluated carefully. The dynamic forces and their direction as well as the degree and firmness of rapport which has been developed must be understood; also whether the patient can be definitely expected to keep in close and regular contact with his physician so that incipient danger can be detected and society protected.

This patient's own attempt at a solution was escape. He is in this respect similar to Rousseau, who fled to England, and although misinterpretations also occurred there, was able to live outside of a hospital. He found outlets in literature and politics which diminished the strength of his delusions. Many paranoic persons succeed similarly or even more thoroughly in a transformation of their unacceptable strivings. To this group belong many fanatics in the religious and social field. It may be correct that sexual desires are of fundamental importance, but in some cases the same reaction has to be explained by different personality factors.

In some patients an outside adjustment is possible because they succeed in ignoring the disturbing projections. This, as well as a more or less successful repression of the material that has broken through, occurs more in the paranoid schizophrenic, than in frank paranoic and paranoid, reactions. Planned efforts at group integration will facilitate repression. Relief along situational lines or the correction of preoccupations of sensitiveness is frequently helpful.

Case 17:

A 49 year old married woman was admitted to the Payne Whitney Clinic on January 30, 1942 because she had delusions that people made derogatory remarks about her. She had noticed these observations since 1938 when she had permitted petting by a man. During the whole year of 1941 she had been treated in another psychiatric hospital where she had great confidence in her physician. Depressive features, guilt feelings, and delusions of reference decreased. She was able to stay away from the hospital for weeks at a time, but was always dependent on her special nurse and never wholly free of delusions. She never mingled with the other patients and was often irritable and rude to the nurses. When coming to the hospital the patient gave a detailed history of her present illness and of her life. In childhood she had been timid and had frequent anxiety dreams. She was the youngest of three children. Her father was an aggressive, successful business man who adored the patient, while her mother preferred her two brothers. The mother was domineering, emotionally ill-controlled, and never showed much affection to the patient. At 20 the patient married against the wishes of her parents, who considered her husband socially inferior. His personality was similar to that of her father, and he made later a considerable success as a lawyer. Shortly after her marriage her father died, and the patient reacted with a prolonged mild depression to it. She became dependent on her husband and devoted her time to the education of her three children, to household duties, social obligations, and charity work. She was socially well liked despite her reserve and snobbishness, hiding her shyness and underlying lack of self-confidence. Her feelings were easily hurt; she tended to bear grudges for long periods of time. For 10 years, she had been suspicious of her husband's fidelity and had felt estranged from him. Her personal standards were high and inflexible. She had always shown great interest in her body, in younger years keeping fit through athletics, in recent years paying much attention to health.

Obtaining this history and paying attention to any physical complaints permitted the physician to establish a trusting relationship during the first four weeks. It was pointed out that her delusional observations might be based on coincidence and she was advised to avoid looking for meanings. The patient had received the same advice from her previous physician and she was willing to accept it. In a review of her previous treatment it was obvious that efforts at socialization had been inadequate. The patient objected to the request to accept a regular routine and to stay with the other patients. When she reacted with fatigue to the emotional strain of being with others, she was carefully examined and the difference between emotional and physical fatigue explained. In March, she recognized that resentment and tension seemed to lead to fatigue. These reactions occurred readily when she was in the company of aggressive patients and similar resentment was caused by her husband's aggressiveness. In April, she noticed that she was more sensitive to the behavior of others when tired. In May and June the discussion led to a review of her social relations during the various phases of her life. She became aware of her resistance to the demands of her husband and daughter, resenting their aggressive independence but unable to overcome her emotional reserve. With her two sons she felt at ease and shared many interests. Her high and rigid standards made her critical of others. In July, the guilt feelings connected with her erotic experience were reviewed in the light of her personality development and marital life. She expressed marked resentment to her husband's behavior which had been especially humiliating to her just before she turned to the man involved, partly for admiration and partly to spite her husband. She was now aware of her reactions of intense and prolonged resentment to frustration. Her delusions became very infrequent after June.

During the months of August to October her increased social ease was utilized for bringing her in contact with a few friends and permitting visits to her home. Considerable time had been spent with her husband to allow him to obtain a better understanding of his wife. He modified his own routine in order to decrease emotional tension in the family. During this period, the patient analyzed the personalities of different patients in her group and recognized similar types in her present and past social life. This was followed by an analysis of the personalities of her parents, her brothers, and her husband. She was able to accept the fact that she should learn to rely on the consensus of opinion and not accept too readily her own emotionally-determined subjective conclusions. Her untidiness in budget matters and her unwillingness to assume financial responsibility was analyzed by her as a device to annoy her husband and punish him for his overbearing attitude. She formulated her love affair as a need to satisfy her desires for being physically attractive and to get even with her husband for his suspected philandering. All these discussions were carefully guided by the physician, usually lasting 45 to 60 minutes, and occurring once to twice a week. She was, however, seen daily in order to discuss any minor problems which might come up, to reassure her with regard to physical complaints and to give her the feeling of receiving interest and attention from her physician. When she left the hospital on October 7, 1942, a concrete plan of living was given to her which balanced housework, volunteer work, social life, and rest. The patient wrote once a month and received practical advice by return mail. She has come for a consultation every three months, and since 1944 twice a year. Several times during the last few years the husband has asked for an interview to review their life. The patient has been free of symptoms since the fall of 1942 and leads an active life.

In many patients the paranoid reaction is, to a large extent, a situational outgrowth. This factor is important in the querulous type of paranoid reaction, i.e., in the person who has a need to receive justice for various injuries. In all these cases the treatment of the individual's personality is of essential importance. Many of these patients are able to lead a successful, although occasionally turbulent, life till some more important difficulties make this impossible and a full-fledged paranoid reaction develops. Physical handicaps and illnesses, disappointments in life, or the realization in later life that it is impossible to reach the hoped-for goal precipitate the reaction. To this group belong many late-life paranoics. The same factors, together with the struggle against unacceptable desires, cause many of the paranoic reactions of unmarried women between 35 and 40 (old maid reaction). Many of these reactions lead to recovery either as a result of successful repression or constructive analytic treatment with correction of physical and situational factors. A new start in a different locality and a different position in life may be indicated.

Difficult therapeutic problems are presented by the paranoid reaction of persons with hearing difficulties. It is more frequent in acquired deafness, especially when manifest in later life. Deafness demands a great social adjustment, especially in persons who have the features which we consider essential in the paranoic constitution. It leads to increasing seclusion and resentment to it and, through self-assertion, to paranoid projections. In fortunate cases, a hearing apparatus may be helpful, but even then a personality adjustment should be attempted. In these and in less fortunate cases regular occupation and interests and participation in suitable social contact must be utilized. Similar factors play a role in paranoid reactions which develop in persons who live in an unfamiliar environment or in a population whose language they cannot understand. In one of our patients, the paranoid systematization cleared up rapidly when he was sent to his native country. The analysis of that case, however, showed a marked underlying desire to return to his country yet feeling duty-bound to remain in the foreign country. Our advice made the impossible decision unnecessary. Only in a few cases will transfer to the native country be possible, but a more congenial and understanding social life can usually be created. Adjustment of the personality is also necessary in those cases. Many times, however, we are greatly limited in our therapeutic approach because these more situationally-determined paranoic reactions usually occur in feebleminded persons. The establishing of good rapport is then of utmost importance.

In some cases the paranoid reaction occurs in the form of a panic. Patients in such states must be considered very dangerous to themselves and to others, and hospitalization is urgent. They are suspicious, feel unable to trust anybody and anything, and are markedly fearful, need constant reassurance and careful repeated explanations of every therapeutic step. To a patient, the hospital environment offers many unusual and puzzling observations to which physicians and nurses no longer pay any attention. Sedatives (barbital .15 gm. — 2½ gr. three to four times a day, at regular intervals) may lead to a control of the panic, but should not be forced on the patient if he refuses them. Insulin therapy (see p. 158) leads to fast improvement in most cases. Prolonged warm baths are usually accepted and are helpful in producing relaxation. Occupational therapy helps a patient to find distraction and ease. Psychotherapy is primarily guided by the need to establish confidence in the physician and the environment, and to allow the acute panic to settle down. Analytic investigation should be avoided, but the patient needs opportunities for ventilation of his fears, delusions, preoccupations, and worries. Each discussion should be terminated with a constructive formulation which the patient can understand at the time and which allows him to find more reassurance and ease based on increased self-confidence. Only after security has been established should the physician attempt to analyze the underlying factors. Even then he should proceed cautiously and take a recurrence of suspiciousness, fear, or delusions as an indication that he deals with still dangerously explosive material. He should then hesitate to push further till a more thorough security has been established. Otherwise, a new panic outburst which may involve the physician may occur. This might necessitate transfer to another hospital or at least to another physician. A recurrent panic may also lead to increased disorganization, making the prognosis less favorable. Minor paranoid panic can be treated outside the hospital, but a physician must realize that he is taking considerable responsibility with regard to suicide. Most of the paranoid panic reactions offer a good prognosis for an adjustment for life. In many cases this is obtained spontaneously through more successful repression and the avoidance of dangerous life situations. In other reactions a thorough constructive analysis allows an adjustment of the basic underlying personality factors. Various dynamic factors are of fundamental importance, latent homosexuality being only one of them. More frequently, a disturbance of financial security, insecure health, ethical problems, and responsibility along various lines are important.

Minor brief paranoid reactions to recurrent life situations in paranoic personalities occur frequently. This accounts for the marked hate which such patients develop toward persons who thwart them. This emotional reaction usually persists and is easily reactivated. Such persons should understand their rigidity and the need to develop plasticity which allows them to become desensitized and to forget hurts. In some, dominant ideas take hold of the personality and force them into fanaticism. Such patients rarely come for help spontaneously. Their environment is tolerant of them, or even becomes infected with their ideas, e.g., in religious and reform movements. There is always the definite danger that a paranoic patient can induce the development of the same conviction in others. Even full paranoic and paranoid illnesses can develop on such an induced basis. They are relatively easily corrected if these patients are removed from the dominating influence of the controlling paranoic figure. Occasionally the paranoic reactions consist entirely of hypochondriacal content. This occurs in patients with a paranoic personality to whom having their bodies intact is of utmost importance. They react with paranoic resentment to operations which disfigure them. I saw such reactions twice after all the patients' teeth had been removed and they were unable to adjust to dental plates. One of these patients wanted to launch a statewide movement to prohibit dental surgery except under medical supervision. The patient was unable to gain an understanding of the uncritical fixity of her convictions but was willing to desist from her plans.

Jealousy reactions are frequent. Freud classified jealousy as normal, projected, and delusional jealousy. Normal jealousy is on a competitive basis. It consists of pain (grief) caused by the losing of the love object, hate of the successful rival, and self-criticism which tries to hold the person himself accountable for his loss. The person's pride (narcissism) is affected and, in a paranoic personality, this wound may never heal completely. Normal jealousy comes frequently to the physician's attention. It is important that jealousy should not be accepted as normal if it is of marked intensity or duration or occurs frequently. In such cases the physician should analyze the various factors and help to achieve a constructive solution with desensitization permitting forgetting. Projected unfaithfulness in both men and women is derived from the patient's own unfaithfulness, either real or in imaginations and desires. Such patients should realize that their personal code does not allow them such indulgences and that they must avoid dangerous situations.

They should therefore know to what they are sensitive sexually (this is meant in its broadest sense and includes many social customs), and that they cannot afford to indulge in actions which may be harmless for somebody else. A brief analysis of the personality is always indicated, not only to expose the frequently unconscious phantasies of infidelity but also the outstanding personality traits which predispose to projections.

According to Freud, homosexual strivings are always the basis for delusional, i.e., definitely paranoid, jealousy. The origin is in repressed impulses toward unfaithfulness with one's own sex. Through transformation the patient develops the attitude: "Indeed, I do not love him, *she* loves him." There is no doubt that this occurs frequently. Other possibilities, however, should be kept in mind, and an analysis of the paranoic personality development and of all possible life experiences and situational factors must be considered if a constructive adjustment is to be achieved. Of special importance are these reactions in late life, e.g., at the involutional age and in early organic (presenile, senile, cerebral arteriosclerotic, and general paralytic) disorders. Instead of elaborating on the various possibilities which can be arrived at by applying the dynamic factors possible in paranoic reactions, I shall present a case which illustrates some of these points and their management.

Case 18:

The 60 year old wife of a successful man entered the hospital because she had suffered from delusions of jealousy for three years. (It is usually most difficult for a physician to decide whether he is dealing with delusions or whether the suspicions are justified. The utmost caution is therefore necessary, and one should not be ready to assure the patient of the wrongness of delusions of jealousy merely based on the partner's denial.) In this case the convictions had reached such intensity and were so widespread that their pathologic character was obvious. This naturally does not preclude that there might not have been unfaithfulness of the husband in the beginning, but this does not enter into the treatment under discussion. After menopause at 57, which coincided with the 58 year old husband's decrease of potency, the patient began to believe that her husband was sexually interested in a young friend. There were times when she accepted his and her children's reassurance. At other times, when she felt depressed, the convictions were unshakable. When financial strain increased (at 59), the delusions became more alarming. The patient formed not only further misinterpretations, but now believed that her husband was trying to poison her, and was therefore advised to enter the clinic where she felt secure.

A brief study revealed that this patient had always lacked confidence in herself. The only safe tie to her husband seemed to her to be her sexual attractiveness to him. Their interests were entirely separate. She was self-assertive and made a success in social life, hiding her concern about the impression she made on others, and her tendency to anticipation. When under strain she reacted with uneasiness and diarrhea, and to prolonged strain with slight depression. Although she had threatened divorce when her husband was unwilling to accept her opinion with regard to her son's choice of occupation (at 52), and had frequently in her life played with such thoughts in her imagination, she became panicky when there seemed to be a possibility that her husband might become interested in somebody else and wish to leave her. Because of her set ideas and ways of carrying out things, she did her best work alone. She was never able to yield to obstacles. She was reserved, inclined to be suspicious, and was unable to forget injuries and disappointments.

The examination revealed no signs of any cerebral organic involvements and she was in good general health. She was immediately urged to join in the full activity of the floor to become distracted from her preoccupations and to develop, if possible, a better socialization. She needed much reassurance about her health and repeated explanations with regard to minor somatic tension and anxiety complaints. The unlikelihood of her ideas was pointed out to her and doubt injected. The patient improved greatly in general, but was unable to correct the delusions of infidelity completely. Her personality insight remained meager although she began to recognize the above-mentioned features as lifelong trends and reactions. Whenever visiting her home, the somatic complaints recurred but no new delusions developed. When the physician gained the impression that the patient was becoming dependent on the hospital, he urged her to leave. The period of hospitalization lasted seven months. She has made a satisfactory adjustment since but still believes that her husband was unfaithful at the time of the onset of her suspicions. She only mentions this when she is under some strain and at that time also has a recurrence of the somatic complaints and depressed mood.

In this patient, in whom marriage was entirely on a sexual basis and never reached the stage of actual family formation, the possibility of losing her only hold on the husband was an unmanageable threat to her life security. She reacted with projections (delusions of jealousy) which revealed her own desires, i.e., to terminate by divorce an unsatisfactory union which now had lost the only bond (sexual relations). Such a result, however, would have put her on her own responsibility and added financial strain and curtailment of her social position. Divorce was therefore unacceptable. It is true that our study did not give us a full understanding of her sexual life but there are no definite indications of a homosexual root. (No follow-up was obtained.)

The frequency of delusions of jealousy in alcoholic patients has attracted much attention. Freud and his school explain it also on a homosexual basis. Some feel definitely that homosexual factors are the root for alcoholism itself. Bleuler stresses that it is more likely that these delusions are projections of the alcoholic's own unfaithfulness, which is so often manifested in minor or full-fledged sexual acts. A careful study in these cases also seems to reveal a paranoic personality which reacts to the toxic and situational factors with projections.

The treatment of symptomatic paranoic reactions is influenced by the underlying fundamental disorder. One should, however, always keep in mind that argumentation or a direct attack on the delusions ought to be avoided whenever delusions appear in the setting of elation and depression. This is advisable whether the delusions are systematized or unsystematized. The patient needs relief from the underlying feelings, which may have a somatic basis, or in which unusual sensations may play a role. This is especially true in depressions where argumentation irritates the patient. One should try to attain a relationship which allows the patient to get away from his attitude of defense or in which he may even be able to unload his strained feelings. The development of neutral common interests, without pressure and urging from others, is most desirable. The injection of doubt will also, in these cases, undermine the fixity of the delusions. After the underlying disturbance has cleared up, a distributive analysis should help the patient to gain an understanding of the factors which caused the projections, especially when they are on a catathymic basis. This is necessary if one wishes to prevent recurrences.

In paranoic and paranoid illnesses with marked anxiety, insulin therapy may prove most helpful in diminishing the intensity of the delusions and making the patient amenable to psychotherapy. When delusions occur in the setting of depressive or manic reactions, convulsive therapy may be helpful. In all these patients, however, psychotherapy is essential to achieve the best results.

Our knowledge of the possible dynamic factors is a helpful

guide to our therapeutic imagination but should never be used dogmatically. We should be guided by the facts and should not force them into a scheme. A distributive analysis always has to be adjusted to the individual case. A physician must be patient, realizing that pushing will result in increased projections, and that an over-zealous interpretation of the illness will cause projections to be extended to him. If the physician is involved in the delusional system, he is not able to be of much constructive help, and the patient should be transferred to another physician if possible. Paranoic reactions, according to A. Meyer's conception, represents an excessive and poorly adapted morbid form of adjustment. The patient has tried to achieve harmony at least within himself. He tends to force the result, if necessary, on everybody else rather than to compromise in any way which might again unsettle him. The paranoic's tendency to become guided by individual dogmatism, however, can also be seen in many persons in normal life. Religious convictions are frequently of a similar type. Many persons dread doubt and have a need to strengthen and expand their convictions through organization. It is essential that a physician try to counteract the development of convictions and paranoid tendencies as early as possible. A. Meyer believes that this can be achieved by cultivating habits of concreteness in thinking and action by developing a healthy type of inquiring mind. Mental activity, which he calls a tentative forerunner of actions, must be considered critically like action itself before one should feel absolutely sure. A philosophy of relativity allows one to combine the ability of firmness of decision and action with clear realization of the limitations of one's knowledge and of the tentative character of most of one's efforts. Training to recognize one's shortcomings and failures, especially with regard to tendencies to doubt and to overassertion, will be most helpful. Many constitutionally predisposed individuals can be helped through such a guidance and protected from developing a paranoic reaction. As in any other illness, much depends on the physician's ability to recognize early unhealthy tendencies and to find ways by which they can be counteracted and modified.

BIBLIOGRAPHY

1. MEYER, A.: The Treatment of Paranoia and Paranoid States. *Modern Treatment of Nervous and Mental Disease*, White and Jelliffe, Vol. 1. Lea & Febiger, Philadelphia, 1913. (Includes discussion of literature, especially Freud and Bleuler.)
2. KEHRER, F.: Paranoische Zustände. *Handbuch der Geisteskrankheiten*, O. Bumke, Vol. 6. J. Springer, Berlin, 1928.
3. FREUD, S.: *Certain Neurotic Mechanisms in Jealousy, Paranoia and Homosexuality.* Collected Papers, Vol. 2. The Hogarth Press, London, 1924.
4. BLEULER, E.: *Affectivity, Suggestibility, Paranoia.* State Hospital Press, Utica, 1912. (Discussion of more recent literature is found in the second German edition — Affektivität, Suggestibilität, Paranoia. Carl Manhold, Halle, 1926.)

Chapter XII

DELIRIOUS AND TOXIC REACTIONS

T HE FULL-FLEDGED deliria, as well as all disorders which are due
to a nutritive or circulatory malsupport of the brain, are included in this group of reactions. Delirium is the outstanding picture, but various types of toxic hallucinations may also occur. These
psychopathologic reactions are always part of another disorder
which must be determined in order to establish a basis for treatment. The two major groups are the toxic, and the organically determined, disorders. Less frequent is a third group, the psychogenic
type — hysterical, epileptic, and occasionally schizophrenic deliria.
Under the influence of leading affects, especially fear, similar, though
less well-defined, reactions may occur. Depressive thinking disorders sometimes lead to confusional states. In these cases the treatment of the depression needs to be modified along the lines which are
discussed in this chapter. Manic excitements with marked confusion
must frequently be treated as deliria. The outstanding symptoms
are clouding of consciousness or drowsiness, poor attention, difficulty in comprehension, and poor orientation.

Delirious reactions always show clouding or drowsiness, de-
ficient grasp, and poor orientation. Fear is usually the outstanding
affect. In some cases, elation may predominate. Visual and tactile
misinterpretations and hallucinations disturb and frighten the patient. Auditory hallucinations occur less frequently but may occasionally assume the leading role. Olfactory hallucinations and
hallucinations of position are relatively rare. The clinical picture is
usually considerably influenced by the personality involved. This,
however, should not lead us to overlook the fact that certain brain
lesions and toxins, especially drugs, may cause specific clinical features. Their recognition allows the physician to diagnose the type
of delirium and to treat the etiological factors which otherwise are
frequently determined only with difficulty. The diagnosis of early
symptoms of morphine delirium is important, e.g., in a patient who
receives morphine during a cardiac delirium. In one case, one may

feel justified in giving the much needed morphine while in another case, its immediate cessation is indicated. The knowledge of specific drug symptoms will prevent us from reading too readily into symptoms meanings which are determined by the personality and from applying too freely and in too general a form what has been learned from the study of the more purely personality-determined reaction, e.g., psychoneuroses and schizophrenia.

The theory that the form and intensity of the delirious reaction are parallel to the degree of the toxin, e.g., the height of fever or the amount of the drug, is no longer acceptable. It is also not merely a case of susceptibility to toxins. Many features of the integrated personality may predispose to delirious reactions. In some personalities, somatogenic or neurogenic factors are most important; in others, psychogenic factors are dominant. The various factors influence each other constantly, with varying intensity, causing new factors to enter into play. Constitutionally predisposed persons may have several delirious reactions of a toxic type during life, frequently to an amount of toxin which the average person seems to stand well. These recurrent delirious reactions usually present a similar picture, with little variation, although in some patients recent life experiences may cause different content. Constitutional tendencies to affective, paranoid, and schizophrenic disorders, can color, or even dominate, the picture. Psychogenic factors frequently cause an increased excitement and unusual symptoms. Poorly organized psychopathic personalities frequently react with fear and outbursts of panic and even violence and are difficult to treat.

The leading affect in a delirium is fear. As the fear increases, it interferes more and more with the support of the brain which leads to an increase of the delirious reaction. Some drugs seem to have a specific fear-producing effect. In other cases, constitutional tendencies predispose to intense fear. Suspiciousness may be the expression of fear, or it may be due to paranoic features of the personality. Full-fledged paranoic reactions may be seen in a delirious setting.

The modern concept of delirious reactions does not permit an independent nosologic entity of toxic hallucinoses. Recent studies of delirium tremens have demonstrated that there is not as sharp a distinction between acute alcoholic hallucinosis and delirium as has been claimed previously. The German nosologic entity "amentia" designates a reaction which is primarily characterized by incoherence of thinking and therefore frequently marked confusion. These cases belong to the toxic-delirious reaction type and should be treated accordingly. "Twilight states" are usually psychogenic deliria. They are most frequently found in psychopathic personalities, epileptic, and schizophrenic illnesses. These highly disoriented and hallucinating patients misinterpret a situation systematically to a varying degree. Fugues belong to the group of oriented twilight states. All these reactions are usually followed by more or less complete amnesia for the period of the disturbance of consciousness and comprehension.

Considering these possibilities, the physician will be guarded in his prognosis in every delirious reaction. He usually is justified, however, in giving a good prognosis for the delirium itself. The average delirium is of short duration, from a few days to two or three weeks, and some abortive deliria may last only a few hours. In some cases, the duration may be considerably prolonged because of various constitutional reaction tendencies. In other cases, the delirium may be the beginning of an illness which will run its course after the delirium has cleared up; for example, a manic excitement or a depression. It is also possible that a delirium may cover up a disorder which had started insidiously before the delirium began, or the delirium may have been only a more or less incidental precipitating factor. Residuals of delirium are rare, but it is possible that certain delusions, especially of the paranoid type, may persist and may not yield even to an intensive treatment.

The treatment of delirious reactions is determined by the etiological factors, the extent of the clouding and difficulty in comprehension, disorientation, and fear, and must be individually adjusted according to specifically determined content and reactions, resulting from special toxic, organic, or constitutional factors. For practical purposes, I mention the distinction between the definite phases which were observed first in infectious deliria but which can be applied to practically all of these reactions: (1) Restlessness, uneasiness, dull headaches, sensitiveness to noises and light, irritability, tendency to emotional instability, frequently fearful dreams and restless sleep, slight difficulty in grasping, slight retention disorder, some distractibility, and often vivid memories of the past. Some patients are definitely euphoric, others are somewhat depressed or slightly suspicious. This first phase may last for a few hours to several days, and lead to complete clearing up or to a more or less sudden development of the second stage. (2) The delirium starts frequently with hypnagogic hallucinations which are recognized as imaginations by the patient and disappear when he opens his eyes. Dreams begin to hang on for a few minutes after the patient is awake. Cloudiness, illusions and hallucinations, fear, and disorientation increase more or less rapidly. During this phase, however, the patients can still be brought into rapport with the environment. (3) Full-fledged delirium with increasing neurologic symptoms. The speech becomes more and more indistinct and slurred, movements are ataxic, and finally the patient lies quietly in bed, mumbling indistinctly. This may lead to stupor and coma. As a rule, however, delirious reactions clear up rapidly. Some authors point out that, especially in young patients, a phase similar to the initial phase may follow the end of the delirium. In older people a Korsakow's picture which clears up after several weeks or months may result. In rare cases, it may last for years. I have seen several such cases after typhoid fever delirium. The final outcome is good, except in alcoholic patients and in old age, where it may lead to a permanent Korsakow's psychosis.

The treatment of delirious reactions has not received sufficient psychiatric attention until recent years because practically all these cases are under the care of the internist. The personality factors therefore usually do not receive enough attention and planned psychotherapy is omitted. In the past, symptomatic treatment of the delirium was considered incidental and all therapeutic efforts were directed to the underlying physical illness. This was a faulty attitude. Correct psychiatric treatment helps to preserve the patient's strength and to prevent complications (infections from minor injuries and pneumonia). In addition, it definitely decreases the intensity and duration of the delirium.

In any delirious reaction, a thorough mental and physical examination must form the essential basis for treatment. The physical examination will not only determine the etiological factors and how they can be influenced but also the present physical status and how the patient's strength can be preserved. Realizing that etiological factors and the intensity of the delirious reactions do not run parallel, it is no longer expected that the delirium will clear up rapidly with the removal of the disturbing factors. Fever, alteration of acid-base equilibrium, and edema of the brain are considered direct delirium-producing factors. Sodium chloride, adminstered orally or parenterally, is used to restore the normal acid-base equilibrium. Large amounts of carbohydrates are recommended because of their beneficial effect on the cerebral metabolism in toxic delirious states. Antipyretics in large amounts usually aggravate the mental picture, and, while lumbar puncture has been advised to relieve the edema, the result is rather doubtful. The use of diathermia should not be advised because of the danger of cardiac collapse. In drug deliria, immediate withdrawal of drugs is always indicated. (In paraldehyde, chloral hydrate, and profound morphine addiction, a delirium may start with withdrawal. One should not expect to influence such a delirium beneficially by the re-administration of the withdrawn drug — see Chapter XVIII). There are few drugs which we are able to force out of the body rapidly (e.g., bromide through chloride). The best way to remove toxins is to stimulate excretion and remove unabsorbed toxins from the bowels through cathartics. Another possibility is to bind the toxins in a harmless form to the body as is now done in lead poisoning. In some infectious diseases serum therapy (e.g., convalescence serum in epidemic encephalitis) influences the delirium beneficially. In infections and brain tumors, surgical procedures may be indicated. In marked delirious reactions, cardiac stimulants (caffeine) should always be kept ready. If some obvious cardiac lesion is present, digitalization is indicated.

The detection and correct handling of early difficulties in grasping and orientation may prevent the development to a full-fledged delirium. Our efforts should be directed to keeping such a patient in a state of ease. Any procedure which might confuse or puzzle the patient should be omitted or delayed if possible. If necessary, these procedures should be carefully explained. Feebleminded or suspicious persons need special attention. Physicians and nurses should be patient and willing to re-explain and reformulate. Removal to a new environment, e.g., to the hospital, or from one room to another in the hospital, or even only into another corner of the ward, is upsetting because the patient is not able to grasp the meaning of the change. Familiar faces of relatives and friends are reassuring, and a few visitors should be allowed. In marked delirious reactions with misidentification of people and situations, relatives whom the patient cannot recognize any longer should be advised to stay away. Frequent change of physicians and nurses is disturbing. The less one has to interfere with the patient, the less will his delirium increase. This explains why so many excited delirious patients quiet down in a short time after transfer to a psychiatric hospital where physicians and nurses are accustomed to deal with restless, irritable, and impulsive patients and where no sedatives are offered to diminish the patient's noisiness. The general rules of dealing constructively with such patients have been discussed in the chapter on excitements. Because of difficulties in grasping, such a patient cannot read or carry on a conversation. Manual occupational therapy, however, such as knitting or basket work can be used to great advantage. Even highly delirious patients may be able to do some work of this kind.

Every delirious patient must be protected against self-injury and suicide. This often occurs because of disorientation or because the patient, driven by fear, tries to escape from an imaginary danger. Restraint should not be used. The patient cannot understand the restraining situation and tries to free himself. This exertion is a greater cardiac strain than if the patient were allowed limited freedom in his overactivity, and frequently leads to collapse. It may be necessary to tie the hands of some patients to prevent the destruction of bandages, although as a rule skilled handling and constant supervision by the nurse makes even this restraint unnecessary. If prolonged baths do not influence the patient favorably or are contraindicated, I would prefer cold wet packs or thin dry packs to any type of restraint used on surgical wards. The general treatment which is used in many surgical wards, together with carefully selected sedatives (see p. 168), will produce sufficient rest.

When fear is a leading emotion the physician should consider the patient as being in distress and in need of reassurance. In the beginning, fearful dreams and nightmares distress the patient. These complaints should never be treated lightly or as an amusing incident. Fearful patients should be reassured and encouraged;

otherwise, panic outbursts which might have been prevented may occur. The fear may be vague and general, or definitely content-determined (e.g., caused by hallucinations or fear of definite persons). The physician should try to inject doubt as to the correctness of these observations instead of merely disputing them. Disturbing persons are best kept away. Delirious patients should never be left alone. At night, delirium is worse and these patients need more reassurance and closer observation at that time. This increase seems to be due to a biologic rhythm and is accentuated by illusions and an increased tendency to projection in the darkness. It is therefore frequently advisable to keep the room lighted until the patient falls asleep.

Mood and content must be considered. Besides fear, a depressive or elated mood is frequent. Many patients are suspicious or definitely paranoid with persistent hates and delusions. The hallucinations may reveal psychogenic factors which should be taken care of during the acute delirium and discussed with the patient after he has recovered. Much of the content, however, is more of a general type or specific to the toxin. Erotic preoccupations, homosexual or heterosexual, occasionally reaching the degree of an erotic excitement, are frequent. Nurses, attendants, and visitors who arouse sexual desires should be kept away or the contact limited as far as possible. Any medical procedure which might aggravate these tendencies, (rectal temperature, enemas) should be avoided. One has to keep in mind that sexual assaults may occur during a delirious sexual upheaval.

During the height of the delirium, the patient is in an excitement, constantly active and frequently inclined toward impulsiveness and combativeness. Prolonged baths are therefore indicated. They also stimulate the general condition and increase free perspiration and with this, the excretion of toxins through the skin. Most physicians hesitate far too much to use baths in delirious reactions. Cold wet packs can be well administered. Sedatives should only be given for the night and in sufficiently high amounts. Preferable are drugs which are excreted easily and do not accumulate in the body. Paraldehyde in high amounts (8 to 12 cc.) and, if necessary, scopolamine-morphine are advisable. Other physicians advise sodium amytal. The other barbiturates should not be used. If one uses hydrotherapy freely, restricting sedatives to the night, without trying to enforce sleep but simply to achieve rest or diminished activity, delirious excitement can be managed without adding more toxin through medication.

The physical condition should be treated carefully. Soft diet and vitamin supplements are indicated. Nourishment should be offered frequently instead of in a few large meals, and the patient should be urged to eat. Milk is especially desirable. Nurses should not try to enforce eating at special times but should make use of the patient's varying condition. Many delirious patients are suggestible and can be easily influenced temporarily. Tube feeding is not necessary as a rule, but should be resorted to without hesitation if the general physical condition demands it. It is usually easier done than was anticipated. Fluids should be given freely. Constipation is usually present and should be treated with cathartics rather than with enemas.

Delirium tremens, which is discussed first because of its importance in psychiatry as well as in general practice, offers a good example of the applicability of the above-discussed therapeutic principles. It shows the characteristics of all delirious reactions with relatively similar content in all patients; i.e., hallucinations of small animals and long thin objects, marked skin paresthesias probably due to peripheral neuritis leading to tactile misinterpretations and hallucinations, and neurologic symptoms. The delirium is usually occupational in character. The leading mood is fear, but in milder degrees is accompanied by euphoria which makes the rapport easier. Auditory hallucinations occur rather frequently and are not always a schizophrenic admixture, as is still claimed. They may be of slandering, threatening content as in alcoholic hallucinosis. Delirium tremens is not a direct reaction to alcohol but is due to the absorption of toxins from the gastrointestinal tract (A. Meyer) or from the liver (de Crinis), both caused by the prolonged and excessive use of alcohol. This toxic condition may lead to brain edema and increased spinal fluid pressure. It is also possible that there is an inability to absorb vitamins, which most alcoholic patients take in insufficient amounts. The sudden withdrawal of alcohol does not cause delirium tremens. Precipitating factors may be physical illness, especially infectious diseases, injuries leading to marked loss of blood, and brain injuries. In the past, the precipitating role of brain injuries has been greatly overemphasized and, in recent years, several authors have disputed its importance. This is of practical interest because many surgeons are afraid of sudden withdrawal and are inclined to offer alcohol to such patients in order to prevent the outbreak of delirium tremens.

In every case of delirium tremens, a careful physical examination is necessary, taking into account the heart condition, liver and renal damage, and signs of chronic gastritis, as well as possible injuries which the patient may have received during his delirium. The necessary physical examination and treatment can readily be done if the physician is at ease, reassures the patient, and does not try to go into unnecessary details. Immediate withdrawal of alcohol is indicated. Cardiac stimulants (caffeine) should be administered as a substitute for the stimulating effect of alcohol. Gastric lavage is indicated, not only to remove the unabsorbed alcohol from the stomach but also because of the chronic gastritis. Carthartics should be given freely (in cases of prolonged constipation, I would give one enema). Fluid intake, especially milk, should be encouraged. If offered in a suggestive way, most patients take enough liquids, whereas they may refuse a soft diet until the delirium has subsided. Carbohydrates should be given in large amounts and a high caloric, vitamin-rich diet should be provided. Intramuscular or intravenous vitamin medication may be indicated. The administration of sodium chloride, orally or parenterally, will help to correct dehydration and restore the normal acid-base equilibrium of the body. Treatment along these lines has been found to be useful in the large number of delirious patients treated at the Psychiatric Division of Bellevue Hospital (New York).

The patient should receive a prolonged bath as soon as possible, unless this is contraindicated by the cardiac condition. These patients usually want to get out of the tub but can, as a rule, be persuaded to remain or to return later. Any kind of restraint is contraindicated. Cold wet packs are rarely necessary. Hydrotherapy is frequently desirable during most of the night. Prolonged bath offers the advantage of good protection against self-injury and suicide. Paraldehyde is preferable to any other drug. In the past, sedatives have been given too freely. The observation that delirium tremens usually terminates in a long sleep led some physicians to advocate the administration of high amounts of sedatives to obtain a long sleep as soon as possible, in the hope of thus terminating the delirium. The result was increased danger of cardiac failure. Since restraint has been omitted and less sedation given, the mortality of patients with delirium tremens has decreased considerably.

Case 19:

A 43 year old man suffered from a perforation of his right eye while cutting wood on December 29th. He received immediate surgical treatment. Both eyes were covered with bandages. On the evening of January 1st, he was restless; at 2 A.M. he became delirous and tore the bandages from his eyes. He thought something was in the injured eye and tried to rub it out, tearing loose the stitches. The delirium tremens lasted several days, after which he recovered. This incident, however, cost the patient his eye. It could have been prevented if the physician and nurses had realized that occlusion of the eyes frequently precipitates delirium tremens in alcoholic patients.

Many physicians advise immediate lumbar puncture to relieve the brain edema. In some cases, it seems to shorten the delirium, but the observations are not sufficient to permit a definite judgment. In increased cerebro-spinal fluid pressure, 30 to 50 cc. are allowed to escape; where the pressure is not increased, 20 to 25 cc. is sufficient. In surgical conditions (fracture), where bed rest is essential, lumbar puncture is best resorted to as soon as possible. In other cases, more conservative treatment is preferable.

Delirium tremens usually lasts three to five days and ends in full recovery. An analysis of the factors which cause the chronic alcoholism is then necessary. This should be done in every case, even though the patient stays only a short time in the hospital. Without offering constructive advice for the future, one cannot consider the treatment more than symptomatic. A high percentage of these patients die from cardiac failure or pneumonia. A relatively small number of the patients who suffer for the first time from delirium tremens develop Korsakow's psychosis. This outcome is more frequent in recurrent deliria.

Case 20:

A 39 year old mechanic, who had been a social drinker for about twenty years, had begun to drink increasingly and had shown symptoms of chronic alcoholism for three years, as evidenced by irritability, anxiety features, loss of libido, and fine tremor. After a marked increase of drinking for several months, the patient suddenly developed (June 23rd) visual hallucinations (shadowy figures threatening him, birds and cats) and delusions that thousands of men were tearing down the city. He felt terrified, but when talked with was usually euphoric. There was marked difficulty in comprehension and usually disorientation to time and persons, mistaking them for his helpers. He reacted with brief sleep to morphine 0.015 gm. (¼ gr.) repeated three times. Admitted on June 27th, he was fearful, resistant, and irritable. His general physical condition was good but the heart was slightly enlarged and the tongue coated. There was a coarse, general tremor and ataxia. Tincture of digitalis, cathartics, and large amounts of fluids and prolonged baths were immediately administered. To reassurance he reacted well for a few minutes, but insisted on having to leave to save his family. Two hours after admission, a lumbar puncture was performed (slightly increased pressure, otherwise normal findings). He was quiet afterwards and two hours later (5 P.M.) went to sleep, waking up at 11 P.M. With barbital 0.6 gm. (10 gr.), he slept for twelve hours, dreaming he was at work. When awakened, he still had some slight difficulties of grasp which cleared up at noon. Afterwards he was clear but markedly euphoric and weak physically. His restlessness always subsided to prolonged bath treatment. Discussion of personality difficulties was refused. Before leaving the clinic (July 3rd) to resume work the next day, the patient had his illness formulated to him by the physician who stressed the effect of alcohol and the need for permanent abstinence, the need for overcoming his reticence and shyness with friends, and to find cogenial non-drinking companionship. Threatened by his employer with the loss of his highly valued position if he began to drink again and realization of consequent financial and social decline, this man has been abstaining totally since discharge, and has found new friends, cultivating church and recreational interests. Such a self-cure of alcoholism is rare, but occurs occasionally in self-assertive persons to whom the delirium was a frightful eye-opener.

A follow-up 10 years later shows that the patient began to drink again after a year, lost his position, and deteriorated rapidly.

The most important drug delirium for the practitioner occurs with *bromide*. It happens more frequently in the United States than in Europe, probably because the lower amount of chloride in the food does not offer sufficient balance to the bromide. Many cases are the result of administration by physicians; another large group are psychoneurotic patients who take one of the many bromide preparations to secure rest and ease. Bromide is a valuable sedative, and the possibility of intoxication and delirium should not interfere with its medical use. One should realize, however, that some persons show a definite susceptibility to bromide which leads to acute intoxication in the form of brief excitements when high amounts are given. Chronic intoxication and delirium occur easily with cardio-renal disorders and structural brain involvement, such as cerebral arteriosclerosis, which diminish the resistance. Chronic alcoholics probably have a lower resistance because of the cardio-renal and cerebral structural damage and the accumulation of two toxins. In all these cases, toxic symptoms or full-fledged delirium may occur when the bromide amounts to 150 mgm. in 100 cc. of blood, while the average person can stand 250 to 300 mgm. Epileptics have a high resistance to bromide. One of my epileptic patients had over 400 mgm. without showing more than sluggishness or ataxia.

The first symptoms of bromide intoxication are fatigue and sleepiness with gradually increasing ataxia. With accurate testing, we may find slight difficulty of grasp, retention, and concentration. With increasing intoxication, the neurologic symptoms increase. Skin changes (especially acne and ulcers) are not an indication of high amounts of bromide but are due to special skin predisposition. Early signs of heart involvement (weakness and irregularity of pulse) are frequent, and severe disturbances of the heart action may occur in cases of myocarditis and endocarditis. Further complications are poor appetite, severe constipation, loss of weight, and cachexia. Broken sleep occurs as an early sign. Most patients develop these signs of chronic intoxication along with apathy and dullness which may lead to deep stupor. A relatively small number develop delirium, characterized by clouding of consciousness, disorientation and difficulty in comprehension, marked fear, and dream-like hallucinations, predominantly visual. Colors, lights, and large animals are frequent as content. In many cases, psychogenic factors color the progress of the delirium and its content. The duration is ten days to two weeks unless constitutional factors (manic or depressive components) have a dominating influence.

In addition to the general treatment for delirious reactions, one eliminates the bromide by sodium chloride administration (6, 8, or 12 gm. — 90, 120, or 180 gr. a day, besides the usual amount of salt in the food), in the form of broth or capsules, and large amounts of fluid. The bromide level in the blood drops promptly with this increased salt intake and after about ten days, reaches 25-50 mgm., a negligible amount. Excretion is mainly through the kidneys and is therefore helped by increased fluid. A small amount is excreted through the skin. Prolonged warm bath is indicated to increase this bromide excretion and also to decrease the excitement and secure rest and sleep. Much attention must be paid to persistent constipation, which in one of our cases led to impaction. The removal of the feces was a serious problem in an emaciated and weak woman. Sedatives should be offered only at night. In most cases, few sedatives are necessary if hydrotherapy is used sufficiently. It is important that the patient take sufficient food. With the decrease of the bromide, the patients usually gain weight rapidly and steadily. In some, cardiac stimulants may be necessary.

A careful study of the factors which led to taking bromide is always indicated. Many patients took the drug to secure sleep or ease which had been disturbed because they were in a depression. After the clearing up of the delirium, the depression becomes apparent and needs to be treated. Others are unstable, psychopathic individuals or patients with hypochondriacal or hysterical complaints.

Morphine delirium is rare. It happens less frequently with the administration of morphine alone than with the free use of Schlesinger's solution which contains, in addition, scopolamine hydrobromide and ethyl morphine hydrochloride. Physicians are frequently unaware of the total amount of these constituents which they administer in twenty-four hours. When early toxic symptoms appear, especially restlessness and broken sleep, the amount of the drug is frequently increased to achieve rest and sleep. This illustrates the importance of being well acquainted with the early toxic signs of the drugs which one uses. The outbreak of a delirium can be prevented by an immediate change of the medication. In opiates (including pantopon, to which many patients are sensitive), restless sleep with fearful dreams increasing to nightmares are early signs. In an *opiate* delirium, marked fear and threatening dark hallucinations predominate. These patients need constant reassurance to prevent panic outbursts. The latter also occur easily with cocaine in very susceptible persons if they are offered the average amount after sinus operations.

Atropine delirium occurs occasionally in patients who have been given atropine for eye conditions. Children seem to be susceptible to it. The toxic symptoms are dizziness, dilated pupils, fast pulse, increased blood pressure, dry throat, skin eruptions, and tremor. When these symptoms are noticed, atropine should be stopped at once; otherwise a delirium may develop with marked excitement, fear and perplexity, visual, auditory, and tactile hallucinations, frequently leading to coma. Injections of pilocarpine and morphine are helpful in acute conditions but of little aid in the delirium which needs to be treated along general lines. If the intoxication is due to oral administration of belladonna, gastric lavage is indicated.

Paraldehyde delirium occurs usually during the withdrawal period but there are described cases which seem to be the direct reaction to prolonged administration of high doses. Because of convulsions, lumbar puncture is usually indicated (see Case 41, Chapter XVIII).

Chloral hydrate offered in high amounts over a long period of time leads to delirium which lasts about two weeks, during which the patient is usually quiet, watching with interest the many small animals and small men which he sees in his hallucinations. These hallucinations usually disappear after the light is turned on. In some, delirium tremens-like reactions develop; in others, affective features (anxiety and depression) predominate. Cardiac stimulation is important. Gastric lavage is indicated because of the irritating influence of the drug on the stomach. Chloral hydrate delirium is rare. This drug is used less frequently than previously but is found in some preparations (dormiol, isopral, hypnal) which are used in psychiatric treatment.

Abuse of barbiturates rarely causes delirious reactions. If they occur, they resemble delirium tremens, often with convulsions. Acute intoxication (usually with suicidal intent) causes coma. The main features of treatment are gastric lavage with use of much fluid, cardiac stimulation, and diuretics. In abrupt withdrawal of barbiturates in patients who have been dependent on this drug, there may result one or more convulsions which can be readily controlled by phenobarbital. As a rule, it is best to consider the occurrence as an incident which should not interfere with the treatment planned.

Among other exogenic toxic delirious reactions, lead and carbon monoxide poisoning are of considerable importance. The earliest symptoms of chronic lead poisoning are fatigue and vague physical complaints. Signs of encephalopathia and epileptic convulsions may not occur until years later. Epileptic convulsions are occasionally followed by delirious reactions similar to epileptic delirium, i.e., marked fear, terrifying and fantastic visual hallucinations, and outbursts of sudden violence. In an epileptic delirium, the patients must be carefully guarded. Prolonged warm baths are helpful. Careful observation is, however, important to protect the patient from drowning in case he has a convulsion while in the bath. Anticonvulsive medication is of little avail during the delirium and is best omitted. If status epilepticus occurs, the treatment outlined in Chapter XIV is indicated. It is advisable to interfere with the activities of an epileptic delirious patient as little as possible because he may easily react with violent outbursts. These patients are usually preoccupied with their hallucinations and delusions. It is striking to note how, under careful psychotherapeutic attention, such a patient can be more or less well managed, while during a previous delirium, when the personality factors were neglected, he was violent and dangerous.

Another type of lead delirium is chronic, often with paranoid delusions and fantastic misinterpretation of paresthesias. When excited and irritable, these patients usually react well to bed rest and hydrotherapy. Otherwise they should be induced to join in a full routine. Occupational therapy and group contact distract them from their hallucinations and paresthesias. In recent years, many authors have urged that every effort should be made to facilitate precipitation of lead in the bones. Some advise the administration of calcium lactate 2.0 gm. (30 gr.) daily and a milk diet. Others stress that improved calcification occurs only if the phosphorus in the diet is proportionately high. As milk contains both calcium and phosphorus, milk diet is most helpful. The older treatment of trying to "de-lead" the body by mobilizing the lead from the bones and accelerating its excretion should not be carried out as long as there is any clinical manifestation of lead intoxication.

Carbon monoxide intoxication occurs in special occupational groups and is increasingly frequent in suicidal attempts. The treatment of the acute intoxication is well outlined in medical text-books. The outcome is recovery, chronic apathetic reactions with memory difficulties, or a chronic delirious or Korsakow state. Less known is that a few weeks after apparent recovery from an acute intoxication, a delirium with excitement and tendency to violence may occur. Hospitalization is then necessary for the protection of the patient and others and for opportunity for hydrotherapy.

Other toxic reactions show little specificity and their treatment is along general therapeutic lines of these psychopathologic reactions. *Fever* delirium is frequent but usually lasts only a short time and is not difficult to manage. In typhoid fever three stages are distinguished: the initial, the fever, and the collapse delirium. The initial deliria show a high mortality. When convulsions occur, lumbar puncture is indicated. The delirious reactions in the various infectious diseases offer no special therapeutic points. Exhaustion deliria are relatively frequent. A discussion of the various other groups is omitted as they do not offer anything new.

Cardiac and uremic deliria are of importance. In these reactions, the physician still shrinks too much from the use of hydrotherapy and offers too many drugs which frequently increase the delirium. In cardiac patients, anxiety plays a considerable role but actual panic reactions are rare when the patient receives individual psychotherapeutic attention. French authors stress that depressive features occur relatively frequently and urge suicidal protection. This is especially important when definite fear, which might climax in a panic outburst, has developed. In the cardiac delirium, anxiety and fear and therefore a tendency to panic reactions with paranoid features are frequent. Most of these climaxes can be prevented by careful individual handling. With improvement of the cardiac condition the patient's delirium often improves rapidly. Frequently deliria do not develop immediately with decompensation but a few days later, often when the edematous fluid is excreted rapidly under the influence of digitalis. In the treatment of cardiac disorders, all these factors should be considered. The physician should always try to prevent marked delirious reactions by adjustment of the hospital routine and increased attention to reassurance. It is frequently impossible to state to what extent cerebral arteriosclerosis is a factor. Such a complication may lead to a guarded prognosis but does not necessarily indicate a chronic organic psychosis.

In renal disorders, delirious reactions are frequent, both the somnolent and the excited types. When convulsions occur, lumbar puncture is advisable.

Eclampsia delirium is usually similar to epileptic delirium. Besides the usual treatment for eclampsia, good results are obtained with the administration of chloral hydrate.

Puerperal psychoses comprise many different reactions besides toxic delirium — depressions, manic excitements, panics, schizophrenic, and psychoneurotic reactions. It is always essential that one study carefully the whole situation and consider the psychogenic factors in the treatment of these psychoses. Pregnancy and delivery frequently present highly complicated situations. The physician will be able to give advice with regard to future pregnancies and childbirth only if he has gained a clear understanding of all the situational personality factors involved. In a small number of cases, there exists a probability of recurrence. Attention to the factors which had played a role will frequently allow the physician to prevent a psychotic reaction to another childbirth.

Postoperative psychoses also form a heterogeneous group, delirious reactions among them. Here again the whole situation must be studied — the patient's attitude to the operation and the various organogenic factors. The treatment is therefore necessarily individually different. In some cases, psychogenic factors play an important role; in others fear is the dominant factor. Drugs aggravate the condition. Infections and the absorption of toxins are only some of the etiological factors in postoperative deliria. Instead of discussing the many possibilities and their treatment, I present the trying illness of the following patient as an illustration:

Case 21:

On a 55 year old widow, a thyroidectomy had been performed after a year of definite symptoms of hyperthyroidism with mild depressive symptoms and slight suspiciousness. A few days after uneventful recovery her sleep became disturbed by nightmares, and increasing fears, grasping difficulties and disorientation, and restlessness with definite elation developed. There were many fearful illusions.

Bromide 1.3 gm. (20 gr.) twice a day and luminal .06 gm. (1 gr.)

twice a day helped a few days but then the patient became combative and screamed. Nevertheless, medication was continued. On admission, the patient complained of being "tested," of feeling as if she were drifting off and going to heaven. Her mood varied but was frequently definitely elated with flight of ideas, often with a tendency to perseveration and marked suspicion to medical treatment, resulting in combativeness. There were often periods of panic in which she feared she was losing her mind. Her physical condition was good. The blood contained 150 mgm. of bromide.

This patient had always been a cheerful and sociable, well-liked person, but because of various physicians' doubtful treatment of her husband's drug addiction over twenty years, which led to a vast expenditure of his previously considerable wealth, she had developed a marked distrust of physicians and medical treatment. There was a definite depressive heredity.

Keeping all these factors in mind (toxic, situational, and personality-determined), we considered psychotherapy of utmost importance to secure ease and co-operation for treatment. Every procedure was carefully and repeatedly explained and when she was combative, physician and nurses tried to alleviate the fears. Visits of one dependable relative were used to increase our rapport but not allowed too frequently because they excited the patient. Nurses with similar interests to hers had been carefully selected according to personalities which would have appealed to her when well. Even during the confused phase, but especially at the periods of relative clearness which occur in every delirium, she was encouraged to participate in occupations and games. Her paranoid misinterpretations were treated by injecting doubt into their correctness and by advising discussions in order to be sure of gaining an objective understanding. Bed rest was advised but not enforced. Continuous baths were helpful for an hour, then usually terminated because of her unwillingness to remain, and were repeated again after a few hours. Cold wet packs, to which the patient reacted well, were rarely given because this type of treatment puzzled her. Fluid diet, offered in small amounts but at frequent intervals and especially when she was less disturbed, was taken in sufficient amount and led to steady increase of weight after the first week. Because of the bromide content, which was considered an aggravating factor, sodium chloride 8.0 gm. (120 gr.) was given twice daily in capsules for two weeks (the bromide had then dropped to 50 mgm.). The bowels were controlled with white oil. Paraldehyde (6 to 8 cc.) was taken by mouth and this, together with baths around 10 P.M., secured rest, and after a week, five to six hours' sleep. Cardiac medication was unnecessary.

After about four weeks, the manic features subsided and were followed by a phase of about six weeks' duration which was primarily characterized by fear, suspiciousness, and aversion to the physicians and nurses. Frequent brief panic outbursts, during which she had hallucinations of men threatening her, occurred. Her mood was occasionally definitely depressed and she expressed ideas of unworthiness. Periods of clearness became more frequent and longer, and were utilized psychotherapeutically. Gradually a rapport which carried into the delirious periods was established. Most outstanding was perplexity which warned us not to expose the patient to any new situation. We were, however, able to let her take frequent brief walks. Small amounts of barbital 0.3 gm. (5 gr.) three times a day were not helpful and were discontinued after a short time. Prolonged bath treatment, especially before retiring, was sufficient to secure good sleep.

During the last four months of her hospital stay, the symptoms gradually cleared up. Until four weeks before discharge, the patient had occasional brief delirious episodes and occasional slight panics. She complained of a tendency to confusion and difficulties in grasp and memory. Occupational therapy was therefore kept on a simple basis and general activities and contact with other patients only gradually increased. Psychotherapy was directed to an acceptance of these symptoms which distressed her greatly, and to a diminution of her great concern about herself, physically and mentally. Recurrent paranoid misinterpretations of hospital procedure were always attended to immediately (see treatment of paranoid reactions). Her illness was repeatedly formulated to her in terms which were understandable and acceptable to her. This was not done in lengthly talks but more by brief remarks which took care of situations as they arose. Prolonged baths were reduced to evenings (stopped four weeks before discharge) and no medication was offered. Frequently slight depressive periods occurred and the patient was therefore kept on suicidal observation. During the first few months she had been almost constantly highly suicidal, afterwards only during her brief depressions which were, however, not predictable. Four weeks before discharge, dilatation and curettage, which we allowed somewhat hesitatingly, were performed. Intensive psychotherapy in preparation for the operation and during the brief convalescence, however, made this an uneventful incident. The patient left in good health, in which she has remained since (eight years). The follow-up study shows that after another 10 years the patient is still in good health.

Organic delirious reactions occur after brain injuries, in the various types of meningitis and encephalitis, and in phases of the organic psychoses. The treatment needs to be modified according to the patient's general condition. Hydrotherapy is helpful and can be safely administered if the cardiac condition is carefully watched. In brain injuries, delirious reactions of various degrees may develop within a few hours or days. Frequently the delirium develops immediately after the surgical intervention. The necessary bed rest should be enforced through administration of paraldehyde and scopolamine-morphine. Careful supervision is necessary. For the preservation of the patient's strength, dietary regime and cardiac stimulants are necessary. Alcohol is contraindicated because the damaged brain is less tolerant of it and brief excitements or alcoholic delirium easily result. These patients react relatively well to psychotherapy which usually makes restraint unnecessary, especially if psychiatrically trained nurses are in constant attendance. In some of the protracted senile deliria with marked motor restlessness or excitement, small repeated doses of scopolamine 0.0004 to 0.0006 gm. ($\frac{1}{150}$ to $\frac{1}{100}$ gr.) three to four times a day are helpful.

The various encephalitic deliria should be treated primarily with hydrotherapy, especially cold wet packs. These patients, especially children, react well to psychotherapy. Some physicians state that restless, slightly delirious children with persistent insomnia obtained good rest with hypnosis. It is best not to offer too much sedation, which often increases the excitement. Scopolamine, which is used freely in postencephalitic conditions, seems to have an exciting effect in delirium. In epidemic encephalitic delirium, convalescent serum is said to effect sudden improvement. Symptomatic treatment is important (cardiac stimulation, diet, and care of the skin condition).

Psychogenic delirious reactions offer no special therapeutic problems which need discussion. Hospitalization is always indicated. Removed from the situation which provoked or fostered the reactions, these disturbances usually clear up within a short time. Psychotherapy is important in the treatment of these reactions but constructive analysis should be delayed until the delirious features have disappeared.

BIBLIOGRAPHY

1. MEGGENDORFER, F.: Intoxicationspsychosen. *Handbuch der Geistes-krankheiten,* Vol. 7, O. Bumke. J. Springer, Berlin, 1928.
2. WOLFF, H. G., and CURRAN, D.: Nature of Delirium and Allied States. *Archives of Neurology and Psychiatry,* 33, 1935.
3. DIETHELM, O.: On Bromide Intoxication. *Journal of Nervous and Mental Disease,* 71, 1930. (Includes an outline of a bromide test.)
4. BOWMAN, K. M., and JELLINEK, E. M.: Alcoholic Mental Disorders. *Alcohol Addiction and Chronic Alcoholism,* E. M. Jellinek. Yale University Press, New Haven, 1942.
5. STRECKER, E. A., and RIVERS, T. D.: Preliminary Report on the Adjuvant Treatment of Toxic States. *Pennsylvania Medical Journal,* 45, 1942.

Chapter XIII

PSYCHIATRIC DISORDERS WITH CEREBRAL DAMAGE

THE PERSONALITY'S reaction to cerebral damage and to brain injuries in general varies greatly. The essential psychopathologic symptoms are disturbances of the functions which are tested in the field of memory of remote and recent events, immediate recall, and knowledge or judgment. In slowly developing cerebral lesions and processes a more or less marked general personality change may precede the appearance of the actual deficit symptoms. In any case, the individual personality reaction to the brain damage colors the psychotic picture and may even overshadow the more fundamental symptoms. Treatment must therefore be individualized, utilizing whatever is available in the personality and environmental setting, and be concentrated on secondary features. One should further keep in mind that the functions of memory and judgment are not independent functions but are integrated in all personality functions and are especially influenced by emotions, attention, interest, and general grasp. Mild toxic factors or dietary deficiencies may add or increase psychopathologic symptoms. The surprising variability of the symptoms is frequently due to these factors and not to changes in the destructive process. Treatment makes use of these interrelated functions to a large extent.

One distinguishes diffuse and focal cerebral destruction and processes. The outstanding diffuse disorganizing processes are the senile, presenile, and allied disorders (presbyophrenia and Alzheimer's disease), general paresis, and Korsakow's psychosis. Other important involvements with more focal and varying diffuse changes are mesoblastic syphilis, arteriosclerotic deterioration, encephalitis, traumatic brain injuries and brain tumors. Many other brain diseases such as multiple sclerosis and Huntington's chorea must be treated along general lines as discussed below and will not receive special attention. The focal destructions and reactions will also be dealt with in the general outline. For practical reasons I discuss elsewhere (Chapter XVIII) that type of chronic alcoholism which leads to structural brain damage. A special chapter is devoted to epileptic disorders. They are not primarily destructive cerebral processes, but secondary lesions occur frequently, and memory disturbances and deterioration are therapeutically important features.

In treatment one must consider the specific features of the structural deficit and the personality reaction. The symptoms of the latter may manifest themselves before the specific organic symptoms become obvious. The patient becomes irritable, impulsive, moody, often anxious and lacking self-confidence, and self-control diminishes. His ability to work begins to suffer because of lack of persistence, apathy, or ill-planned push of activity. Complaints of fatigue and hypochondriacal preoccupations are frequent. Hysterical symptoms occur occasionally. Tics and stuttering, which had disappeared in adolescence, reappear. Relatively frequent are obsessive and compulsive symptoms and anxiety reactions. With the development of obvious defects in memory and judgment, these symptoms may increase and only begin to drop out with apathetic deterioration. In other individuals, euphoric elation with rather aimless overactivity appears early. Sleep disorders occur frequently. The patient often loses weight; sexual desire may be increased but potency declines. Head sensations and paresthesias may be disturbing. To further progress of the illness, some patients react with depressions of various types whereas manic excitements are rare except in the paretic group. Paranoid developments occur frequently. Schizophrenic pictures are rarely observed except in the presenile group. Delusions and hallucinations of any of the sensory organs depend on the personality involved but are rarely due to specific localizations, and are occasionally elaborations of specific deficits and physical symptoms. Epileptic convulsions are usually of the simple automatic type, with or without predominant involvement of certain parts of the body. Secondary development of alcoholism is relatively frequent. The course is progressive, leading to deterioration, but often because of its slow development, the patient may die before this stage has been reached. In paresis, spontaneous remissions may occur (4 to 5 per cent) and in cerebral arteriosclerosis a temporary disappearance of symptoms (lucid intervals) may take place. Our therapeutic approach should be guided considerably by the change of symptoms.

Etiological and specific treatment is possible when definite exogenic factors are at work. Syphilitic psychoses should always be attacked by specific therapy. In general paresis, fever therapy, especially malaria treatment, has proved to be of specific value. In both the mesoblastic and parenchymatous type, results depend on the degree of structural involvement and on the nature of scar formation. In brain tumors and brain injuries, the surgical approach is of essential importance. The hope of specific attack on arteriosclerosis has little support in modern medicine. In toxic conditions which have led to structural brain damage, e.g., advanced chronic alcoholism, the withdrawal of the toxin is important but most likely will not influence the histologic changes. The improvement is the result of the disappearance of general toxic and delirious symptoms. The treatment of organic psychoses is therefore completely, or to a large extent, symptomatic, adjusting physically what is possible and stressing psychotherapeutic modifiability with emphasis on re-education and occupation.

Much attention should always be paid to the somatic features. A healthy diet, adjusted to the patient's needs, and regular meals with additional nourishment in undernourished patients are important. Vitamin deficiencies should be corrected. Bowel movements should be regulated by diet and physical activity, and cathartics should be used freely whenever indicated. Abdominal massage may prove to be helpful in stimulating the activity of the bowels. Neglect of attention to elimination may cause impaction, especially in senile cases. Manual or instrumental removal of fecal impaction brought about by neglect may be hazardous in such cases. The weight should be maintained as closely as possible to the ideal weight with due consideration, however, to the patient's constitutional tendencies and general condition (e.g., cardiovascular condition).

Sleep disturbances should be treated by means of a healthy routine, physiotherapy, and psychotherapy as well as sedatives. We should not expect to obtain seven hours' sleep in every case, and should formulate to the patient the need to accept the idea of sleep reduction with advancing age and especially early awakening in the morning, advising him, however, to stay in bed to obtain sufficient physical rest. Many patients show a tendency to sleep during the daytime. This must be corrected through a well-planned routine. As a rule, when no special physical factors argue for the need of rest or sleep during the day, a patient with insufficient sleep at night should be urged not to lie down except for brief periods of rest. In senile cases with definite sleep reversal, i.e., sleep in daytime and no sleep at night, sleep education by means of hydrotherapy may be helpful. In other cases, a well-planned routine during the day and small amounts of opium in the evening, 0.03 gm. (½ gr.) by mouth at 8 P.M., or at 6 and 8 P.M., may produce sleep at night but should be discontinued after the desired result has been obtained. In restlessness and poor sleep a combination of scopolamine 0.001 gm. (⅟₆₀ gr.) with chloral hydrate .5 gm. (7½ gr.) or codein 0.03 gm. (½ gr.) is frequently useful. In the average case, occasional administration of barbital 0.3 to 0.5 gm. (5 to 7½ gr.) should be sufficient especially if one makes use of prolonged baths in the evening. Bromides (sodium bromide 0.5 gm. — 7½ gr.) are of value in minor sleep difficulties in old age, but are a toxic risk and therefore only advisable under careful supervision. One should always keep in mind that the tolerance of the damaged brain is greatly diminished and that toxic symptoms occur readily with otherwise normal dosage because of diminished tolerance as well as insufficient elimination.

Head sensations and dizziness, various pains, and gastro-intestinal complaints may necessitate symptomatic attention. It is wise, however, to avoid physical symptomatic treatment as much as possible, to use a well-planned routine of living and occupation for distraction, and to try to modify the patient's attitude to his complaints. The undesirability of symptomatic treatment, on the other hand, should not lead to hard and fast rules and to the refusal of relief by medication if the seriousness of the complaint necessitates it or when the patient's condition is such that no better results can be expected. Apoplectic attacks should be attended to by general medical treatment. The resulting hemiplegia necessitates attention to the general condition and to careful hygiene. Treatment by prolonged warm bath is of great value in all these cases. In all cases with partial paralysis, exercise and massage should be used methodically. This is also important in Parkinsonism, in which scopolamine 0.0006 gm. (1/100 gr. four times a day) seldom helps much (in contrast to its good influence on postencephalitic Parkinsonism).

Convulsions are best treated with phenobarbital 0.03 to 0.06 gm. (1/2 gr. to 1 gr.) three times a day, dilantin a daily amount from 0.2 gm. (3 gr.) to 0.6 gm. (10 gr.), or mesantoin 0.2 gm. (3 gr.) twice to three times a day. Attention should be paid to dietary adjustment, and prevention of constipation. Bromides should be given very carefully 0.3 to 0.5 gm. (5 to 7½ gr. of sodium bromide three times a day) and in combination with phenobarbital if this drug alone is insufficient (because of diminished tolerance the treatment varies from that of the idiopathic epileptic disorders). Precipitating factors should always be investigated carefully, especially the possibility of the use of alcohol to which the structurally damaged brain shows marked intolerance. Complete abstinence is preferable in all psychopathologic disorders caused by cortical damage and is indicated whenever the process has advanced to the point at which alcohol tolerance is markedly diminished. Nicotine should also be strictly limited. However, the physician has to remember that nicotine has a stimulating influence on peristalsis and that constipation may result from the reduction of smoking.

Nocturnal brief delirious reactions and excitements frequently react well to the administration of prolonged warm baths and small repeated doses of scopolamine 0.0003 to 0.0005 gm. (1/200 to 1/120 gr.) hyperdermically twice to three times with a two-hour interval, or 0.0004 gm. (1/150 gr.) four times a day by mouth. In some patients, reassurance helps to diminish the fear, while others react little to it. Protection against accidental self-injury and suicide is necessary. In prolonged deliria and excitements, the general treatment of these reactions is indicated. (Chapters VIII and XII.)

In habit training an attempt is made to correct or at least to improve and to prevent general habit deterioration and the more specific functional deficits. It is necessary to supervise and to correct lapses of general hygiene, and to regulate personal cleanliness, regular bathing and washing, change of underwear, normal attention to, and care of, elimination, and care of the teeth and hair. The patient should be urged to dress neatly and to be tidy in general. Table manners suffer early and interfere with normal group adjustment. In his general behavior, the patient should be made aware of difficulties and urged to correct them. He should learn to control irritability and impulsiveness and all the reactions which interfere with a healthy social life. Training, i.e., learning and repetition of newly acquired habits until they become more or less automatic, is valuable when definite functions have been impaired. Most frequent is the need for speech training which may take a considerable length of time and much patience. This training must be carefully adjusted to the patient's personality. Speech training is highly valuable in more focal involvements but should also be utilized in modified form in the other less generalized brain processes. In apraxia and localized paralysis, training of the functions involved, with utilization of interrelated functions, is frequently valuable. These procedures are discussed in detail under brain injuries and brain tumors (p. 339), where it is frequently of utmost importance to correct the impaired functions which are the residuals after trauma or surgical intervention.

Patients should be urged to follow a well-planned routine which utilizes their interests and capacities and takes into consideration their mental and physical handicaps. Planned occupation is important in early and deteriorating cases of brain disease. Keeping a patient interested will prevent a slump in his habits and distract him from his shortcomings. In advanced cases of organic brain disease, a simple but well-regulated life prevents more rapid deterioration and cultivates previous interests in general hygiene. Occupation should be very simple, but well-planned large hospitals show that some tasks can always be provided. Group life stimulates these patients in a healthy form. Supervision which can be easily carried out should always be combined with activity, play, and re-education. Taking care of these patients demands active and individualized planning.

It is desirable to keep the patient in his accustomed routine as long as possible, if he is willing to accept the necessary modifications. If this is not possible, e.g., where the patient is unable to accept curtailments which are necessary because of impaired judgment or because of danger to his physical health, or when the progressive deterioration makes it impossible for his family to bear the burden any longer, hospitalization is urgent. On the whole, especially in arteriosclerotic and senile cases, relatives shrink from hospitalization and try to live up to their high concept of duty. The physician must explain to them carefully the need for better planned treatment and must correct the impression that the patient is being "put away." Otherwise, many families will have their lives disrupted and will be unable to offer the patient as much as a state or a private hospital can. In many cases, outside adjustment is possible if voluntary or legal guardianship is carried out. Immediate hospitalization is urgent when a patient is a danger to himself (suicide, lack of attention to physical treatment and sufficient nourishment, poor judgment with unwillingness to accept restraining influences), or to others (uncontrolled anger, paranoid dangers, especially jealousy and sexual aggression). Occupations in which the patient exposes himself or others to danger must be prohibited. Patients should not be isolated except for brief periods, if necessary, or when uncontrollably dangerous to others, which is rare. Even then, attempts at re-socialization should be constantly undertaken. Bed care is indicated only for the treatment of physical involvements.

There is still too great a hesitancy in utilizing prolonged baths, which are helpful and not dangerous if the necessary precautions are taken. The temperature should be kept around 97 degrees Fahrenheit. Many patients react better to lower temperatures (95 to 96 degrees Fahrenheit) and the optimal temperature should therefore be determined individually. Constant supervision is necessary, and the patient must be removed if any cardio-vascular disturbances develop. The patient should never be kept in the bath by force. His physical weakness and neurologic involvements, often accompanied by restlessness and overactivity, necessitate constant protection from self-injury. Thermotherapy is usually contraindicated except in paresis. Physical exercise, walks, and games are desirable even in deteriorated cases, but are naturally adjusted to the physical, especially the cardiac, condition.

This entire outline of treatment must be combined with all the necessary psychotherapeutic considerations. An understanding of the personality involved allows the physician to utilize the patient's interests and to prevent many frictions by protecting his sensitiveness. It is therefore always important that one find time to analyze what causes irritability, anger, and impulsiveness and what increases excitements. Reassurance, based on a careful physical study and carefully explained symptomatic treatment, will temporarily alleviate hypochondriacal concern and many minor complaints. Obsessive-compulsive symptoms are best helped by occupational therapy and re-education, in which, however, one needs to be elastic. One should never merely prevent the carrying out of compulsions but should offer the patient, through brief and carefully spaced interviews, an outlet for his tension. Direct, and even better, indirect, suggestions are greatly helpful and may lead to success whereas an open discussion may produce arguments or antagonism. In few cases is hypnosis possible or successful. The best active psychotherapy is based on distributive analysis, which makes use of general life adjustment and utilizes "persuasion" (Dubois) and suggestive influences whenever possible.

Active psychotherapy along fundamental lines is rarely possible but should be tried in early paranoid and jealousy reactions. In depressions, the general principles for their treatment have to be applied. In expansiveness an elastic treatment, as in hypomanic and manic reactions, is necessary but with due attention to the poor judgment involved and the question of the patient's dependability. The symptomatic treatment of more incidental personality involvements demands much attention and, if successfully managed, makes the general treatment easier. I refer here briefly to anxiety states and panic reactions. Anxiety is frequently relieved by hydrotherapy or, when this is refused because of fear of it, by small amounts of tincture of opium. In panics the patient needs reassurance and protection and temporary separation from other patients and, if possible, hydrotherapy. Small amounts of barbiturates, which are helpful in younger patients in states of tension and panic, are usually of little avail in organic cases, but may be tried.

CEREBRAL ARTERIOSCLEROSIS

Arteriosclerosis of cerebral vessels and resulting deficit reactions may be one of the earliest symptoms of general arteriosclerosis. I have seen manifestations as early as at 42 years. The average age of these patients is 55 to 65 years. The earliest symptoms are frequently general nervousness, personality changes, head sensations, or convulsions. Sooner or later a careful sensorium examination reveals definite deficit symptoms which, however, vary greatly at different times. The memory deficit is usually more patchy than in the senile deteriorations and the progress less steady, interrupted by lucid intervals and sudden aggravations. These patients are generally treated outside of the hospital, more frequently by general practitioners and internists than by psychiatrists.

It is always wise to keep these patients in their work routine as long as' possible but with attention to deficits in judgment and ability to cooperate. Responsibility should be diminished to the maximum extent possible. It may be possible to relieve a patient from responsibility inconspicuously and to have it shared by somebody else. This procedure should be kept in mind with regard to financial responsibility. If it is necessary, a voluntary guardianship should be advised which should, however, be plastic enough so that the patient will accept it. When the patient is unable to accept the need for this legal guardianship, hospitalization may have to be enforced. If lucid intervals occur this arrangement may be modified but not given up entirely, as exacerbations may occur suddenly. The physician must emphasize these possibilities to the family and to the court, and must warn against offering the patient unlimited freedom of action and decision.

In the adjustment of routine, shorter working hours, if possible interspersed with rest periods, are advisable. Such a patient may well be able to do his accustomed work for two hours in the morning and in the afternoon even when the organic process is quite advanced, if the other time is well spent on planned recreation and physical rest. Social recreation during the daytime and in the early evening, e.g., playing cards, chats, walks with others, keep the patient's general interest alive. Hobbies of past years and various interests which have been neglected in a busy life may be stimulated. The patient should be urged to pay attention to personal appearance and habits. Constipation and sleep need to be regulated. Many patients must be warned against overeating. Alcohol should be prohibited (convulsions on an arteriosclerotic basis are precipitated by small amounts of alcohol) and smoking reduced to a reasonable amount. The sexual life needs to be discussed in detail, with due consideration of the partner's sexual status. In increased libido with decreased potency the patient needs to be advised, after careful explanation of general sexual physiology and hygiene, to use sufficient spacing in sexual activities and to avoid indulgence in sexual play or phantasies or frustrated attempts at intercourse. Avoidance of stimulating literature and separate sleeping quarters help to decrease the sexual urge. Cold sitz baths, especially in women, are frequently helpful. When danger of sexual aggression exists (exhibitionism; extra-marital relations; ill-advised marriage, especially one to a young person), hospitalization is usually necessary. Jealousy reactions are frequently distressing occurrences but may yield to psychotherapeutic discussions, at least to a degree which permits life outside of a hospital. This may be more easily possible if the patient can be persuaded to stay with another member of the family. On the other hand, a physician should not allow the healthy members of the family to suffer beyond reasonable limits. Impulsive and irritable patients may be a definite danger to others, which the physician has to evaluate carefully.

This brief discussion demonstrates the importance of psychotherapy in the consultation treatment of cerebral arteriosclerosis. Treatment may not only offer symptomatic relief but may prevent a more rapid decline. Situations which precipitate an increase in symptoms — strong emotional reactions (especially depression and worrying), mental strain, and physical exertion — can thus be prevented. The insidious onset of the personality reaction may be easily overlooked and minimized and the best therapeutic chances missed.

Nocturnal excitements, caused by outbursts of fear and brief deliria, necessitate constant supervision which, in the average case, cannot be carried out successfully outside a hospital. In such states, the patient may commit suicide. This danger is also considerable in arteriosclerotic depressions and depressive mood swings. When such a patient has an occupation in which transient disturbance of consciousness involves danger to himself and others, changes must be demanded (e.g., certain occupations in railway systems). Driving a car may frequently have to be prohibited.

Convulsions are best treated with phenobarbital and an adjustment of routine. Headaches and dizziness deserve attention, because the patient may be inclined to worry greatly about them or to make them the center of hypochondriacal concern. Cardio-renal involvements must be treated and special attention paid to the tendency of accompanying anxiety and fear reactions. Besides somatic treatment, all these symptoms should be influenced psychotherapeutically.

Hospitalization is usually less frequently necessary because of deterioration than because of inability to co-operate. Beginning apathy and rut-formation are treated more successfully on the outside than in the hospital, but to interrupt more advanced reactions of this type, re-education in a psychiatric hospital during a period of two to three months is helpful.

PRESENILE, SENILE, AND ALLIED REACTIONS

Presenile illnesses occur in the early fifties and are similar to the senile reactions of late life. The tendency to deterioration is usually more marked, according to the personality involved. Elated (euphoric) and depressive features may be dominant. Other patients react with acute excitements with fear and hallucinosis, leading to deterioration or death. Late catatonic reactions are not infrequent. In paranoid pictures one usually finds poor systematizations. Some paranoid delusions originate in misinterpretations of delirious hallucinatory experiences at night. Depressive delusional formation is usually accompanied by marked anxiety. Most presenile cases show an insidious development, mistaken for mere irritability, nervousness, or hypochondriasis.

Senile changes first become obvious in the increasing rigidity of the personality features and habits. The outstanding characteristics are inability to accept other viewpoints, a narrowing of interests and of the mental horizon, resistance to new ideas and the holding on to old ones. Orderliness increases to pedantic and set attitudes and habits, caution to suspiciousness, anxiousness to marked anticipation of difficulties and fear of the future, a tendency for saving to miserliness. The mood becomes labile, and marked negative suggestibility in general is combined with increased suggestibility to ideas and persons which appeal to certain strivings and interests. This is of special importance because money may therefore be spent ill-advisedly and the patient may be influenced in disposing of his estate in his will. Sexual urge frequently increases and because of decreased inhibition and defect of judgment leads to exhibitionism, sexual play with children, involvement with prostitutes, and ill-considered marriages. Because of such personality tendencies, relatives often ask for medical help, and hospitalization may be necessary when patients are unable to cooperate.

The increasing defects in memory for recent events may often be corrected to a considerable extent if the patient makes notes on scratch pads. With marked defects in memory, hospitalization may be necessary because the patient becomes irritated by it or blames it on the interference of persons in his environment. Many patients hide their deficit through confabulations. Impaired judgment is dangerous because it leads to poor decisions in business and investments, especially if it is combined with an urge to activity.

While some senile patients become apathetic, others become more active. Restless activity is frequently more marked at night and prevents the patient from retiring or staying in bed. A strict routine of living and small amounts of scopolamine 0.0004 gm. ($\frac{1}{150}$ gr.) before retiring or also during the day are helpful.

Persistent, marked emotional reactions, e.g., hate, yield poorly to psychotherapy but settle down readily if the patient is removed to a neutral environment (to a different family or a hospital). Irritability and impulsiveness or depressive moods are less disturbing when the patient is removed from the home.

Disturbances in orientation to time and place demand protection of the patient by supervision. If the family cannot afford this or if the patient is unwilling to accept it, hospitalization is indicated.

The practitioner must be able to deal with all these reactions. The psychiatrist is usually called only when the reactions are markedly advanced, or when obvious psychopathologic features play a role. Most frequent are depressions, with agitation or apathy, which involve considerable suicidal danger. Manic reactions are less frequent. Treatment then deals primarily with a secondary affective disorder (see Chapter VIII and IX). Delusions of a persecutory nature (e.g., ideas that somebody is stealing one's belongings), and of hypochondriacal type, are usually very set and are best treated by ignoring them in a well-planned routine and through reassurance whenever necessary. Anxiety and fear demand much reassurance. Small amounts of opium are occasionally helpful. Some patients react well to carefully adjusted prolonged warm baths. The restless activity of protracted deliria is occasionally lessened by administration of repeated amounts of scopolamine or prolonged warm baths. Such patients may often be occupied with simple tasks of a repetitious type, such as cleaning and dusting. In underactivity, which is usually accompanied by apathy, the patient should be continually urged to participate in some simple routine. Much can be done to occupy senile patients if nurses are untiring in their efforts and if the patients are grouped carefully. Patients who irritate each other should be separated. Isolation should be avoided except for brief periods of time. Re-education is important to correct increasing habit-deterioration in eating, dressing, and use of the toilet. Hoarding, uncleanliness, and untidiness should be prevented. It is frequently surprising to observe a marked improvement along these lines after such a patient has been in a well-managed hospital for a few days. Physical weakness and awkwardness may lead to self-injury if the patient is not carefully watched and helped. Various arteriosclerotic symptoms need to be treated, especially cardiovascular and renal complications.

The treatment of senile patients should be modified considerably according to the social and occupational setting. It is not wise to overlook these factors because the patient does not seem to be interested in them any longer. Environmental influences may be helpful or detrimental, and visitors desirable or undesirable.

Presbyophrenia and Alzheimer's disease present the distressing problems of chronic delirious disorientation and increased, apparently aimless, activity which persists even in bed. In some cases, scopolamine administration has proved to be helpful. With increasing deterioration these patients need much general nursing attention. In all these cases treatment in an open ward, with temporary separation when they are disturbing because of shouting or impulsive outbursts, offers the best opportunity for careful supervision.

GENERAL PARESIS (DEMENTIA PARALYTICA)

The invasion of spirochetes leads relatively frequently to parenchymatous changes in the brain, manifesting itself in the clinical picture of general paresis. What predisposing factors are essential is not known, and various investigators are inclined to different viewpoints, some stressing the probability of a special strain of spirochetes, others constitutional factors and special modes of living. Prophylaxis therefore has to be directed toward the prevention of syphilitic infections and to their early treatment.

The clinical picture varies according to the personality involved. The expansive (manic) form which was considered most striking at the end of the last century is perhaps becoming less frequent, and the most frequent clinical picture is now the euphoric and simple dementing form. Some patients react with a depression, others with paranoid and catatonic symptoms. Especially in beginning cases, the diagnosis of neurasthenia and hypochondriasis is often made. These symptomatic differences may frequently prevent an early diagnosis, which is essential for successful treatment.

In the average case, a personality change is noticeable early. The patient becomes irritable, restless, and often has excessive ambitions which he may show in business and in social life. He begins to take risks which he would not have done before. Some show a weakness of will and have a let-down of ambition and interests. Criminal acts may attract the attention of the family to the slowly developing personality change. Frequent complaints which bring these patients to their family physician are sleep disturbance, irritability, "nervousness," and depressed moods. Others complain of attacks of dizziness or fainting, transient double vision, and speech difficulties. Neurologic and spinal fluid examinations allow early diagnosis.

From about five to fifteen years after the syphilitic infection, the illness becomes manifest. This interval may vary greatly. There are described patients who reacted with an acute general paresis within two years of infection. The course is always progressive, although occasionally interrupted by more or less complete remissions of varying duration which may suggest recovery. In rare cases, the illness progresses rapidly and leads to death in a short time without being influenced by treatment.

The treatment of choice is fever therapy, the outstanding form of which is induced malaria. In recent years some authors have advocated a combination of malaria and penicillin therapy. This treatment is indicated in all cases of paresis and taboparesis where the patient is in good general health. If the patient is weak or undernourished, a brief period of upbuilding may be necessary. Contra-indications are marked malnutrition, marked obesity, active pulmonary tuberculosis, advanced nephritis, cardiac decompensation from any cause, and aortic aneurysm. Syphilitic aortitis with good cardiac reserve is no contraindication. The results depends on the extent to which the cerebral structural changes have advanced. Slowly developing cases of the simple dementing or euphoric form frequently reach the physician late. The manic-depressive forms offer the best prognosis. Paranoid and schizophrenic features frequently persist after the paresis has cleared up and such patients may then need life-long hospital care. In some cases, these features appear only after otherwise successful treatment. In the prognostic evaluation, the personality setting therefore needs to be considered. Juvenile paresis and rapidly advancing paresis are less influenced by malaria. Old age has frequently been considered a contraindication but the Viennese group has often obtained good results in well-preserved old people.

The infection of choice is benign tertian malaria, transferred from patient to patient. The necessary intravenous injection of 5 to 10 cc. of blood can be done at once by merely changing the needle to a sterile one if the patient and donor are in the same room. Otherwise, citration is necessary (1 cc. of 2.5% sodium citrate solution to 10 cc. of blood). Citrated blood may be shipped by air mail to other places. There is therefore no longer any obstacle to the wide use of malaria therapy. It is not necessary to take the blood at the time of a paroxysm. The average patient reacts well. Occasionally a second inoculation is necessary. In Negroes who are often immune to tertian malaria and in previously treated patients, quartian malaria may be used. One should always guard against accidental inoculation with tropical malaria and reject donors who may have suffered from it in the tropics.

The average incubation period is three to eight days, and patients should be kept in bed when fever starts (during the incubation period excited patients can be put in continuous baths). Many patients react first with a low grade irregular fever before tertian or quotidian paroxysms start ($104°$-$105°$ F.). If fever reaches beyond $106°$ F., it should be reduced by tepid sponges. Malaise, headaches, and in taboparetic patients, exacerbations of lightning pains may be controlled by codein and acetylsalicylic acid repeated not oftener than every four hours. Digitalization is indicated if signs of congestive heart failure appear. It is always necessary to watch the blood pressure carefully, and termination of the malaria is necessary if the systolic pressure remains below 70 between paroxysms. Marked persisting tachycardia during afebrile periods, indicating myocardial damage, also demands termination. Hemoglobin estimation and erythrocyte counts should be taken every third or fourth day, and the treatment should be terminated if the hemoglobin falls below 50 per cent. Nausea and vomiting may cause interruption if they lead to exhaustion, dehydration, and starvation acidosis. Enlarged spleen is frequent. In regular urine examinations, one must look for red cells (albuminuria and cylinduria are common during the febrile period). Catheterization, which may be necessary because of retention, has to be done with utmost precaution. It may occasionally be necessary to interrupt treatment because the patients develop marked delirious reactions with frightening hallucinations. Such patients may refuse food. In others, food refusal is due to delusions or suicidal desires. The frequently considerable loss of weight is quickly regained and no special diet is necessary.

Successful treatment is obtained with eight to twelve paroxysms. The malaria is then terminated by giving quinine 0.3 gm. (5 gr.) by mouth three times a day for two weeks. It is of no importance what quinine preparation is used and the inexpensive sulphate is satisfactory. Many physicians feel that a smaller amount of quinine (the above amount for only one week or less) is sufficient. If temporary interruption for a few days is desired, quinine 0.12 to 0.15 gm. (2 to 2½ gr.) for only two to three doses is sufficient. During convalescence bed rest for seven to ten days is indicated. Four to five days after completion of the fever therapy, Moore advises giving six injections of neoarsphenamine 0.3 to 0.6 gm. (5 to 10 gr.) at five to seven days' interval for antimalarial and general tonic effect. The whole treatment takes about six weeks. If the cases are carefully selected the death rate is low (1 to 2 per cent).

The clinical and serologic results are not parallel. The spinal fluid begins to change to normal after six months but this improvement may be delayed to eighteen months. The blood Wassermann may or may not change. The patient may show immediate clinical improvement and the best results are obtained within six months. There is still considerable discussion whether complete recovery occurs, but even the most skeptical physicians admit that with malaria therapy, remissions occur more frequently and are much longer than in untreated patients. In cases of relapse, the fever therapy may be repeated, but the prognosis is more unfavorable.

It is wise to be cautious in allowing a successfully treated paretic patient to resume full responsibility. Patients who do more or less simple routine work should return to work as soon as possible. One should, however, arrange with patient and family for supervision, especially in financial matters. Patients who occupy responsible positions should start on a modified routine and should not be allowed to carry out their previous duties for one to two years. A voluntary guardianship should always be advised, and legal steps urged if the patient is unwilling to cooperate. The marital partner must be told of the disease. In sexual relations, contraceptives should be used if sterilization, preferably of the patient, is not accepted.

In many cases, definite defects persist and necessitate further hospitalization or guardianship. The outstanding symptoms are lack of interest and spontaneity, dullness, emotional lability, irritability, slow motility, and difficulties in retention. In a few cases, paranoid pictures with hallucinations and delusions develop. This is a personality reaction to the fever therapy and comparable to similar observations after toxic-infectious psychoses. A large percentage of this group are chronic alcoholics. Definite individual prognostication is therefore not possible with malaria therapy, but this treatment should always be advised if no definite contraindications exist. In many advanced cases, the treatment leads to symptomatic improvement which makes hospital management much easier.

Among the numerous workers in this field, there are many who believe that the favorable influence of malarial therapy is due to the elevation of temperature above the thermal death point of the treponeme and its direct destruction by heat. Mechanical methods to produce artificial fevers utilize diathermy, short-wave radio, the electric blanket, the "hot box," and hot baths. With all these methods of producing mechanical fever, there are some favorable results secured in paresis. Some physicians using diathermy or short-wave radio, particularly, claim that these results are as frequently produced as with malaria. Other observers, however, believe that the incidence of complete remission in paretics treated with induced mechanical fever is slightly less than in malaria; that the remissions are not so long-lasting, and that the pathologic findings in treated patients do not show the favorable alteration of the psychologic process in the direction of a change from parenchymatous to mesoblastic involvement, as with malaria-treated paretics. The various mechanical methods are to be regarded as still in the experimental stage in so far as the treatment of neurosyphilis is concerned, with the weight of present evidence indicating that they are less advantageous than malaria. They do, however, serve a very useful purpose as a method of administering fever to certain patients in whom malaria is, for some reason or other, contraindicated, or who may be immune to tertian malaria, either racially (as in Negroes) or because of a previous natural or induced attack.

In recent years, penicillin has given satisfactory results in the treatment of general paresis, but not superior to those of fever treatment. Its administration has the advantages of shorter duration than malarial therapy, less danger in case of cardiac complications, less nursing care required, fast convalescence and therefore an earlier return to an active life. At The New York Hospital the total amount of 4 million units of partially purified sodium salt of penicillin in aqueous solution is given during the course of treatment. Individual doses of 25,000 units every two hours are injected intramuscularly during 7 to 14 days. Some physicians obtained best results in a combination of malaria with penicillin. In combined treatment, penicillin is given in the same dosage and started with the appearance of fever.

In advanced cases, permanent hospitalization has to be considered. It is justifiable to keep a quiet paretic at home if there is no possibility that he may squander money and if there are no symptoms which might indicate the possibility of criminal acts or sexual dangers (e.g., assault). Such patients should, however, be under voluntary or legal guardianship. The general treatment is then the same as in a hospital.

Hospital treatment of such paretics is entirely symptomatic, changing with the progress of the illness. Attention must be paid to general hygiene and diet. In the beginning of the illness the patients lose weight. After some time, they regain their normal weight and with the progressing dementing process they may develop obesity. The final stage is indicated by marasmus. In this stage the patients are helpless. Much attention should be paid to the condition of the skin, which is considerably helped by the free use of prolonged warm baths. In taboparesis, exercise combats atrophy of the muscles and ataxia very often to a remarkable degree. Trophic disturbances lead frequently to bed sores. Hematomata of pinna occur readily and are not an indication of maltreatment as relatives may be inclined to believe.

In the final stages, speech is not understandable and nurses and physicians must take care of all the needs which these patients cannot express. They lose sphincter control and frequently become unable to swallow. Intercurrent diseases such as pneumonia and skin infections caused by decubitus lead to an earlier death. Tube feeding may become necessary, and aspiration pneumonia readily occurs in completely paralyzed cases.

In juvenile paresis, hospitalization is usually desirable. Not only will the patient receive better care but his family should not be expected to carry this burden.

In mesoblastic syphilis, specific and fever therapy are indicated, at home if the patient has enough insight and ability to cooperate completely; otherwise in a hospital. The technique of treatment is so well presented in textbooks (Moore) that it can be omitted here.

INCAPACITATING NEUROLOGIC DISORDERS

In progressive neurologic disorders the patient's attitude to his incapacitating disease is most important. In these conditions, one is only able to offer symptomatic relief. Most important therefore is a psychotherapy which helps the patient to understand himself to such a degree as to allow him to lead a normal life as long as possible. With the progression of his disease he must learn to maintain an attitude of acceptance which is not defeatism or optimistic self-deception. He must have a routine which keeps him as active as his disabling physical disease and possibly-developing psychopathologic symptoms permit. It is essentially the internist and general practitioner who treat these patients. A long-term plan of treatment, which is adjustable to occurring changes is necessary.

The physician needs to study and understand the personality of the patient and of those in his immediate environment, as well as the meaning which the illness will have to them psychologically and practically. A good understanding of the living conditions is important. As long as possible useful occupation should be maintained and suitable social and physical recreation urged. Plans must be made early for the time when the patient is forced to retire to semi- or full invalidism. Interests which can be satisfied during this period of life must be developed.

In many of these illnesses, e.g., multiple sclerosis, psychopathologic deterioration will make the final phase easier for the patients but painful to the relatives. In other illnesses, e.g., the chronic stage of postencephalitic Parkinsonism, the patient must suffer through a long physical decline with full preservation of his personality. It seems indicated to discuss here the treatment of only this latter group, as the previous discussions in this chapter pertain to the deteriorating disorders.

The chronic stage of epidemic encephalitis is characterized by progressive Parkinsonism. The personality reaction may be that of the individual to his neurologic symptoms. In some patients psychopathologic reactions develop, e.g., reactive depressions which yield well to appropriate psychotherapy. In others, hysterical features, manic, depressive, paranoid, and schizophrenic admixtures occur. Apathy and attention disorders may present the picture of slight deterioration which decreases with suitable routine activities. Most distressing, and not very amenable to present therapeutic methods, are the lack of inhibition, leading to overeating, sexual overactivity and misdemeanors, lying, cheating, stealing, vagrancy, and increased impulsiveness which causes such patients to be restless, impudent, and frequently cruel and brutal. Many are in a euphoric mood which aggravates these symptoms. It is possible that prefrontal lobotomy may give relief in these patients as well as in those who are distressed by compulsions and compulsive laughing and crying. In all these patients, however, psychotherapeutic help should be offered first, followed by any neurosurgical procedure.

Treatment by drugs is well presented in textbooks of medicine and neurology, but not enough stress is laid on the need to study the individual personality. In advanced cases, re-education, which makes free use of planned suggestive therapy, is frequently easier in the neutral environment of a hospital than at home where many frictions exist. Hospitalization is always indicated where impulsiveness and lack of inhibition make dependable cooperation impossible. In other patients, distributive analysis and synthesis by means of brief psychotherapy is desirable.

Case 22:

A 16 year old boy had epidemic encephalitis, the acute fever stage lasting about three weeks. The month following he was restless, especially at night, and slept during the day. A year later he developed frequent attacks of dyspnea, especially when excited, and Parkinsonism (rigid, bent posture with diminished accessory movements, the jaw hanging down). Stuttering, which had been present since the age of three, increased somewhat. The patient was treated with endocrine preparations (thyroid and pituitrin), but showed no improvement. He left school and stayed at home, doing little, and only what pleased him. The mental examination (at 18, 1926) revealed intact intelligence and memory. He was a somewhat immature adolescent, considerably spoiled, without plans for the future, affectionate, his feelings easily hurt, inclined to sulk, and although sociable, having only few friends. The parents were greatly overconcerned and willing to cooperate.

During four weeks' hospital stay, the patient improved considerably with scopolamine 0.0004 gm. ($\frac{1}{150}$ gr.) four times a day, increased after one week to 0.0006 gm. ($\frac{1}{100}$ gr.) four times a day. At this time he complained of marked dryness in his mouth, difficulties in swallowing and reading, which promptly disappeared after the administration of pilocarpine 0.006 gm. ($\frac{1}{10}$ gr.) three times a day. His rigidity disappeared completely and posture and facial expression became normal. His attacks of dyspnea, however, persisted until the scopolamine was increased to 0.0008 gm. ($\frac{1}{75}$ gr.) four times a day (after another week). From the beginning, the patient had been put on full ward routine. In brief discussions in which difficulties in adjustment and undesirable personality reactions were discussed, the patient gained an understanding of his selfish and inconsiderate attitude, his lack of social ease and self-confidence, his sensitiveness to criticism and adverse attitude to others, excitability and impulsiveness. Plans for the future were made with attention to the need for a healthy routine and socialization. He was urged to take a job and not plan to finish high school and college, for which he was not fitted. The possibilities of and need for adjustment were thoroughly discussed with his parents. Stuttering which had diminished during the treatment was explained as a personality reaction.

After discharge the patient began to work in a garage, with the goal of having his own garage later. He felt well but the attacks of dyspnea still occurred about once in three months, usually when he was excited. Stuttering also persisted to a slight degree. Since 1928 he has been symptomatically well. He is now a well-adjusted person who is financially independent, successful as a garage owner. He still needs, however, to take the same amounts of scopolamine and pilocarpine regularly. On several occasions he tried to reduce the medication and twice stopped entirely but had to resort to it again because symptoms of rigidity and attacks of slight dyspnea appeared within a short time. Until 1935 the patient was seen once in two years for a control examination. Since then, he has been treated by his family physician along the above lines. In 1945 (age of 35 years) his Parkinsonism had progressed so that he began to feel tired, but maintained his activities. In 1947 (37 years) he was still able to work all day. Seen in several consultations he was able to to plan for a future with reduced activity. It was difficult to change his wife's attitude of hopelessness and distress to an acceptance of the inevitable fate.

The postencephalitic behavior disorders of children warrant special discussions. Such children are frequently in a state of overactivity. They may be euphoric, with persistence of desires and lack of restraint, doing impulsively whatever they like. Some are apathetic. Irritability and explosiveness make group adjustment difficult. Their amoral and asocial behavior should not be mistaken for constitutional deficiencies. Sexual overactivity is accompanied by marked lack of shame, which makes education to restraint more difficult. Intellectual deficits do not seem to develop except in the very young; where they seem to be present, one usually deals with lack of attention, restlessness, and forgetting of the previously acquired knowledge.

Education is of utmost therapeutic importance. Good results have been obtained by placement in carefully selected foster families, preferably on farms, and in schools, especially formed for such children. Such education should never take a disciplinary aspect. Many children are highly suggestible and suggestion is frequently helpful. Hypnosis, which has been advised to combat the sleep disorders of the acute and subacute states, is claimed to be occasionally valuable. More important, however, is the general atmosphere with a spirit of optimism which exerts its influence continuously. E. D. Bond and K. E. Appel, who outlined treatment in specially formed schools, stressed the need for long-time planning for nurses and teachers. Personality understanding is the basis for establishing rapport and education. In a hospital, schooling and recreation can best be supervised and adjusted to the child's needs. Constant super-vision, which necessitates a large personnel, is essential for good results. The teacher should correct lack of initiative by stimulating, rather than pushing; lack of originality by creating situations which offer opportunities for exercising it; inattention by frequent inter-ruption and avoidance of dwelling too long on the same topic, and overactive restlessness by keeping busy with extra work.

Correction of behavior needs to be carried out continuously. A well-regulated schedule offers substitution of activity or occupation when bad habits are observed. Tantrums and anger outbursts should be analyzed individually. Cruelty against animals can be turned to interest in animals. Sexual instruction, offered on a natural basis, and active group life will lessen the child's preoccupation with sexual problems, diminishing his desires, and making control more easily attainable. Sterilization is indicated only after educational means, carried out over a period of years, have failed. Castration is contra-indicated in children because of the undesirable eunuchoid person-ality reaction. It is difficult to find suitable schools for children with postencephalitic behavior disorders. It is not fair to send those with good intelligence to a school for feebleminded children. The above-outlined teaching procedure is fundamentally different from that of the feebleminded group.

Placement in foster homes, preferably on farms, is advocated by E. L. Richards, who has obtained good results in the training of such children, with a gradual development of a sense of responsi-bility to people around them. By explaining the child's personality and difficulties to carefully selected foster parents, there can be created an environment in which the difficulties which might arise are understood and a consistent but sufficiently plastic policy of train-ing adopted. Supervision by the psychiatrist, together with regular but usually widely spaced interviews with the children, allows cor-rections and modifications in the educational program. After years of such treatment these children will frequently reach a degree of stability which allows them to return to their homes and to assume an ordinary life. It is at present still difficult to evaluate what has been achieved with children who show marked personality changes but, in the average case, the prognosis is not so bad as has been claimed. In most instances, it is difficult to predict clearly what can be expected because one cannot determine how much is caused by structural brain damage and how much by poor training during convalescence. Constitutional tendencies (e.g., psychopathic personality trends) and early acquired deficiencies (feebleminded settings) will frequently make the treatment more difficult. Permanent hospitalization is therefore not rare. It is, however, undesirable to have children on adult wards. Children's departments have become an increasing need; each state should have at least one hospital equipped to take care of such children. Markedly psychopathic children, early schizophrenic, difficult postencephalitic and feebleminded children frequently must be treated in closed institutions. Routine and re-education ought to be adjusted to their age.

BRAIN INJURIES AND BRAIN TUMORS

In many of these conditions, acute as well as chronic, psychiatric attention is frequently of major importance. After successful surgical treatment one may deal with a focal deficit which needs specific and psychobiologic treatment. Similar therapeutic considerations are frequently indicated after lobotomy. (See p. 164). It is essential that a careful psychiatric examination determine the actual deficit and a brief personality study evaluate the resources and interests which can be utilized. An examination during convalescence is insufficient in many cases because the difficulties may not become obvious until the patient is again subjected to the demands and strain of his ordinary life.

Minor localized brain injuries rarely lead to marked psychopathologic involvements. Many personality reactions to the accident (fright, psychogenic, and hysterical reactions) and compensation neuroses are erroneously explained by a structural damage. It seems possible that transient local damage, localized in the frontal or occipital regions may manifest itself in apathy and the need for sleep. Treatment consists of bed rest. If epileptic convulsions develop later, phenobarbital is indicated. In all these cases, attention should be directed to prevention of the development of hypochondriacal and other personality reactions. In marked focal brain damage in head injuries, there may develop serious localized symptoms (e.g., aphasia), which need considerable psychiatric treatment during convalescence as outlined below. In the acute stage, excitements and delirious reactions are not uncommon. Concussion is characterized by disorders of retention and grasp, or delirious reactions which may result in the Korsakow's picture. Delirium tremens may be coincident with concussion. The factor of fright must be considered in all cases of brain injury.

The treatment of the acute condition is primarily surgical. Active surgical procedure is considered indicated by many surgeons while others prefer an expectant treatment. All such patients need rest and quiet. If delirious reactions develop, they may be treated with paraldehyde (10 to 15 cc.), chloral hydrate 1.0 to 2.0 gm. (15 to 30 gr.), and scopolamine-morphine injections hypodermically (scopolamine 0.0005 gm. — $\frac{1}{120}$ gr. and morphine 0.01 gm. — $\frac{1}{6}$ gr.). The maintenance of the patient's strength is achieved by soft diet and sufficient fluids offered at frequent intervals. Alcohol is contraindicated. Restraint is resorted to much too freely but cannot always be avoided if a patient tries to remove the dressings of his injury.

After-treatment rarely receives correct attention. The most important symptoms which should receive psychiatric attention are diminished mental and physical performance which may even reach the degree of deterioration, personality changes connected with the structural deficits, and personality reactions to them. Under personality changes are included irritability which easily tends to result in anger outbursts with lack of emotional control, impatience which is especially marked to the patient's own family, labile mood, euphoric and hypomanic moods, or apathy. The latter is marked if the injury leads to blindness and the patient becomes absorbed in his preoccupations. Because of sensitiveness to light and noises, patients refuse to go out on the streets, to movies, or social gatherings. Because of disorders of attention and inability or unwillingness to make a constant effort, reading may be difficult. In addition, there is frequently genuine apathy with lack of strivings and interests. Many have various subjective complaints, referring to hearing or visual disturbances, dizziness, nausea, sleep disorder, anxiety symptoms, and to the symptoms of mental deficit (retention and memory difficulties, lack of interest, attention and persistence in planning and actions). Intolerance to alcohol, and less frequently, to tobacco and heat are important. Some patients become sensitive to emotional excitement and strain. Among the somatic symptoms should be mentioned vasomotor disorders, whereas tremor and exaggerated tendon reflexes may be due to a traumatic neurosis. It is difficult to distinguish between what is directly referable to structural damage and what to personality reaction and general setting. The above-mentioned symptoms are not parallel to the amount of structural change and little is known about their relation to special localization. The development of the following are designated as personality reactions: affective and schizophrenic reactions; hysterical, compensation, and fright reactions; epilepsy, and reactions related to a psychopathic constitution. All these possibilities must be carefully studied if one wishes to carry out constructive treatment. Careful psychologic studies with special attention to vision, reading, writing, intellectual functions, actions and reactions are essential.

Treatment consists of attention to the somatic condition, re-education, and physical training. An individual plan should be outlined and there should be established a routine which is stimulating but does not demand more from the patient than is possible for him without feeling under strain. When minor reactions exist, treatment by consultation is successful. In advanced cases, psychiatric hospitalization is necessary.

Constant somatic attention is necessary and one-sided re-education ought to be avoided. Medication may be indicated for headaches. Sleep disorders are best treated with hydrotherapy. Psychotherapy should always be used to influence the somatic symptoms. Reassurance and encouragement are necessary and should be combined with suggestion and explanations as described under Dubois' "persuasion." For the treatment of convulsions see page 347. Structurally damaged brains are less tolerant to bromide and intoxication may occur. Some of the somatic symptoms may be relieved by surgical intervention.

Re-education utilizes learning and training. This is important for disorders of speech, writing, reading and arithmetic as well as for disturbances of retention, memory, attention, and intellectual functions. It is obvious that a physician is not equipped to carry out such re-education without the help of specially trained personnel. Special centers where this treatment can be offered are desirable. A careful charting is necessary so that one may see the progress, or how lack of progress can be corrected. These charts serve also to encourage the patient by offering him objective proof of his progress.

In an institution, group teaching with individual attention should be the rule and individual teaching the exception. In such institutions in Germany which were built for veterans, various methods have been well worked out. Re-education of occupation can be carried out in well-planned shops.

Physical training involves active and passive movements, exercise and athletics, with stress on group activity but carefully selected for the individual case.

In the postoperative treatment of brain tumors, the psychobiologic reactions should always be considered. Dependent on the results of the operation, these reactions may be of merely incidental or of major importance. Re-education and personality adjustment must deal with localized defects and personality reactions. The treatment outlined above with regard to brain injuries may be applied to brain tumors. Much better results may be obtained if these principles are utilized. Many apathetic postoperative cases and many circumscribed defects which the surgeon is inclined to discharge with a shrug of his shoulders can be influenced beneficially by re-education and life adjustment, carried out, if necessary, in a psychiatric hospital where a planned routine and occupational training are offered according to the individual's defects and his previous interests and strivings. In all these post-operative cases, attention to somatic complaints is necessary. Symptomatic treatment is, for instance, advisable to diminish head sensations. This is of even greater importance in inoperable, slowly progressive cases where palliative operations are also frequently indicated.

BIBLIOGRAPHY

1. MOORE, J. E.: *The Modern Treatment of Syphilis.* Charles C Thomas • Publisher, Springfield, 1943. (Includes a thorough discussion of the treatment of general paresis.)
2. KOTEEN, H.; DOTY, E. J.; WEBSTER, B., and McDERMOTT, W.: Penicillin Therapy in Neurosyphilis. *American Journal of Syphilis, Gonorrhea, and Venereal Diseases,* 31, 1947.
3. BOND, E. D., and APPEL, K. E.: *The Treatment of Behavior Disorders Following Encephalitis.* The Commonwealth Fund, New York, 1931.
4. PFEIFER, B.: Die psychischen Störungen nach Hirnverletzungen. *Handbuch der Geisteskrankheiten,* Vol. 7, O. Bumke. J. Springer, Berlin, 1928.

Chapter XIV

EPILEPSY

CONVULSIVE disorders, whether they be symptomatic or belong to idiopathic or essential epilepsy, must be studied and treated from a psychiatric as well as a neurologic point of view. Although the diagnosis is now usually made on a neurologic basis, psychopathologic findings should always be considered. They may be slight, or marked, or even present the leading issue. Convulsions are very disturbing symptoms but do not present the essential feature of epilepsy. Their suppression is in general highly desirable but the goal of therapy should be the adjustment of the patient to his illness as well as to his other problems, and to make him a self-reliant individual who can fit successfully into his environment.

Treatment must be based on the individual's psychopathology as well as his convulsive symptoms. Psychotherapy is therefore an essential tool. The plan of treatment should cover a long period of time and be dependent on psychopathologic changes or psychodynamic, somatic, or environmental factors. Modifications in treatment are evaluated.

The main symptoms causing the patient to seek help are convulsions and petit mal attacks. In considering epilepsy, one must exclude convulsive disorders which are symptomatic in toxic and neurogenic disorders (e.g., brain tumors and cerebral arteriosclerosis). In the toxic group, exogenic factors may play a role. In these symptomatic conditions, the treatment should be directed at the underlying causes. Personality factors are usually precipitating and not causative. It is wise to keep hysterical reactions separated from epilepsy. When they occur simultaneously, the different manifestations should be distinguished and treated accordingly. One of my epileptic patients, for example, developed hysterical blindness as a reaction to an unpleasant marital situation. This reaction was treated by hypnosis and a brief study of the factors involved, the whole phase lasting two weeks. Afterwards, however, the treatment of epilepsy was again the dominant issue. If such a distinction is not carried out, treatment will become unclear.

Etiological treatment is possible only where definite openings exist and will lead to relief along certain lines. This treatment, however, should be connected with a general treatment of epilepsy. The surgical removal of cortical scars in order to lessen the frequency of the convulsions and to control the persisting convulsions more easily is a symptomatic treatment which deserves to be considered in any case where there are indications of scar formation. It is considered important that one remove not merely the scar tissue but also a considerable amount of the surrounding cortex. Craniotomy for the extirpation of the lesions should be performed only when there is definite evidence of scar formation. Reflex epilepsy should always be treated by operative removal of the stimulating cause. Yet this is rare, being more frequent in children than in adults. On the whole, one should guard against surgical optimism and only resort to surgical intervention when definitely indicated. Metabolic and endocrinologic disorders are rarely of etiological importance, and many, hopeful for cures by such specific treatment, have been disillusioned.

Treatment deals primarily with management and control of the epileptic manifestations, and the adjustment of the personality along general and specific lines. During a convulsion, one should interfere as little as possible. It is best to let the patient lie in a position in which he will not injure himself, e.g., on the floor if he cannot reach a couch. To put a pillow under his head or a towel between his teeth will not always be possible. Whenever one tries to interfere too much, especially by holding the patient, the seriousness of the convulsions may increase and the patient become combative. Some patients fall into a sleep at the end of the convulsion and then need no special attention. Others are dazed and wander about aimlessly or have an urge to move about (epilepsia procursiva). These states are usually of a few minutes' duration only. The patient needs to be watched and, if necessary, urged kindly to sit down for a rest. He should not be held by force because interference with the automatic activity might lead to dangerous outbursts of anger. Hospitalization should be considered only if the patient exposes himself to serious danger during these brief states. Petit mal attacks at the time of their occurrence are best ignored by persons in the environment. All these patients, even children of school age, should be made aware of their manifestations and advised strictly to avoid exposing themselves to situations in which the sudden occurrence of an attack would produce a serious hazard. Occupations and athletic recreation have to be planned accordingly. No patients with attacks of loss of consciousness or of muscular control can be allowed to drive a car. This is probably the most annoying restriction upon which the physician must insist. It would be wrong to permit driving on the basis that an aura would allow sufficient time to stop the car. Most epileptic patients are inclined to take these hazards lightly. On the other hand, one should guard against making the patient an invalid. He should learn to deal with his epileptic manifestations in the best possible way.

The personality and environmental setting therefore have to be considered carefully. Many of these patients show a combination of general hypochondriasis and carelessness with regard to the dangers in which they may involve themselves and others through an attack. Others have a tendency to moodiness and discouragement. Their mood reactions have a tendency to persist and to lead to rut-formation. Reactions of sulkiness, envy, and resentment need constant psychotherapeutic attention. Sensitiveness to the behavior of others, often combined with tactlessness on their own part, makes group adjustment difficult. Impulsiveness and poorly controlled outbursts of temper are not as frequent as one would gather from literature. It is well to keep in mind that the textbook epileptic usually represents the more difficult cases of the hospital group. Consideration of the whole personality will prevent the physician from reaching too readily the conclusion that epileptic manifestations occur primarily in psychopathic personalities. It is essential that one investigate briefly all personality features and determine what can be used constructively for re-education through psychotherapeutic discussions and training. Each consultation must be utilized accordingly. Psychotherapy is important in every epileptic patient. It leads to a diminution of emotional factors which affect the epileptic condition unfavorably and helps the patient to gain a healthy attitude to his illness. He should become reconciled to suffering from a handicap which in the average case is not important enough to prevent a satisfactory life.

The environment may stimulate or increase personality difficulties. An understanding of the various personalities in the household and one's place of work is important. A change to a new environment may be beneficial when sufficient modifications are impossible. Suitable work should be found to avoid undue strain which precipitates or increases attacks. This does not mean that one should omit investigating the situation carefully to determine whether or not some adjustment is possible.

Much has been written about epileptic intellectual changes which incapacitate patients seriously. There is no doubt that slight memory and retention deficits of a progressive nature occur, often accompanied by increasing apathy and habit deterioration. These cases, however, form a minority. Whenever these symptoms are found, toxic factors resulting from medication have to be excluded. In some, aggravations of a temporary nature are due to postconvulsive lesions. There seems to be, however, a definite group with progressive deterioration in which hospital treatment or guarded family care is indicated. It is interesting to note that some intelligent epileptic patients develop intellectual characteristics which should be taken into consideration; i.e., a definite slowness in grasp and a frequently relative sluggishness of the associative functions, a tendency to overattention to detail, and an inclination to become lost in details of execution. Conscientiousness or insufficient self-confidence may increase these tendencies. In childhood and adolescence, difficulty in learning may be related to an insufficient ease in changing from one topic to another. These students are limited in being unable to incorporate new, with established, knowledge. A narrowing of interests, daydreaming, and essential attention disorders impede learning and may give the impression of inadequate memory functions. Self-centeredness and decreased spontaneity may be present. All these features should guide the physician in leading the patient to find the position in life for which he is suited.

Factors in the patient's personality and environment which precipitate epileptic manifestations and aggravate the illness must be carefully studied in every consultation. Some factors causing strain were stressed above. In addition, attention should be paid to chemical and physiologic changes, infections (especially in children), fatigue resulting from physical or mental exertion, and constipation. In many patients, one deals with spastic constipation which should be treated with atropine and enemas. In others, atonic constipation necessitates frequent cathartics and dietary adjustment (see p. 212). In many patients, fewer seizures occur during periods of freedom from constipation. On the whole, the physician should pay considerable attention to regular bowel movements but guard against fostering an attitude of overconcern to the functions of the body. Alcoholic beverages of any kind should always be strictly prohibited. Before and after menstruation, and during the pregnancy and lactation periods, symptoms are apt to increase.

Dietary and endocrinologic treatment has attracted a great deal of attention. Careful investigations in recent years have brought about some clarification. It seems certain that the influence of specific foods in producing convulsions has been greatly exaggerated, probably as a result of the tendency to generalize into broad principles observations on those foods which seem to have precipitated attacks in a few cases. A well-balanced diet containing plenty of fruit and vegetables and a moderate amount of meat is to be preferred. The belief that meat induces attacks cannot be supported. Specific restrictions of diet are necessary in rare cases where certain foods constantly bring on an attack, and when attacks occur only after specific foods have been eaten, or when bromide medication demands the avoidance of highly salted food. Over-eating is a more frequent problem than insufficient food intake. Starvation and the ketogenic diet treatment are valuable in some cases, although it must be admitted that the results at present are far less promising than had been anticipated. These procedures will be discussed at the end of this chapter under the section on epilepsy in children. In the adult, results have been, on the whole, discouraging. Endocrinologic treatment has been applied too freely. Here again, findings and therapeutic results obtained on a few cases have been generalized. It should be constantly urged that the physician be guided by indications which are based on clinical findings and not by theories. There are cases where calcium administration, thyroid, or pituitary treatment is indicated. In a few cases with morning attacks, we found a low blood sugar in the early morning, and that glucose administration (three lumps of sugar in a cup of coffee) before getting up decreased the frequency of attacks. These, however, are rare exceptions among the vast number of epileptics.

Therapeutic overactivity is dangerous because it distracts the patient and physician from what is essential and prevents the continuity of treatment which is necessary for success in these cases.

Anticonvulsive medication is indispensable. The control of attacks allows the patient to lead a more or less active and self-dependent life and prevents possible damage to the brain in the form of postconvulsive lesions. The disadvantage of making drug-sensitive patients sluggish can usually be avoided by individualized dosage. The possibility of permanent damage caused by histologic changes is rare, if it exists at all. The outstanding drugs in use are bromide, phenobarbital, dilantin, and tridione. All these drugs deserve separate discussion.

Bromide, the oldest anticonvulsive drug, controls seizures only after a certain level of bromide has been obtained in the blood. This level varies individually in a considerable degree. Bromide is retained in the body until a balance is established between intake and output. Chloride is replaced by bromide. The finally resulting chloride-bromide equilibrium, which is therapeutically effective, is easily disturbed by the increased intake of sodium chloride and by polyuria. It is therefore essential that a diet containing only a moderate amount of chloride be used to establish a sufficient bromide deposit in a short time and that marked variations in salt and fluid intake be avoided to prevent marked fluctuations in the body bromide. It is best to start with small amounts, 0.5 gm. ($7\frac{1}{2}$ gr.) three times a day, increasing after two weeks to higher doses, 0.6 gm. (10 gr.) three times a day, and after two more weeks to 1.0 gm. (15 gr.) three times a day if the bromide level in the blood is still below 200 mgm. in 100 cc. and the clinical symptoms are not well controlled. Through repeated bromide determinations every two to four months, one should be able to keep a steady bromide level, with medication given two to three times a day. It is desirable to keep the bromide as low as possible. In some patients, seizures are controlled by as low a level as 100 mgm.; in others, it is necessary to reach 280-300 mgm. One should not go higher, as otherwise intoxication symptoms might result. The amount of bromide to be administered to reach a sufficient level varies individually and according to diet.

Bromide medication has the great advantage over other anticonvulsive drugs of being eliminated slowly. If the patients, as so frequently happens, omit taking the medicine regularly, a slow drop in bromide occurs. At such moments, seizures may reappear but before they have reached a disturbing degree the patient will return to his medicine. There seems to be little advantage in using bromide combinations. The most satisfactory results are obtained by administering sodium bromide with some water before meals.

Bromide intoxication is characterized by sluggish thinking, sleepiness, and ataxia. Delirious reactions seem to be rare in epileptic patients. By adding more salt to the diet, increasing the fluid intake, and controlling constipation these symptoms disappear within a few days. In skin-sensitive persons, bromide acne occurs readily even with small bromide deposits. It is not a sign of intoxication and can frequently be corrected by applying salt water to the skin, preferably before retiring and in the morning, or by offering Fowler's solution (3 minims three times a day). In especially sensitive cases, ulcers may occur. In all cases of persistent acne or ulcers, bromide should be discontinued.

Phenobarbital (luminal, gardenal) is a most effective anticonvulsive drug. As a rule, convulsions are more easily controlled by drugs than are petit mal attacks. Average doses are 0.03 to 0.06 gm. (½ to 1 gr.) twice to three times a day. It is usually useless to go beyond 0.1 gm. (1½ gr.) three times a day. Phenobarbital is excreted relatively fast. The medication must be taken regularly. Status epilepticus may result if phenobarbital is omitted over a few days. Toxic symptoms with these small amounts of phenobarbital are not to be expected, even if taken over years. Some observations to the contrary, however, demand further studies.

The combination of phenobarbital and bromide may be desirable. In starting treatment, phenobarbital is necessary to stop the convulsions. When a sufficient bromide deposit has developed, phenobarbital can be reduced and then completely withdrawn. In some cases, continued treatment with relatively small doses of phenobarbital and bromide is most efficacious. Medication should not be diminished until the patient has been free from seizures for at least a year. Even then, however, one should not consider the patient cured. Many patients have free intervals from several months to years and then a recurrence. In evaluating improvement, attention should be paid to the general personality adjustment as well as the epileptic symptoms.

Sodium diphenylhydantoin (dilantin, epanutin) is an excellent drug for the control of convulsions, but is not effective with petit mal attacks. The drug is given in capsules containing 0.1 gm. (1½ gr.), the daily amount varying individually from 0.2 to 0.6 gm. (3 to 10 gr.). If burning sensations in the stomach are noticed as a result of the drug's marked alkalinity, the capsules should be taken between meals. A mild toxic symptom, which usually disappears in a few days, is dizziness. Fever and rash in children, and hypertrophy of the gums are considered by most authors an indication to change to phenobarbital. In recent years methylphenylethylhydantoin (mesantoin) has been recommended because it lacks the danger of gum hypertrophy and muscular incoordination. The doses are 0.1 gm. (1½ gr.) two to four times a day in children, and 0.2 gm. (3 gr.) twice to three times a day in adults. It will, however, be wise to start in adults with 0.1 gm. three times a day and increase gradually to higher dosage by adding 0.1 gm. a week. Skin rashes may be a toxic symptom. Trimethyloxazolidinedione (tridione) is effective in the control of petit mal attacks, pyknolepsy, myoclonic jerking, and akinetic seizures. The results in psychomotor attacks are less satisfactory. The amounts administered are 0.3 (5 gr.) four to five times a day. Toxic symptoms are mild, consisting of fatigue, drowsiness, occasionally blurring of the vision, sensitiveness to light, or skin eruption. The therapeutic significance of these symptoms depends on the patient's reaction to them.

In cases where convulsions occur during sleep, chloral hydrate 0.5 gm. (7½ gr.) is helpful. I have given it for months without observing any damage. Other drugs which are advertised so freely can be dispensed with completely.

In status epilepticus, on the neurologic pavilion of The New York Hospital sodium phenobarbital 0.26 gm. (4 gr.) is administered intravenously at once, and 0.13 gm. (2 gr.) given intravenously every half hour for a total of six injections. If this procedure does not bring about cessation of the convulsion, the patient should receive a general anesthesia (ether or avertin). After termination of the status epilepticus, sodium phenobarbital in doses of 0.06 gm. (1 gr.) or 0.03 gm. (½ gr.) should be administered subcutaneously. The dose should be lowered gradually over a period of several days until a maintenance dose has been obtained. As soon as possible one should transfer to oral therapy.

In fugue attacks and twilight states, protection of the patient is necessary. An increase of drugs does not influence them much. At night, hypnotics are indicated. Most patients can be handled well on the outside and hospital care is only indicated if they are of long duration or if the patient commits dangerous acts in them. Patients in delirious excitements, on the other hand, should be treated in a hospital (see Chapter XII) because they may harm themselves, and especially because they are frequently dangerous to others. Impulsive and automatic acts of psychopathic individuals necessitate prolonged, if not permanent, hospital care. Some of these cases react well to drugs, others little. In the latter, the main emphasis should be laid on re-education which is successful if a good and lasting rapport can be established.

Psychotherapy is essential in every epileptic condition. In many patients, dynamic factors are of considerable importance. An analysis which is distributed along the lines of the difficulties, together with careful investigation of the personality is indicated. In the analytic procedure, one should be guided by the personality setting and guard against going into material with which the patient cannot deal constructively. This warning is especially important in the sexual realm. As a result of claims that the basis for some epileptic conditions is found in sexual maladjustments, many physicians have pushed their therapeutic investigations in this direction as far as possible. The result is frequently a sexual upheaval or stirring up of sexual preoccupations which do not subside later and which give a peculiar and aggravating picture to these cases for years. There are cases where such an analysis can be carried out constructively but they are far less frequent than is assumed by many. As a rule one should combine a study of the personality with continued efforts at re-education. A routine which balances work and recreation and does justice to somatic necessities is of utmost importance. Much attention should be paid to the environmental and work settings, evaluating the various personalities with whom the patient comes in contact regularly, and showing how friction or sympathetic and solicitious overattention can be avoided.

Brief or infrequent psychotherapeutic interviews are frequently the best method in dealing with particular problems which should be corrected. The psychopathologic findings will guide the physician in pursuing his long-term therapeutic plan and in modifying his technique. Dynamic analysis may have to be curtailed because of the patient's intellectual difficulties. Pathologic persistence of emotions may prevent a satisfactory catharsis. One should guard against repetitious discussions which might strengthen undesirable emotions. A physician will have little difficulty in establishing a durable relationship if he shows patience and sympathy and understands the patient's personality. His interviews should be directed to an understanding of the patient's personality development and the personality features present during the varying phases of a treatment, which may last a life time. Factors of interpersonal relationships referring to family, community, and work conditions deserve constant scrutiny. Depending on the patient, advice may be offered in the form of suggestions or in direct form. At the end of a lengthy interview, a concise summary is indicated because of the patient's difficulty in distinguishing between the essential and non-essential. The persistence of his emotions and interests makes him forget readily such conclusions which have to be brought to his attention again and frequently re-analyzed in subsequent interviews. Shortened interviews are possible when the physician has become intimately acquainted with the patient's life, the personalities in it, and repetitive emotional reactions. Although treatment over a period of years is necessary, undue dependence on the physician should be avoided and constant effort maintained to have the patient assume increasing responsibility. The gradual change from apparent immaturity to self-reliance with increasingly better socialization represents genuine improvement. The discussion of brief psychotherapy on page 111 gives an outline which can be used in a long-term therapeutic plan if one recognizes the changing psychopathology. The following case offers an illustration.

Case 23:

The case of this 39 year old lawyer is presented as a demonstration of long-term treatment in which brief psychotherapy is combined with bromide treatment. If treatment had been started in recent years, tridione would have been administered. Considering the satisfactory adjustment with relatively small amounts of sodium bromide, no advantage would have been gained by changing the drug.

In 1930, the patient, then a 22 year old college student was referred to me for the treatment of convulsions. The attacks started at the age of 8, occurring for a few years only at night but in later years also in the daytime. Several times a week he experienced brief petit mal attacks. At other times these attacks were more marked, when his head would turn to the right and he had the experience of strangers appearing familiar to him. Convulsions occurred about four times a year and were always preceded by a vague aura which permitted him to protect himself. Phenobarbital helped little. The patient used laxatives freely because constipation seemed to provoke convulsions. He avoided pork and carbohydrate-rich foods.

This intelligent patient presented his illness and the pertinent facts of his life in a very circumstantial way. He spoke slowly and his voice lacked modulation. His understanding of his own personality was very slight. Although he gave illustrations which revealed him to be overly exacting in his work and very sensitive to slights by others, he denied these features. He did not recognize his inability to differentiate satisfactorily between the essential and non-essential. Although he was somewhat tactless, he was well liked and sociable. Usually cheerful, he had noticed a tendency to moodiness in the preceding two years. He was a good athlete. His illness had led to marked body overconcern. He began to feel inadequate in work and social situations whereas previously he had been self-confident. His sexual life did not present a problem. After an adolescent period of masturbation, at 18 he began to have infrequent sexual intercourse with friends. When he entered college at 17, he had considerable difficulty in adjusting to campus life. After a year he felt part of the group and studied well, entering law school at 22. His father died when he was 10 and he and a brother, who was two years his senior, were brought up by a self-reliant mother who has always worried a great deal about the patient's health.

Although the patient had been studied satisfactorily by a neurologist the previous year, a careful general physical and neurologic examination seemed indicated in order to establish the basis for a good patient-physician relationship. The completely negative examination permitted the physician to offer strong re-assurance and to advise the patient to eat a normal diet. It was stressed that more bulky food and physical activity with moderate amounts of laxative would permit control of his constipation. A careful psychiatric examination was used to point out his good intellectual functioning and recent difficulties in studying were related to anxiety about his condition. The undesirability of self-analysis was brought to his attention. Based on life incidents he had mentioned, a discussion ensued as to what extent attention to details and over-exactness as well as social sensitivities might not be important features. Recognizing his defense attitude in these psychologic discussions, the physician pointed out possibilities in his personality and avoided singling out his readiness to react with resentment.

The patient was seen in three one-hour interviews. In the last interview, the therapeutic goals were formulated as a change in his attitude to his illness, a better integration with the group, a need to recognize his emotional reactions, and a control of his convulsions by medication. He returned to school where he was seen irregularly by the college physician. The patient wrote on several occasions with regard to taking his sodium bromide 1.0 gm. (15 gr.) twice a day which controlled his convulsions well with blood level of 175-200 mgm. of sodium bromide in 100 cc. of blood. He returned every summer for two or three interviews, in which his personality adjustment was reviewed. His mother's financial losses forced him in to law practice earlier than had been anticipated. From 1931 to 1935 his relationship to his over-concerned mother was studied and he gradually became self-reliant but remained too attached to her. It was necessary to urge him into a healthy and expanding socialization. He became aware of his tendency to be too saving because of his insecurity and his anxiety to offer his mother as much comfort as possible. In 1934 he reached a point in which he considered his illness a handicap which would not allow life success. He learned to be less self-centered and to disregard minor body discomfort. The occurrence of a convulsion after an appendectomy in 1934 did not upset him. The advice was given to postpone marriage plans until he felt competent to have a family without too great a strain. Heredity influences were minimized in his case, but the increased amount of responsibility, financial and otherwise, was stressed.

In 1936 he felt ready to take part in public affairs. After a period of strenuous court trials he reacted with several convulsions on the evening of the last day of court. The need for a better balance of recreation and rest and for a curtailment of his high ambitions was reviewed. He had become desensitized to the occurrence of the convulsions and recognized that even this unfortunate handicap did not affect his professional and social standing. Advice was usually put to him in the form of questions for which he was to find his own answers for a basis of his decisions. In 1937 several interviews were devoted to analyzing the girl he thought of marrying. He recognized that he had selected her because she had a protective attitude like his mother but had little in common with him. This marriage would have rendered unnecessary his constant efforts at the modification of undesirable personality traits. He had become aware of the tendency of his emotions to persist a long time, leading to unwholesome resentments and to becoming too devoted to those whom he liked. Although he had learned to guard against undue attention to details, this trait made him slow in his legal work. In 1939 therefore he gave up certain types of trials and became increasingly interested and successful in his office practice.

In this period of his life he began to analyze again his excessive amount of loyalty to his mother and friends.

After having been free of convulsions for two years, in 1942 he had an attack with a fugue state lasting twenty minutes. It seemed possible that his neglect of recreation over a period of nearly a year and a great burden of work which he had ambitiously assumed contributed to his attack. He reviewed these episodes constructively in two interviews, and made an effort to obtain physical and social recreation. The latter was especially important because he had again become self-centered and led an increasingly seclusive life with his mother because he felt tired in the evenings. Another discussion dealt with his being classified 4F. During the war years when he devoted his spare time to extra work on public duties it was especially important to review his mode of living. In 1944 he began to lead a well-planned life, working steadily but taking regular time for physical and social recreation. He became interested in a young girl with whom he felt he had much in common although she was less educated than he was. His marriage in the spring of 1946 has been successful. His wife, who comes from a healthy family, has accepted his epilepsy. In the last four years he has had petit mal attacks once to twice a week but they are so brief that others do not notice them. He had a convulsion a year ago. The bromide in his body does not seem to produce any undesirable effect. He has become alert to his thinking, talks freely and faster than previously with a better, although still insufficiently, modulated voice. There is little circumstantiality noticeable in his conversation.

Hospital treatment may be necessary in order to allow the patient to find ease and self-confidence in a neutral environment. In some cases, it helps to establish a healthy routine and re-education of faulty habits. These cases can be benefited greatly by about two months' hospitalization. In deterioration, or in patients who cannot live on the outside because of irritability or because they need too much attention for self-protection, prolonged or permanent hospital care is indicated. Some of the so-called epileptic colonies offer an exceedingly well-planned life. In well-to-do families, such patients can usually be well taken care of by placing them on a farm with an attendant. The danger of criminal acts and homicide has been greatly exaggerated. Such possibilities, however, should never be dismissed lightly when indications are present. They are most serious when epilepsy occurs in a psychopathic setting. In the hospital, these patients are frequently most trying. In the average case, treatment does not vary from that on the outside. It is frequently wise, however, to avoid offering anticonvulsive drugs in high amounts. It is an old observation that many irritable epileptics show a marked decrease of tension after a convulsion and can be managed easily for the following few weeks. Such patients are much more difficult if their seizures are suppressed by medication.

A special discussion of epilepsy in children is warranted because of the frequency of this illness in childhood and because its treatment demands specific consideration of the childhood setting. It is important to recognize the ease with which some children react with convulsions to infections. In these cases, one does not usually deal with epilepsy. In all childhood convulsions, a thorough physical examination is indicated. The control of convulsions is best obtained by sodium bromide, dilantin, and phenobarbital; the control of petit mal attacks and akinetic seizures by tridione or phenobarbital. In some children a combination of these drugs gives best results. "Ketogenic diet" treatment, which was found to be helpful in convulsions and to some extent in petit mal attacks, is used little because the difficulties in carrying it out are so often insurmountable. This treatment uses a high fat, low carbohydrate and protein diet, to be administered for about one and a half years. During the last few months, the ratio of carbohydrate and protein to fat is systematically changed until it reaches 1:1, then, an ordinary diet can again be offered. The production of ketone bodies and acidosis seems to be therapeutically important. It was also proposed to start the treatment with a starvation period of four to six days, which leads to rapid ketosis and dehydration, and to follow this with the ketogenic diet. It is obvious that any treatment which includes a dehydration regime should be carried out in a hospital where one is prepared for emergencies (danger of cardiac failure). This treatment is the first attempt at offering dietary advice on a scientifically established basis. The older dietary considerations were usually empirically determined and general conclusions were drawn from a few cases.

Attention to personality functions is most important in children. Educational and environmental influences can foster or correct the undesirable tendencies which one observes so frequently in epileptic children. They are usually sensitive, self-centered in their interests, often irritable, and inclined to sulkiness. These characteristics, which vary greatly in degree, make adjustment to the group difficult. They need to be encouraged to adjust to others and led to understand their behavior. One frequently notices a marked need for order and a sticking to details and rules. At the same time, such children are not necessarily orderly in their habits. Similar personality features are ethical-religious needs, an exaggerated desire for justice, and resentment of any slight injustice, especially minor insults which touch their personalities or what is important to them. They are critical of others but are usually unable to develop a constructive criticism. Many show early a wealth of imagination. With increasing personality changes, a poverty of ideas and association develops, leading to monotony of thinking and interests. Teaching should therefore be stimulating and varying. On the other hand, there is a definite difficulty in giving up a topic readily. To hurry such children and time them is therefore usually undesirable. Other intellectual difficulties have been discussed previously (see p. 344). Emotions persist longer than in the average person (affection as well as hate and resentment). These children stand teasing poorly, although they enjoy teasing others. Keeping these points in mind, it is not difficult to establish a strong rapport which allows the physician, parents, and teacher to exert a strong influence without provoking stubbornness and resentment. Their quick temper with poor control may lead to impulsive outbursts. These outbursts can easily be handled if one understands the child. Cruelty is a feature which has been greatly exaggerated and offers a far less therapeutic problem than is frequently assumed. Delinquency plays a minor role. More important is the frequent overconcern to their bodies which can develop into an attitude of invalidism to their illness early in life. Some of the more self-assertive patients react with an attitude of spite. This is more frequent in adolescence than in early childhood. It is essential that even the child learn to live as normal a life as possible with his handicap. Teachers and school authorities need to develop an attitude of constructive understanding and not ask to have epileptic children removed except if it is absolutely indicated.

If possible, the children should be adjusted to the ordinary school. For children with disturbing symptoms, such as frequent convulsions or marked personality peculiarities, epileptic schools should be founded. Many of the unintelligent epileptic children could be taught in special groups in such schools. Only markedly retarded children, in whom the epileptic convulsions are mostly a symptom of constitutional cerebral deficits, should be admitted to institutions for the feebleminded.

There is an essential difference in the teaching of epileptic and feebleminded children. The epileptic child needs to be stimulated by the teaching but should not be pushed into abrupt changes of topic. Rules need to be carefully explained. When they are understood thoroughly, the child will be able to use them. Because of a poorly developed retention function, they can depend less on memory than other intelligent children (in addition, sedatives increase this difficulty). A child with frequent petit mal attacks and absences may miss certain words or sentences of the teacher's explanation. In preparing for a life occupation, the personality and the clinical picture should be considered. Instead of going into further detail, I shall present a case which illustrates the educational aspect.

Case 24:

A 9 year old boy was taken to a psychiatrist in 1927 because of his inability to adjust to school. He was sensitive to teasing and unable to accept even mild criticism without bursting into tears; he was timid and felt generally inadequate. This feeling was increased by his family's high standards of scholastic achievement. His parents were greatly concerned about his health and frequently kept him away from school because of constipation and colds. At that time, he began to develop a tic of throwing up his right or left hand when looking at the sun. The patient was considered unintelligent by his teacher because he was slow in grasping. His Binet-Simon test, however, gave a mental age slightly above his chronological age. The family was advised to put the patient in a small school where the teachers seemed to have a good psychologic understanding. He improved somewhat in his school performance, but little otherwise. A year later, at 10 (1928), he had his first convulsion. He was seen at that time and the Binet-Simon test repeated. The mental age was again slightly above his chronological age. During the test, the boy was shy, lacked confidence in himself, constantly repeated the answers in a low voice to make sure he was correct, and took much time in working out the problems. When urged to proceed faster, he became confused and tearful. He was very poor at questions in which school knowledge entered, but good in offering spontaneous interpretations and in topics in which he was interested, such as history and geography. His vocabulary was large and he used it well. It was felt therefore that the test could not give an accurate indication of his intelligence and that he was intellectually well equipped. The parents were overanxious and wanted assurance that his condition had nothing to do with epilepsy.

As the physical examination was entirely negative, the patient was put on bromide medication, starting with 0.3 gm. (5 gr.) three times a day, which was increased to 0.5 gm. (7½ gr.) after three weeks. After two more weeks, the blood contained 175 mgm. of bromide and four weeks later, 200 mgm. To be able to take the medicine more conveniently, the medication was changed to 1.0 gm. (15 gr.) after breakfast and supper. He had no convulsions but on one occasion, a petit mal attack. There were no symptoms of bromide intoxication at any time. On my advice, the patient was transferred to a larger boarding school with good scholastic standards where the headmaster was especially interested and talented in dealing with children who presented difficulties. This school was also chosen because its standing encouraged the child, who had begun to consider himself feebleminded. It also helped him to socialize better and to develop in a more neutral environment than his home. The illness was carefully formulated to his parents in order to gain their intelligent help. It was pointed out to them that not all convulsive disorders lead to deterioration and invalidism. They learned to recognize the unfortunate influence of their overconcern and anxiety and to correct these tendencies.

The boy found friends in his new environment and became interested in games and athletics. During this first year, he was seen on an average of once a month. On these occasions, blood examinations were carried out regularly. The therapeutic discussions dealt with his adjustment to the group and his hypochondriacal concern. In the beginning, he complained much of constipation, which was easily regulated by adding prunes to his breakfast, occasionally bran cereal, and on rare occasions, cathartics. He learned to keep track of his bowel movements and to report increased constipation to the school nurse, without becoming unduly concerned. There were often complaints of indigestion, which he was advised to disregard as gastric analysis had been negative. With physical training, his general health improved. However, the tendency to throw up his hands diminished little. His school difficulties were considerable and demanded attention in discussions with, and advice to, the teachers. There were marked difficulties in reading. He was slow in grasping words and had a need to understand their meaning before he could proceed with ease. He was also slow in arithmetic, often forgetting the numbers and having to start all over again. Private tutoring for arithmetic was advised in order to allow him to learn rules by careful understanding and to offer him greater opportunity for the training of his memory and logical thinking. He was good in geography, which stimulated his interest and imagination, and in discussion (the epileptic enjoys criticizing others, arguing, presenting his point of view, and convincing others.)

In the summer of 1930 when exerting himself too much at camp, he had another convulsion. The precipitating factors were carefully reviewed with patient and parents. The patient was now a well-liked and lively boy without undue body concern. Returning to school, he experienced difficulties in spelling. This was primarily due to a lack of interest and attention. Presenting aspects of spelling which appealed to his interests, one was able to correct this in two of the consultations, which now occurred every six to eight weeks. His interest in arithmetic had increased and he was able to get along without a tutor. His memory functions had improved considerably through training. He now had the normal ambitions and interests of a boy of his age (12). There was, however, still a tendency to day-dreaming during lessons which did not interest him. This was made the topic for repeated brief discussions. He dropped back in history because too much stress was laid on names and dates. He did well later with another teacher who discussed more situational and cultural factors which simulated his interest and allowed him to find interrelations. French and English were difficult because not enough rules were taught by which he could be guided. On the other hand, he did well in Latin with its rules and order. He was frequently ashamed to ask the teacher questions. He learned to overcome this after repeated discussions of his shyness, his intellectual ambitions, and his unwillingness to expose himself to failure. Self-reliance increased after he had begun to recognize his tendency to depend on others (the school, individual teachers, and his physician). He became more willing to accept his limitations.

In October 1932 (at 13½), in a period of rapid growth and when working too much with insufficient sleep and recreation, another convulsion occurred. A review of the precipitating factors resulted in a better balance of work and recreation with sufficient sleep and time to eat. Recreation had been cultivated too much on a competitive basis instead of one of pleasure. Another attack occurred in the spring of 1933. At this time, physical exertion on a fishing trip and indulgence in sea food were precipitating factors. The sea food was of importance because it led to an increase of salt in his diet and caused a drop in his blood bromide, which all these years had been remarkably constant between 200 and 250 mgm. This boy (at 15) was doing well at school. The Binet-Simon test gave him a mental age of 14. The outlook for recovery is not good, but even if, after having reached maturity, occasional convulsions occur, he will be far from being an invalid. He has learned to accept his illness without making it the center of his preoccupations. His school training will allow him to find an occupation for which he is fitted with his talents and interests. Three to four consultations a year are now sufficient. They are utilized for a checking-up on his medication and for psychotherapeutic discussions.

The patient has now (1947) become a well-adjusted man who runs a large farm very effectively. Medication has been changed by his physician according to currently recommended drugs. Best results seem to have been obtained by phenobarbital, which controls his attacks except for the occasional return of his tics when in bright sunlight.

It is important that one preserve a healthy therapeutic attitude with epileptics, guarding against pessimistic nihilism with entire dependence on drugs, and yet against optimistic overactivity. One should look at this illness as the orthopedic surgeon does at many of his problems. The patient may be under a considerable handicap all his life, but this should not necessarily lead to invalidism. If the development of deterioration reaches a degree at which hospitalization is necessary, an active interest in these cases should be kept alive in order to be helpful to them. The establishment of epileptic colonies has been a great therapeutic step. It allows socialization and cultivation of interests with individual modifications. The mere segregation of epileptics in special groups in a state hospital is usually undesirable. It leads to neglect of these patients, who then receive merely custodial care.

Little is known about hereditary factors in epilepsy. There seems to be a small group with a definite hereditary tendency. In this group, marriage is contraindicated and, if it has occurred, sterilization is indicated. In the average epileptic, advisability of marriage depends on the personality setting and how the patient is able to deal with his handicap. Permission to have children should be viewed from a similar point of view. One should consider the patient as well as the prospective children.

BIBLIOGRAPHY

1. PENFIELD, W., and ERICKSON, T. C.: *Epilepsy and Cerebral Localization.* Charles C Thomas • Publisher, Springfield, 1941.
2. BRIDGE, E. M.: *Epilepsy and Convulsive Disorders in Children.* (Includes treatment, diet and drugs.) McGraw-Hill, 1949.
3. DIETHELM, O.: The Bromide Treatment for Epilepsy in the Dispensary. *Archives of Neurology and Psychiatry,* 21, 1929. (The technical procedure for determination of bromide in the blood is presented in the *Journal for Nervous and Mental Disease,* 71, 1930.)
4. LENNOX, W .G.: Two New Drugs in Epilepsy Therapy. *American Journal of Psychiatry,* 103, 1946. (Discussion of tridione and mesantoin.)
5. DIETHELM, O.: Brief Psychotherapeutic Interviews in the Treatment of Epilepsy. *American Journal of Psychiatry,* 103, 1947.

Chapter XV

PSYCHONEUROSES

A WIDE VARIETY of disorders must be discussed under this unsatisfactory heading. I chose the term because it is most widely
used, although its meaning has changed greatly. "Psychoneurosis,"
"neurosis," "hysteria," and "neurasthenia" originated when an organic basis was assumed and their treatment was relegated to the
neurologists. Even now, psychiatric textbooks do not offer enough
space to their thorough discussion.

The *subdivisions* deal with the generally recognized reactions of
anxiety, neurosis, obsessive-compulsive neurosis, hysteria, and phobias. Many psychoneurotic reactions, however, have been discussed
in other chapters: under sexual disorders are mentioned impotency,
frigidity, and menstrual disorders; under epilepsy, psychogenic factors and reactions; as well as a chapter on stuttering, tics, compensation neuroses, and psychopathic reactions. In the introduction of
this chapter, psychoneurotic reactions which are less well defined
than the above-mentioned groups are discussed, as their treatment
should be guided by the more general principles of psychotherapy
and not by specific considerations. The terms "neurasthenia" and
"hypochondriasis" are omitted because these two reactions do not
present psychopathologic entities. Dynamic psychopathology has
demonstrated that the direct influence of anxiety is the cause of
the symptoms in both. Anxiety neuroses, hysteria, obsessive-compulsive neuroses, and phobias receive special attention under their re-
spective sub-headings.

In every psychoneurotic reaction a careful diagnosis should be
established, so that the type of the reaction, the individual features,
and all the possibilities of correction can be considered in the therapeutic procedure. The physician should use the most suitable psychotherapeutic procedure with analysis and re-education as the main
methods as well as opportunities for somatic environmental correction and adjustment of work. In the vast and from the symptomatic
point of view highly bewildering field of psychoneuroses, a de-

plorable tendency has developed to adhere to specific therapeutic means with disregard to definite indications. Some believe in exclusive analysis without much discrimination. Others stress re-education above all other methods. There are groups which state frankly that all these reactions should be treated more or less alike and that the division into sub-groups is a mistake. In recent years psychotherapy has often been used exclusively with a purposeful neglect of organic implications. There are, on the other hand, physicians who believe in an organic basis and treat their patients accordingly with endocrinologic preparations or physiotherapy. It is essential that treatment be carried out according to the facts as they are presented and not according to scientific bias.

The diagnostic evaluation should establish whether one deals essentially, or in part, with reactions to organic or toxic factors or to specific life situations, or primarily with personality-determined neurotic developments. Episodic recurrences necessitate the exclusion of the presence of an underlying depressive disorder. A careful understanding of the make-up of the personality is essential to determine utilizable assets and to what extent obstacles to therapeutic correction exist. It is well known that neurotic reactions occur readily in psychopathic personalities. In those cases the treatment of the personality as outlined in Chapter I is essential and the correction of the specific neurotic reaction frequently only of incidental importance. The claim that all psychopathic personalities are neurotic personality developments cannot be sustained when one considers not only special groups but all of the personalities belonging to the category called "psychopathic." There is, however, no doubt that many of these developments of personality are of a neurotic nature. Yet even then, a treatment primarily by analysis is highly problematical. Psychotherapeutic enthusiasts who propose this course overlook the ingrained nature of the habits of early life. Even in later childhood and in adolescence, reaction tendencies and habits become a part of the personality to such an extent that only prolonged individualized re-education produces satisfactory therapeutic results. In other psychopathic personalities even this does not lead far. I refer here especially to reactions in set personalities with tendencies to persistent emotional reactions and projections. On the other hand, to deny the value of a primarily analytic procedure, with special attention to synthesis in some of the neurotic manifestations in psychopathic personalities, would lead to overlooking therapeutic opportunities. The claim of some psychiatrists that all psychoneurotic reactions occur in psychopathic personalities is incorrect. This formulation originated with physicians who see hospital cases primarily, disregarding all the less severe cases which the practitioner has to treat.

Many psychoneurotic reactions are early manifestations of depressive and schizophrenic illnesses and structural disorders. The neurotic manifestations require attention, but the treatment of the underlying fundamental disorder is of primary importance. It is a safe practical rule to consider hysterical and compulsive symptoms occurring in a fairly stable personality for the first time after the age of thirty as manifestations of an underlying illness. These two psychoneuroses start in childhood and adolescence. Anxiety with regard to physical functions and to physical appearance is determined by the personality to such an extent that forerunner tendencies can be seen in the whole development, even if no marked hypochondriacal reaction becomes manifest before certain life situations arise. The first occurrence of hypochondriacal concern is frequently associated with toxic or endocrinologic changes. To the latter group belong occasional menstrual, pregnancy, and involutional reactions. It is occasionally difficult to determine whether a depression is of psychoneurotic origin and should be treated primarily by psychotherapy. Hospitalization of such cases is no doubt the safest situation for aggressive psychotherapy. Suicidal possibilities in even short depressed moods, which are reactions to psychoneurotic symptoms or to disturbing psychotherapeutic discussions, should always be taken seriously. When psychoneurotic reactions develop in the setting of an organic illness, psychotherapy is important. These cases are diagnostically difficult, primarily because physicians still have too great a tendency to consider an illness either of organic or psychoneurotic nature and are guided accordingly in their treatment.

The treatment of psychoneuroses is directed at finding the fundamental factors which are primarily psychogenic or personality determined, and offering the patient an understanding of their dynamic importance and of the possibilities for correction. Psychotherapy is therefore the most important mode of treatment. Opportunities for the correction of somatic factors, however, should never be overlooked. Symptomatic treatment and adjustment are frequently the only possible goal. Every critical physician will try to recognize the limitations of therapeutic possibilities and guard against definite and far-reaching promises. He must be willing to judge from the outcome of his investigations that his original optimistic assumptions were not justified, and be content with imperfect results, instead of going on doggedly for months and years. This should not be construed as meaning that intensive treatment over long periods of time may not be justified in some cases.

Psychotherapy (see Chapters II, III, IV, V) consists of a study of the individual personality, its development, and its reactions to specific life situations. As a rule, the best procedure is distributive analysis and synthesis. It can be adjusted to the individual case and problem and leads to an understanding of the dynamic factors of involved as well as simple psychoneurotic reactions. Psychoanalytic and allied methods are desirable in well-selected cases, especially in phobias, hysteria, and obsessive-compulsive reactions. In the average type of psychoneurotic reaction with which the practitioner has to deal, a less time-consuming and less expensive treatment will lead to satisfactory results. Psychocatharsis may also lead to a fundamental adjustment but is usually not sufficient without additional analysis and synthesis. This procedure is mainly indicated in the treatment of symptoms to which considerable affect is attached. Reeducation, based on a personality study, is of fundamental importance in most cases and should never be regarded as mere symptomatic treatment. An inquiry into the patient's general hygiene is always indicated. Frequently the patient is not aware of the fact that he makes impossible demands on himself and tries to live up to so-called normal standards which may be quite disproportionate to his make-up.

In some psychoneurotic patients, constitutional tendencies are open to correction through physiologic treatment. In recent years, endocrinologic treatment has been urged. Unfortunately, current methods of investigation of endocrine functioning are still unsatisfactory. Even with well-developed laboratory methods, the interpretation of the results in psychoneurotic patients is frequently difficult. Disturbances of the functioning of the thyroid gland can be fairly well determined when they are of marked degree. In psychoneurotics, however, one is concerned with minor changes. It is no doubt always wise to try thyroid therapy where signs of hypothyroidism are found. Some authors believe that minor complaints are frequently due to some thyroid deficiency and can be readily corrected. Signs of mild hyperthyroidism are more difficult to evaluate. They are frequently the expression of anxiety and fear. A study along these lines should always be indicated, especially if no definite improvement occurs under planned internal medical treatment. Much has been expected from treatment with sexual hormones. The results as published in literature are not satisfactory yet, and many cases which could have been helped by psychotherapy have developed into chronic conditions. Neither castration nor the implantation of testicles is of value in these conditions. Insulin has become a valuable therapeutic tool in many personality disorders. Ambulatory insulin treatment may be used to alleviate excessive anxiety which impedes the progress of psychotherapy. One can summarize the usefulness of endocrinologic treatment briefly. If there are definite signs of specific endocrinologic disorders the appropriate treatment is indicated, but one should never be guided by symptoms which may be psychoneurotic without a careful study of the personality involved. Specific treatment of sympathicotonia and vagotonia which German authors had recommended has not been found to be efficacious. In some psychoneurotic patients there is a beneficial influence of hydrotherapy, climatic influences, and planned physical exercise. There are, for instance, certain constitutions which react to a more or less marked extent with fatigue and slight anxiety symptoms to excessive humidity during the hot season. Acting on the advice to take a prolonged vacation during this uncomfortable period in Baltimore, two of my patients have been free from these symptoms, which disturbed them greatly and to which they had reacted with hypochondriasis and anxiety. One may occasionally have to advise change of location in such cases. Dietary correction may be of similar importance.

Symptomatic treatment and adjustment are frequently the best one can expect. A far-reaching analysis, leading to a fundamental adjustment may be impossible when one deals with inadequate personality assets, insufficient intelligence, or lack of time. In some an analysis may not lead far because one deals primarily with habit formations and set attitudes as observed in overconcern to physical functions and reactions of anxiety and tension. In others the patient lacks sufficient assets to utilize what the analysis has elicited and is not able to carry out what he can recognize as essential. This occurs in psychopathic personalities of various kinds. In all these patients symptomatic treatment is important. Some may need help only over a short period of time, while others may need to come off and on for years, or even during their whole lives. It is important that the physician plan his interviews carefully so that each terminates constructively and does not lead to mere reassurance or somatic treatment. An understanding of the personality is always necessary if one wishes to understand and correct reactions to strain of various kinds. Psychotherapy is important but so is attention to somatic features and correction of social factors.

Symptomatic psychotherapy is based on an analysis of the personality and a study of various neurotic reactions in the individual setting. It does not mean an analysis of symptoms but of reactions which are singled out because they are important to the patient or to the physician. The understanding which has been obtained by the patient is utilized for his re-education. In these constructive discussions, much stress should be laid on the working out of a life plan which the patients can use for guidance. They must learn to accept long-term treatment for symptoms which may recur but this should not lead them into a reaction of invalidism. The recurring symptoms will become indicators of a disturbance in their personalities. These patients should learn to look for the underlying causes, correct them, and ignore the symptoms. If they do not succeed in recognizing and correcting the causes or if the symptoms persist or disturb them, an interview with the physician is indicated.

In symptomatic treatment, suggestive therapy and, in carefully selected cases, hypnosis are of great importance. In order to avoid repetition, reference is made here to Chapter III in which the technique is outlined. Outside influences should be studied in order to correct the unhealthy suggestive influence of others or tendencies to irritation. Formation and re-formation of habits are important. Among them need to be cited the patient's attitude to his body, his concern about the impression he makes on others, anticipation of mishaps and indulging in unhealthy fantasy life in general, reactions to failure and various kinds of mood influences, attitudes of apathy and boredom, lack of perseverance, and tendencies to envy and resentment. A re-education of the volitional tendencies is important. This necessitates a careful study of the causes of his lack of persistence or of anticipation, lack of courage, overanxiousness, which may prevent his getting started. Emotional factors may interfere with the progress or dissatisfaction, caused by too high expectancy, may not allow him to get the satisfaction of achievement. Re-education must work on the patient's weak links in the chain of performance. "Persuasion" (see p. 106) is frequently helpful, allowing the patient to gain an understanding of dynamic factors in a simplified form. Discussion of errors, bias, resentment, and envy will modify attitudes and make the patient more plastic in general.

It need hardly be mentioned that the production of fear is not an acceptable therapeutic tool, whether this be achieved through suggestive, mechanical, or chemical means.

A study of the actual conditions in the patient's life through the help of social workers is indicated, not only because one feels that one cannot depend on the patient's own evaluation of his life, but also because the physician might produce changes beneficial to the patient through this intermediary. Thus social workers are necessary not only for the poor in our dispensaries; the wealthy patient may be just as much in need of a social investigation and advice from a trained worker.

Somatic symptomatic treatment ought to be administered only after consideration of the total personality and under the guidance of psychotherapy. It can usually be avoided. A careful physical examination, carried out as soon as possible, should establish complaints of organic origin to be treated somatically, and those which are physical expressions of personality disorders to be treated with psychotherapy. It is important that this physical examination be carefully planned in order to avoid subsequent re-examinations which will disturb the patient's confidence in his body which one has tried to build up. When re-examinations or later consultations with specialists are unavoidable, the physician should make these occasions for therapeutic discussions of the patient's attitude to his body and the purpose of the new examination. Whenever feasible, patients should be advised of physical complications, described, however, not in technical terms, which may be disturbing, but in a formulation which they can understand and which will prove to be helpful.

It is rarely advisable to offer medication for anxiety and its cardiovascular expression. Gastrointestinal disorders of a functional type deserve correction of faulty diet. It will be best if the psychiatrist plans the diet together with an internist. Special medication for hyperacidity and hypoacidity as well as for hypermotility is usually offered by the general practitioner or internist. As a psychiatrist I have rarely had need for such medication, and I am convinced that most of it will become superfluous when physicians treat this reaction with correct psychotherapy. In headache, analgesics are indicated if it is disturbing and not the main, but an incidental, complaint. In persistent psychogenic headache, suggestive and hypnotic treatment is indicated. In this connection, I wish to stress that many cases of migraine are especially amenable to psychotherapy.

Weir-Mitchell's rest cure treatment, which stressed the need for environmental change, rest, high caloric diet, massage, and mild exercise, was based on physiologic considerations which can barely be considered adequate any longer. From a psychiatric point of view, his original treatment, which included isolation in a darkened room, is unacceptable. When treatment by rest cure is still used, psychotherapy plays a considerable role. Even so, this method distracts the patient from what is essential in the treatment of his condition and too readily offers him opportunities for excuse when symptoms recur later in life. Some psychiatrists use a modified Weir-Mitchell treatment, considering it indicated if signs of definite exhaustion are present (generally poor physical condition, marked fatigue, or caradiovascular hypotonia) or if the patient is run down after a physical illness (infections, toxic conditions, metabolic disorders, marked loss of blood, and physical overexertion). There is no doubt that every physician should pay careful attention to the building up of such patients. This does not, however, imply the evolvement of an elaborate routine in the sense of a rest cure. It is important that occupational therapy be used in such neurotic patients even while they have to stay in bed.

Sleep disorders require special attention. Most frequently one is confronted with difficulties in falling asleep, or restless and broken sleep in which dreams or nightmares are disturbing. In the first group, discussion of the disturbing factors and re-education are essential. Many of these patients with sleep disorders must learn how to relax. The method which is used to induce psychocatharsis (see p. 108) has proved to be quite satisfactory. The patient is led to assume a passive attitude, letting thoughts and sensations appear and disappear without paying special attention to them. Topical preoccupations are thus relegated to the background. He is warned against attempting forceful relaxation, which entails effort and therefore prevents relaxation. Many patients with anxiety and hypochondriacal overconcern can learn readily to overcome difficulties in falling asleep. If dreams are obtainable when a patient's sleep is disturbed, their brief analysis is indicated. Regulating a patient's sleep is an individual problem. Some patients need to retire later than others, or secure optimal results from a relatively short sleep. In some patients who work under persistent marked tension, a brief midday nap, preferably after luncheon, helps to prevent afternoon fatigue and is preferable to a long sleep at night. Such a procedure should always be tried if working conditions allow it. Irritability and difficulty in getting started after awakening in the morning can frequently be corrected by a brief cool shower, stimulants (coffee, tea), and brief exercise. Reading as a means of becoming sleepy is generally undesirable. Few people are able to put a book aside immediately when they get tired, and by reading another page may become wide awake. Sedatives ought to be limited to only a few days, if they are necessary at all.

Faulty eating habits may contribute to emotionally-determined gastrointestinal disorders. Regular meals in a comfortable setting, with sufficient time, are important. Distention occurs readily in patients who gulp their food, thereby swallowing considerable air. When salivary secretion is diminished because of emotional (anxiety) factors, fluids should be taken freely with the food.

Clothing should be adapted in patients who have unsatisfactory thermic regulation. Patients who are sensitive to cold temperatures have many complaints during the cold season and in the spring and fall. This discomfort can be corrected by warm underwear. Fashion often presents an obstacle to such simple advice, and therefore the whole problem deserves careful discussion. Electric pads may be a necessity for inducing sleep in such patients.

General hygiene demands the physician's constant attention. Sexual hygiene is discussed in detail in Chapter XVII. A healthy balance of work and recreation has been stressed in the introductory chapter on treatment in general. The choice and time of vacation is especially important in patients who react with minor physical complaints and general nervousness to prolonged strain. A plastic routine should always be discussed thoroughly with cyclothymic patients. They need to know how they can best get through mildly depressed periods. At such times suitable recreation and companionship which will be helpfully distracting should be available. Friends who participate in pessimistic discussions which increase the patient's depressed mood, and others who irritate through their buoyancy should be avoided. Reading should be guided accordingly.

Pharmacologic treatment plays a minor role. Roborant treatment with preparations of arsenic and strychnine is rarely necessary. A well-regulated routine will usually correct the psychoneurotic lack of energy, fatigue, and weakness much more effectually. The same holds true of medicine prescribed to increase appetite. Nevertheless, when a physician feels the need to resort to these medications, their administration should be carefully worked into the general therapeutic plan.

Sedatives are undesirable but unavoidable in the consultation practice of the general practitioner. The psychiatrist will rarely resort to them even in consultation treatment. In hospital treatment they are contraindicated. Hydrotherapy and psychotherapy replace them effectively. The simplest sedatives are most desirable because the physician can understand and master them readily. Small amounts of phenobarbital (0.06 gm. — 1 gr.) and barbital (0.12 gm. — 2 gr.) once to twice a day are advisable in tension and anxiety states. Sodium bromide 0.5 gm. (7½ gr.) once to twice a day has been recommended by older authors. The skillful practitioner can readily dispense with the innumerable samples of patent medicines which are constantly sent to his office. In contrast to some psychiatrists, I feel definitely that opium has no place in the treatment of anxious psychoneurotic patients and would also warn against combinations which contain codein. The psychoneurotic patient is predisposed to addiction. There is no drug on which he may not become dependent or for which he may not even develop a craving, as recent clinical observations have demonstrated.

In children the treatment of minor behavior disorders and psychoneuroses is fundamentally the same as has been outlined above. Modification of the psychotherapeutic approach to fit the child's personality with stress on healthy education, careful attention to environmental factors, and removal from undesirable settings are important. Specific psychotherapeutic methods have been discussed in Chapter V.

The treatment of psychoneurotic patients in the in-patient service of the Payne Whitney Clinic has demonstrated the desirability of hospital treatment in a limited group of patients. Whenever the patient is persistently unable to follow the plan of treatment, especially with regard to well-planned work and recreation, or when he is unable to achieve a minimum of socialization or self-dependence, treatment in a hospital should be considered. Another indication is the inability to accept therapeutically necessary frustrations. Hospital treatment, however, should not merely provide the necessary psychotherapy but should also create an atmosphere in which the philosophy of work and recreation and needs for socialization are strictly maintained, where freedom is restricted by the recognition of limitations, and genuine self-reliance is constantly sought.

CONCERN ABOUT BODY APPEARANCE
AND SOMATIC FUNCTIONS

Everyone's attitude to his body and its functioning is important. Some people have a more or less constant attitude of overconcern to it, usually starting in childhood and greatly fostered by a similar attitude in the environment. These anxiety reactions are recognized by every physician who realizes the need to consider the patient's overconcern in any somatic treatment. Many physicians, however, have considerable difficulty in recognizing and treating this reaction in persons who have apparently never been concerned in the past about their health, but show undue concern to a current physical illness. A careful review of such patients' lives usually reveals a definite interest in their bodies which may have manifested itself in physical training through athletics, marked pride in their good health, interest in health problems, special attention to cosmetics, or attractive ways of dressing. Many persons have not expressed frank body concern merely because they have always been in good health. Such persons frequently show undue concern or frank anxiety at the beginning decline of aging.

In all reactions of anxiety to somatic functions and body appearance, the personality and its development in life should be studied and utilized in treatment. In a relatively small number of cases, specific life experiences and dynamic factors play a role. To this group belong circumscribed and specific hypochondriacal complaints which are on a dissociative-substitutive basis in hysterical and schizophrenic reactions or linked with convictions and early delusional formation in a paranoic reaction. Some patients show a marked progressive and spreading tendency of their hypochondriacal complaints, leading to an increasing invalidism; whereas in others, the complaints remain stationary and monosymptomatic. These differences are related to psychodynamic factors in the patient's early development which may lead to well recognizable personality patterns. The progressive reactions occur readily in immature individuals and in persons who depend on others or impose on them. They often resemble the make-up which predisposes to hysterical reactions, and the hypochondriacal reaction may consciously or unconsciously serve a purpose. Monosymptomatic hypochondriasis is frequently a reaction of disappointment and inadequacy in the setting of a rigid personality. Constitutional tendencies toward depression actuate hypochondriacal reaction as a result of the general feelings of inadequacy. Circumscribed attacks of hypochondriacal overconcern, lasting from several weeks to months, are usually the outstanding manifestation of an unclearly expressed depression. These cases must be considered as suicidal dangers and treated primarily as depressions.

The treatment of these reactions to one's body is guided by the assumption that one deals with a personality reaction with different degrees of psychogenic material. Investigations of the psychodynamic factors therefore assume a varying importance. They are, however, the necessary basis for the re-education of the more or less well-formed or even set habits of observation of sensations and the anticipation of their occurrence and increase in intensity. This principle of treatment remains the same whether body concern forms the essential disorder or is merely a symptomatic feature in another disorder of the personality.

It is most important that the physician obtain the detailed complaints at the beginning and try to group them according to their significance. Patient listening in the beginning offers assurance that every complaint is taken seriously and not pushed aside because of the physician's bias. It forms the basis for confidence and rapport. The next step is to gain a clear understanding of the development of the various complaints. Most patients are able to give the dates accurately enough to allow the physician to see whether connections with specific life situations exist. In order to determine such relationships, a careful brief history of the person's life development must be obtained. An orientation with regard to school and work record, general health, living conditions, responsibilities of marriage and children readily reveals the outstanding life situations. An inquiry into the personality reveals why certain situations had been a strain on this patient, causing him to react with his complaints. The family history is helpful because it discloses outstanding inherited traits and the environmental influences to which the patient had been exposed in childhood and later. The attitude of the present environment should be investigated so that unwholesome or too freely expressed sympathy and overconcern can be corrected. If relatives are present or can come to see the physician later, a careful formulation of the undesirability and dangers of overconcern and too much interest in one's body will help a great deal in creating a healthier home atmosphere. I usually offer part of this formulation in the patient's presence so that a husband may know, e.g., that his wife's change in attitude is not due to wanting sympathy and affection but is part of the medical treatment. A careful and detailed physical examination should be made as soon as possible. It is wiser to carry out a physical examination which does not seem absolutely indicated to offer the patient a proof of the lack of a somatic basis than to leave the patient dissatisfied. Otherwise he will insist on it, and, in most cases, the examination will have to be done later. Re-examinations should be avoided. They shake the patient's confidence in his physical health and disturb the suggestive influence of the previous negative examination. If, because of any unforeseen development, another physical examination is necessary, the reason for making it should be explained carefully. In other words, each re-examination presents a psychotherapeutic situation. The physician who plans his initial examination carefully has a great advantage in the treatment of these patients over the physician who is impatient or too self-assured in the beginning, or who suffers from over-anxious scruples during the treatment.

A formulation which includes all the somatic and psychobiologic findings and presents their interrelations in a form which the patient can readily grasp is offered after all the investigations have been completed. Any somatic illnesses are best mentioned frankly in a form which takes into consideration the patient's tendency to over-concern and anticipation. The necessary physical treatment will not interfere then with the psychotherapy which is attempting to develop bodily security and to turn interests into other directions. I feel that a formulation based on the principle of A. Meyer's life chart (see p. 502) is most easily grasped, and is convincing to the patient. The physician's formulation should make clear to the patient the difference between symptoms which are on the basis of a physical illness or those caused by emotional factors and the development of symptoms to specific life situations as a result of the make-up of his personality. The explanation of the interference of emotions with the smooth functioning of the body leads to a discussion along the lines of Dubois' "persuasion" (p. 106). This understanding, together with the accompanying strong suggestive influence, re-stores the patient's confidence in his body and makes him willing to disregard disturbing sensations. The need for a well-balanced hygienic life ought to be stressed. Physical recreation is naturally desirable but should not be overemphasized. Otherwise the patient's bodily overconcern will find an outlet in athletic overcompensation which will crumble easily and be replaced by hypochondriacal concern when strain and disturbing emotions shake the patient's ease and confidence. In many cases which one sees, such management is sufficient for the time being, and the patient does not need to return at all, or not until he reacts to new strain and is unable to correct his reaction. In other cases, prolonged treatment in repeated consultations is indicated.

Prolonged treatment of these reactions attempts to re-educate the patient's attitude. To achieve this, a study of the emotional factors which played a role in the past is necessary. The patient's routine is adjusted along the lines of general hygiene. He is urged to cultivate regular sleeping and eating habits and well-planned recreation (physical, social, aesthetic) according to his needs and interests. This offers a healthier training than physical exercise. The patient is advised to work; if no sufficient work routine exists, the physician will have to resort to volunteer work of various kinds. A physician should therefore know the occupational opportunities which a community offers. In the consultations, an increase of complaints is utilized for an investigation into the factors which caused the increase. Recapitulation of complaints is not allowed because it augments the patient's doubts as to his physical health and makes him aware of his body. The goal of his re-education is to learn to guard against the awareness of sensations and, especially, against indulging in such observations. By them he is made aware of numerous sensations which average people do not notice, and the intensity of normal sensations of fatigue, various kinds of pressure, etc., is increased to the point of aches and pains. Such formulations should be offered briefly after the constructive analysis of disturbing situations. Gradually the patient's attitude of thinking changes. He becomes aware of his preoccupations sooner and can push them aside before they have led to a marked increase of intensity of his sensations. He learns to appreciate the need for distraction and the value of well-planned recreation to which he can resort. It is unnecessary to mention all the possible symptoms and how one should deal with them. The main principles remain the same. In some cases habits of eating need to be corrected, e.g., hasty eating which leads to swallowing of air and digestive difficulties; in others, faulty bowel elimination, insufficient or too much rest, faulty breathing, or poor posture have to be corrected. These hygienic remedies are helpful if they are not made the keynote of treatment as, unfortunately, usually happens.

Many hypochondriacal patients find it necessary to return for occasional consultations the rest of their lives. This need not discourage the patient or the physician. The latter can perform continuous constructive treatment to keep the patient in satisfactory health. All these consultations should be carefully planned so that the best results can be obtained in as short a time as possible. Like every other neurotic patient, the hypochondriacal patient should learn to value time, so much of which he has wasted in his own and other people's lives.

Far-reaching analysis, e.g., psychoanalysis, is rarely indicated. The essential problems can usually be obtained readily through skillful and planned questioning. The exception might be monosymptomatic hypochondriacal reactions. Little work has been published on such reactions, which frequently offer a poor prognosis. Freud's formulation of hypochondriasis as a narcissistic neurosis has not led far in therapeutic directions.

Hospital treatment is indicated in cases of marked invalidism which makes the carrying out of a well-planned routine impossible. Frequently hospitalization is advisable to remove the patient from an undesirable environment. In the first case, the treatment should be carried out in a psychiatric hospital. In the second case, a general hospital or nursing home may prove satisfactory if sufficient facilities for occupation exist. Most nursing homes, however, are unsatisfactory. The following case illustrates these points and also the fostering of invalidism through ill-advised medical care.

Case 25:

A 20 year old college student was sent to me by an internist who had found her to be in good physical health. She had many complaints which had developed during the last three years. She had, however, always been concerned about her health and had frequent indigestion. After graduation as the first in her class from high school, she went, during the summer (1930), to a business college which she disliked. She felt under strain and tired. That fall, when entering college, she became irritable, restless and her sleep was broken. Her appetite was poor and occasionally she suffered from nausea. Menses became slightly irregular. After the final examinations she felt worn out and listless. During the summer vacation she was improved. During her second year in college, a feeling of general fatigue and stomach complaints developed and her parents were disturbed by her complaint of marked thirst. She was treated for anemia. During the next summer vacation (1932), there was no improvement in fatigue and appetite but she felt better otherwise. Her symptoms were diagnosed as a possible pituitary disturbance. After tonsillectomy and appendectomy in the fall (1932), she showed temporary improvement but after a few weeks, her symptoms returned. The patient became restless and cried frequently, feeling sorry for herself. In February 1933, she was kept for three weeks in a general hospital where the diagnosis of ptosis of the stomach was made. A rest cure was advised, and insulin for insufficient appetite and hormonotherapy because of cessation of her menses since the operation were administered. The patient developed increasing invalidism and on her physician's advice did not return to college. She again improved somewhat during the summer of 1933, spending it outdoors on a beach. Returning to college, she became worse and spent most of the fall in bed. When I saw her, her complaints were "weakness and a funny feeling" in her stomach and a quivering feeling in her throat. These, as well as dizziness and her dry throat which caused her to drink so much, were apparently feelings of anxiety. She often noticed numbness in her face, limpness in her hands, and was disturbed by a detached feeling in her head and sluggish thinking. Her symptoms disturbed her greatly and she cried when she described them. The patient recognized her overconcern and blamed her mother for having stressed health too much to her since childhood, but did not see what she could do about it. She had been told that feeding had presented considerable difficulty until the age of 8 months and had been urged to pay attention to her food and take a rest whenever she felt tired. She was willing to accept the fact that situational and emotional factors played a role and that it was best to enter a psychiatric hospital to gain a better understanding of herself and re-educate her faulty way of thinking and living. I did not feel that the depressive features were more than incidental. Her general vagueness, her persistent complaint of something being wrong with her left eye, and her feeling detached suggested a schizophrenic factor but the hypochondriacal concern seemed the outstanding therapeutic problem. Her numbness was apparently due to bodily awareness and not an hysterical manifestation. Her marked degree of invalidism made hospital treatment necessary.

The patient impressed me as immature physically and in her personality. She was an intelligent, sociable, but shy girl, cheerful but easily worried over her health, proper diet, and her standing in school. She became easily enthusiastic but her interests never lasted long. She was suggestible and dependent on her parents and friends. Her mother was of a similar make-up and always paid special attention to this only girl, who was the second of four siblings. The father was a kind man, interested in his business and family. At the time of admission, the patient was 20 pounds underweight. Her hands perspired freely and her pupils were dilated.

The first week after admission (11/25/33), the patient improved fast and made a good adjustment to the group. This was due to her being encouraged by the attitude of physicians and nurses. The second week her symptoms returned and she was ready to give up. She became bored and listless. It was stressed to her that the newness of the situation had begun to wear off and that she should learn to develop a genuine interest in what she was doing and in other people. She was encouraged to participate in athletics which offered her body much needed training. In the occupational hours, she was allowed to paint, which she enjoyed, but was requested to perform the required general work first. Playing the piano was allowed as a regular recreation. Reading was encouraged on only a limited basis because she used it as a means to avoid games and conversation with others. A discussion of interests proved of little help. She wanted to become a nurse or to be active in charity work. It was pointed out to her that such contacts would make her more aware of illnesses and lead to bodily concern. Her desire to do something for others was on an immature basis and also seemed to her an easy way to meet people. In the discussion of her family setting we stressed the need for healthy emancipation and self-reliance. During these brief discussions, the patient was vague and evasive with little desire to find a constructive solution, expecting the physician to offer the answers. This was carefully avoided. When reassurance and encouragement were necessary, they were offered in definite and even emphatic terms, making use of her marked suggestibility. Persuasion was used to formulate the symptoms to her. She was advised not to repeat her complaints but to find out what caused variations in their intensity. This led to a gradual recognition of the undesirability of insufficient occupation, her habit of self-observation, and her tendency to discouragement. She felt depressed when thinking of a futile future or when feeling lonely. It was repeatedly pointed out that she had to make an effort to offer something to others if she wanted to become part of the group. When she had entered college, her family had objected to her social activities because they might interfere with her scholastic success and because of financial reasons. This curtailment led to considerable dissatisfaction, and her feelings of social inadequacy increased. Joining a sorority in her second year proved unsatisfactory because she was too shy and self-centered to make a sufficient effort to become part of the sorority life. She had few interests in common with other girls. Greater effort than in high school was needed for satisfactory scholastic achievement and even so, her standing was merely average. At this point, the possibility of turning to some occupation rather than acquiring an aimless college education was discussed but no definite decision was reached.

The patient improved steadily but not beyond a moderate point during six weeks' treatment. I felt that other factors were also disturbing her and urged a more thorough discussion of the setting in which her illness had started and also of her sexual life, which had been described as quite unimportant. In the middle of January, greater attention was paid to these factors. The patient then discussed her resentment to having had to attend a college which she considered inferior socially and scholastically. She had marked social prejudices and a desire for being admired by others. Her mother's affectionate domination was unbearable to her and she had hoped to gain emancipation by going to college in another town. She was worried by her seemingly ungrateful and unkind attitude to her mother and tried to conceal it from her. In college her naïve childhood beliefs were shaken and she was unable to find a satisfactory religious attitude. Sexual discussions worried and stimulated her. Since 13, she had indulged in masturbation and had tried ever since, unsuccessfully, to overcome what she considered a sin. Being sex-shy, she had never confided in anyone. She remembered her reaction of disgust to the onset of menstruation for which she had been unprepared. At that time (13), she had suffered from vomiting and nausea for a year, which she now considered a reaction to disgust and worry. These discussions upset the patient considerably, but were nevertheless continued until the essential material had been obtained. Her complaints increased, especially the sensations of anxiety, and the patient became listless and slightly depressed. She was urged to continue her activities in order to become distracted from her preoccupations and her body. During the following two weeks, she needed considerable encouragement and reassurance with regard to her physical health. In occasional brief interviews was stressed the need for a constructive solution of her problems. Any further analysis which would have merely bewildered her was avoided. Her request for repeated physical examinations was refused because it would weaken her self-confidence and stir up more doubts and concern.

During February and March, the patient showed steady improvement. She was advised to visit her family and an increase of symptoms after such visits was discussed with her. She reached the conclusion that she should stay with relatives for a period of several months after discharge because her mother's attitude had changed little. She expressed a desire to accept stenographic work, which she might enjoy because it gave her a feeling of usefulness and financial independence. She wanted, however, to stay longer in the hospital. We stressed the need to leave as soon as possible because she might become dependent on the hospital. When making definite plans for leaving (April), she again had an increase of symptoms. This was partly due to an acute illness of her father. She was urged not to dwell on his illness and the possible complications. To his sudden death (May 5th), she reacted with a normal amount of depression. This situation was used therapeutically. Her normal reaction was formulated as an encouraging sign of her emotional stability and self-reliance. She was urged to leave soon in order to lessen the financial burden and to encourage her mother. Several week-ends at home proved successful and she left at the end of May. Her complaint at that time was slight dizziness and feeling detached. She was, however, willing to accept the fact that nobody's health is perfect and to recognize the increase of the intensity of her symptoms when watching them. A carefully outlined routine which included work and recreation, with special attention to Sundays, gave her a feeling of security. She improved during the summer with only an occasional brief consultation. In October, she secured a secretarial position and has been working steadily for two years without need of psychiatric help. She is still aware of the above-mentioned feelings when not being fully occupied, but they are unimportant to her. Although living at home, she has been able to guard against body concern and leads a more independent life. Her mother has learned to see the need for this and guards against expressing solicitude. There is little doubt that the patient's adjustment is none too stable, and it is most likely that she will be in need of further psychiatric help when she has to carry undue strain. Her family physician realizes this and will promptly attend concern about her health and renewed symptoms. Correct psychotherapy should therefore be able to prevent another far-reaching hypochondriacal reaction. (No information regarding her health has been obtained in the last ten years.)

In children, therapeutic attention is primarily directed at the re-education of habits of overconcern and healthy education in the future. Placement in a foster family or boarding school helps greatly by creating a healthy atmosphere. One should, however, consider very carefully such a step, which affects family life and family formation so strongly.

ANXIETY NEUROSES

The outstanding complaints are anxiety attacks which occur with greatly varying frequency. In the interval between attacks, the patient may feel entirely well. More frequently, however, tension, which expresses itself in restlessness and irritability, minor symptoms of anxiety, and so-called anxiety equivalents, is present. The causes of anxiety neuroses are manifold. Any situation which causes considerable strain over a sufficient length of time may be a causative or contributory factor in some personalities. Freud's original formulation which reduced anxiety to sexual frustration is not broad enough. His final theory applies to anxiety as such and is not a therapeutic formulation. It is wise to keep this in mind because some of his pupils had a tendency to accept as facts and therapeutic principles statements presented by him as theory.

With the progress of the illness, the attacks become more frequent and the tension increases to a disturbing degree, manifesting itself in various somatic symptoms, which easily become the nucleus of hypochondriacal concern. Uneasiness and anxiety about the recurrent attacks lead to apprehension and anticipation of attacks, which in turn precipitate their occurrence. Minor incidental panicky reactions may occur and are usually easily managed by reassurance. In some cases, anxiety and tension are the beginning of a serious panic reaction. If such a complication occurs (see p. 220), the necessary precautions and therapeutic steps must be taken at once. A frequent mistake is to consider phobias (see p. 401) as anxiety attacks and to overlook the correct therapeutic procedure. Anxiety attacks occur frequently in depressions with marked tension or in psychopathologic reactions associated with cortical damage. A possible relation to toxins always should be investigated carefully. Drugs, alcohol, and excessive nicotine may be important factors. The diagnosis of hyperthyroidism still occurs too frequently and a high basal metabolic rate is taken as sufficient proof of its presence with utter disregard of the possible influence of strong emotions. Anxiety is an emotional reaction which may complicate and aggravate any somatic illness. Its treatment is therefore important, and every physician should be well acquainted with its manifestations and management.

The treatment can be divided into two aspects — the management of acute anxiety and anxiety attacks, and the treatment of the anxiety neurosis. For the latter, one has to study the individual. This investigation may reveal little or much pertinent psychogenic material.

During acute anxiety, the patient refers his symptoms to the heart. To obtain full reassurance, a thorough cardiac examination should be made at once. If laboratory studies and a more detailed observation seem indicated, it should be advised without hesitation as soon as the patient has regained his ease. Sedatives or the administration of alcohol should be avoided.

When the physician is called for repeated attacks, a new cardiac examination should be avoided because it would shake the confidence which the patient developed after the first examination. Confidence will be easily re-established by the physician's quiet and convincing reassurance. The patient is urged not to call the physician, thereby increasing self-dependence. He is advised to see the physician only in appointed consultations and try to neglect the symptoms. A formulation of how uneasiness, worry, and anticipation increase his activity and precipitate attacks is helpful. The increase in intensity of sensations, especially cardiac symptoms, when the patient watches himself should be stressed. From the start, every effort should be made to prevent a hypochondriacal reaction to anxiety symptoms (see previous discussion). Sufficient time should always be taken to inquire into precipitating factors. As little time as possible should be spent on reassurance. Otherwise, the patient becomes dependent on it and will demand it whenever he feels uneasy. The therapeutic goal is to establish self-reliance.

The treatment of anxiety neurosis consists of a study of the patient's personality, of possible psychodynamic factors, and the re-education of faulty habits. It is best to scrutinize the onset of the illness and to pay less attention to the recurrent attacks. Less and less strain will be sufficient to produce an attack as the illness progresses. Special attention is paid to personality factors which produce anxiety, such as standards which may come in conflict with reality, and attitudes which cause tension. Situations causing frustration and tension should be investigated. The desire to do something against one's standards and the need to live up to too high standards frequently play a role. An attitude of overconscientiousness or pride, which does not allow one to recognize defeat, causes a struggle against obstacles to which others can adjust. The same high standards are applied to health, and tension symptoms are viewed by the patient with uneasiness and alarm. The tendency to anticipate difficulties is frequently an ingrained feature in such patients. They should be made aware of this tendency through treatment, reducing it to one constructive foresight. Whenever a problem of the future presents itself he should settle it at once, try to dismiss it from his mind, and not allow himself to go over it again. He should learn to take a chance on making mistakes, realizing that anticipation will undermine his self-confidence and ease and prepare him less for an emergency than if he had given little thought to it. An ability to react spontaneously and to trust spontaneity to a reasonable extent will develop. Reactions to strain and responsibilities are investigated and the patient's attitude to them modified. Reality and imagination are of like importance. The best known examples of frustration of wishes and desires which are not overtly expressed are found in sexual life. Similar indulgence in unhealthy preoccupations exists, however, along many other lines and easily produces symptoms of anxiety. An understanding of oneself and control of one's thoughts and actions are necessary in a healthy life.

Frustraneous sexual excitement, especially coitus interruptus, is undesirable but does not necessarily lead to anxiety symptoms. It depends on the personality setting and the meaning of those reactions to the individual.

Anxiety reactions are frequent and well known to any practitioner. Most of them can be treated by him in consultation. It is best to have the patient continue his work. When this is impossible, a well-planned routine needs to be substituted. Sedatives ought to be avoided. If the physician feels that the patient has need for it, I would advise bromide 0.3 to 0.5 gm. (5 to 7½ gr.) or barbital 0.15 gm. (2½ gr.) once to twice a day. If difficulties in falling asleep exist, the teaching of relaxation is indicated. When the sleep is disturbed by fearful dreams and nightmares, a study of the dream material will offer important clues. Increased physical recreation — long walks, golf, swimming — is desirable and helps to correct fatigue caused by tension. As attacks occur readily in crowded rooms or in places where the patient is unable to get away easily, the patient usually limits his activities. He should be advised to disregard the symptoms and, after having improved, even to expose himself to such situations. Anticipation brings on these attacks, which should not be confused with actual phobias. At least temporary abstinence from alcohol and sexual activities is indicated. It is otherwise most difficult to determine what role these factors actually play. In most cases, I also advise a two weeks' abstinence from smoking, because it is usually done to excess to overcome symptoms of tension and restlessness. The persons in the patient's environment need a reassuring statement from the physician because they are usually alarmed by the attacks. They have to help in creating a wholesome atmosphere. When this is not possible, or when the patient is so disturbed that he is unable to carry out the routine prescribed, hospital treatment is indicated.

The following case illustrates the importance of psychodynamic factors and the need for their adjustment. As in many cases of this type of anxiety neurosis, insufficient psychogenic material was obtained through questioning along the usual lines. The patient was understood and helped only by determining the cause of his anxiety reactions during his hospital stay and through the discussion of sensitive topics in the personality study, in his letters, and in dreams.

Case 26:

A 41 year old business man who was treated in 1927 for an anxiety neurosis offers a good illustration of treatment which utilized an analysis of the setting of his anxiety reactions as they occurred during our observation, the study of his personality, and the re-education of his tendency to anticipation and physical concern. This patient had been unable to work for several months because of anxiety attacks, sensations of pressure in his neck and occiput, and great worry over his condition. The first few consultations revealed that he had become tense and restless in the spring of 1923, and had his first anxiety attack in the summer of 1923. He improved after five weeks' vacation but never lost the sensations of pressure in his neck and had occasional anxiety attacks during the following years. After an attack in July 1927, he developed increasing anxiety. His physician urged him to ignore his symptoms. This advice irritated him considerably, as he felt there must be a cause for his emotional and somatic reactions. He had always been an active, self-reliant man who enjoyed good health.

A thorough physical examination was the basis for our reassurance with regard to his physical health. A formulation which stressed the need to obtain an understanding of the factors causing his reaction was offered, and he was told to learn to disregard the symptoms. He was put on full-day routine and advised to continue whatever he was doing, notwithstanding anxiety symptoms. Socialization was cultivated and this allowed him to become part of the group by sharing the various interests of others and communicating his own ideas.

The initial survey revealed that we dealt with a cheerful man who, however, had always been inclined to pay too much attention to his health and to become readily apprehensive. He was liked but had little need for social contact outside his business. In work, he was conscientious and cautious and drove himself hard. Since 15, he had been self-supporting and successful. At 25, he married a spoiled woman who had little interest in his business and spent money rather freely. This did not worry him much during his prosperous years (33 to 36, 1919 to 1922), but distressed him increasingly when financial losses (at 37, 1923) demanded curtailment. His wife was frankly discontented with their need to save on household expenses. At this time, the patient entered into a love affair with one of her friends but broke off after a few months because he was afraid of being discovered. Intercourse with his wife had been unsatisfactory for several years as she had suffered severe lacerations from nine pregnancies (six children living). Despite attempts at precaution (douches), pregnancies had occurred. In this setting of considerable worry, the patient had two anxiety attacks (June 1923). He became greatly upset, afraid he might have appendicitis, and stayed in bed a week on his physician's advice. After five weeks, he returned to his office. Since then, he had been disturbed by drawing sensations in his neck, being emotionally easily upset, and he gave up most outside activities because he felt tired. When a friend committed suicide in July 1927, the patient had another anxiety attack. Further attacks and minor anxiety symptoms occurred. He stopped work and was admitted to The Phipps Clinic three weeks later.

The patient improved rapidly after having been reassured by the physical examination and our formulation of his illness. He was, however, little inclined to look for disturbing factors beyond those which had been mentioned before. He insisted that a fall in 1905, when he had slipped on ice-covered steps and hit his back, was the primary cause of his illness. At that time, he had been unable to move or speak for an hour. Discussing this incident and the immediate setting of his anxiety attacks, the patient began to realize his tendency to react with anxiety and apprehension whenever there seemed to be a possibility of an impending operation or a serious illness. The accident had produced considerable fright and apprehension. The first anxiety attack occurred when he had been concerned over some transient abdominal pain and feared appendicitis. Another attack, which he had forgotten, was due to the fear of having a gastric ulcer (March 1927) and the increase of symptoms before admission occurred when the possibility of having a brain tumor was discussed with him by friends. The first few days after admission, he had been anxious and apprehensive because he wondered what the physicians might do next. His sex life was accepted as an additional factor. Because of fear of impregnating his wife, he had not been able to relax during intercourse, and had obtained little pleasure. In addition, he tried to protect his wife who suffered intensely during intercourse. On this basis, he tried to rationalize the need for extramarital relations. His nervous symptoms to these experiences was explained by his fear of public opinion. In 1927, when he had extramarital relations for the first time, he had also been nervous and restless because he feared discovery. The patient showed little curiosity about the personality factors involved and felt that he had improved fast and was nearly well.

On August 9th, he reacted with marked "fullness" in his neck to a letter from his superintendent at business. He stated that relations in his office upset him frequently because of this man's self-assertive arrogance and lack of dependability. Many minor points of friction in his business were now discussed, the patient's sensitiveness to criticism and rudeness from others, and his exaggerated need to assume full responsibility for the mistakes of his subordinates. When another patient discussed tongue kissing in his presence (September 13th), the patient experienced slight anxiety symptoms. He then talked more of his unsatisfactory sexual life and expressed marked resentment to his wife's sexual behavior, her lack of understanding, and unwillingness to cooperate with him in general. Two days later, he mentioned recent and past dreams with sexual content in which he had satisfactory intercourse with friends. A discussion of these dreams led to a more inclusive review of his sexual life. In 1922, he had intercourse several times with a friend, in 1923 with a visitor, during the winter of 1922-23 with a married woman. When having intercourse with his wife, he pictured those other women. The last extramarital intercourse happened with a friend in 1924 and since then, sexual play with her. A study of his ethical standards brought out that promiscuity was unacceptable to him. He was brought up with rigid sexual, as well as ethical, standards in general.

On September 22nd, he reacted with an anxiety attack to a letter mentioning that his wife was ill from flu. This reaction was due to his tendency to hypochondriacal fear and exaggerations, and resentment to his wife (hoping that her illness might be serious). A dream about making mistakes in business led to another discussion of business difficulties. Two days later, he volunteered uneasiness about being discharged too early because he had improved so fast, and fear that he would not be able to deal with business and marital difficulties. At this time, his anxiety symptoms increased. He first explained it by his not being able to stand the teasing and self-assertive behavior of a hypomanic patient, discussing in full his sensitive reactions to such behavior in daily life, and later in mentioning with expressions of disgust, an attempt at intercourse with his sister at 14. At this time, sexual tension became obvious. He felt that he needed social contact with women, and that he could abstain from intercourse. Therefore, he asked for the privilege of taking nurses out. The need to be able to control his sexual desires was now discussed in full. He again brought up his unsatisfactory married life, especially the lack of companionship and his wife's fretting against financial curtailment. He resented this especially because he had always been proud of taking care of his family well. In 1924, he had thought of separation but felt obliged to live with his wife because of the children. He had worried over his inability to control his promiscuity, which he considered a sin. Fear of aging and invalidism had increasingly become a topic of concern. During these two weeks of treatment, the patient had again felt nearly well. On October 16th, he had an anxiety attack when cancer was found in another patient. It proved to him his still insufficient confidence in his health and his tendency to anticipate illnesses. It also made him aware of his tendency to feel too sympathetic toward others and his need for sympathy, attention, and affection from others, which he had missed at home and in the hospital.

On October 23rd, he had some anxiety features. Against the rules, he had accompanied a nurse downtown. He recognized his persistent unwillingness to accept full sexual control, which his standards demanded, and now saw clearly the need to control his tendencies to indulge in thoughts along those lines. He began to see the need to pay more attention to a healthy family life and to find possibilities of common interests and activities with his wife and children. Recreational activities (social and physical) had proved to be highly helpful in the hospital and needed to be cultivated at home. At this time he became aware of his lack of confidence in handling his sexual and social life well, although he had become aware of circumstances which constituted risks for him and of his tendency to invite dangerous situations, to anticipate difficulties, and to watch his body too closely. Around this time his exuberance changed to a more sober mood. His interests turned to an understanding of his personality and, during the last three weeks in the hospital (discharged November 26th), a satisfactory constructive survey of his interests, assets, and liabilities was accomplished. From childhood, success in business and community life and as a supporter of his family had been his main goal. His wife had been his sexual companion and the mother of his children, but little else had bound them together. With her waning physical attractiveness and complaints about painful intercourse, desires for other women became dominant. There was considerable flirting among married couples in his social group and opportunities for indulgence presented themselves frequently. Although he disliked the behavior of his wife's social group, he accepted invitations because of his sexual desires. He had never had time for his family or for recreation, which he enjoyed in the hospital, and made plans now for regular golfing, fishing, and hunting. A methodical man, he was too easily upset by disturbance of routine in the office and especially at home where his children became a source of annoyance to him. He recognized the danger of increasing ridigity in his habits and attitudes. Being cautious, he worried too much about decisions which had to be made when he was not certain of all the facts. On the whole, however, he carried responsibilities well, even when under pressure. He had been too concerned about the impression on others and had too great a desire for being praised. Although affectionate and sympathetic, he had not much real love for his wife and children because he had been too self-centered. His need for security, financially and otherwise, had become increasingly exaggerated. Fear of disease had been present since childhood and caused excessive cleanliness. Sexual life had been taken as merely physical and the personality factors in it neglected.

A visit by his wife three days before discharge offered him an opportunity to study his reactions to her and discuss them with his physician. When he left the hospital, he realized that anxiety symptoms might occur when he was emotionally disturbed and that their appearance ought to urge him to look for the disturbing factors. He returned to work immediately and arranged his life according to his outline. For the first week, he noticed some tension in his neck. Afterwards, he felt entirely well. Intercourse with his wife became satisfactory. The physician had several discussions with her which included her attitude to sexual intercourse. Much of her pain had apparently been due to her fear of it and her constant watching for the occurrence of pain during intercourse.

In January 1928, the patient had a slight anxiety attack when having to live for two days in the house of a business friend with whose wife he had had sexual intercourse. He recognized this reaction as being caused by remorse about his behavior to a friend and fear that he could not trust himself yet. In March 1928, he noticed restlessness and some tension as a result of friction with his wife, but experienced fast improvement when he began to pay more attention to recreation, which he had neglected. Both these episodes were adjusted in consultation with his physician. He felt well until the summer of 1929. At that time, he asked for readmission. He had suffered from marked anxiety in the preceding two weeks and was greatly hypochondriacal. He was advised to stay in town a few days, carry out a carefully-planned routine to become distracted from himself. The main factor had been his resuming flirtations and, on three occasions, extramarital intercourse, to which he had reacted with considerable guilt. Having been well for a year, he had felt secure enough to disregard what he had considered a hygienic life. This episode reaffirmed the need to live up to his standards. In the summer of 1930, he had some anxiety and marked hypochondriacal concern when a friend, with headaches similar to his, was found to have a brain tumor. He was readily reassured by a brief examination. Since then, he has been well, never in need of consulting a physician, and leading an active life. Correspondence with the patient reveals that he has remained in good health (1946).

HYSTERICAL REACTIONS

The older descriptive formulation of hysterical reaction has been replaced by a dynamic one which forms the basis for therapeutic approach. Previously, the ability to produce, on a psychogenic basis, somatic symptoms which resemble various illnesses was considered essential. We know now that an hysterical symptomatology is impossible, and that the understanding of the individual personality and the individual reaction is essential. A. Meyer points to the main dynamic principle by speaking of a dissociative substitution reaction. Others stress the motivation (wish to be sick, flight into the illness). Some authors are especially interested in an hysterical personality make-up. This point is stressed because of the well-known fact that so-called unstable personalities develop hysterical reactions most frequently. In accordance with this is the fact that such reactions occur readily in childhood and accumulate in puberty, adolescence, and during the involution period. Hysterical reactions also occur in the setting of illnesses which disorganize the personality — schizophrenic illness and psychopathologic reactions to cortical damage.

Modern treatment attempts to find the dynamic factors involved but stresses the need to investigate carefully the personality setting. It is not a symptomatic, but an etiological, treatment. This, however, does not exclude attention to symptoms and their use as a means of attack on the personality factors when opportunity arises. An analysis of symptoms in the older sense, i.e., an analysis in order to find the meaning of the symptoms, is not desirable.

An understanding of the personality setting is desirable before one decides on a definite therapeutic plan. One must distinguish between the well-organized personality in which analysis will be the usual choice, and the psychopathic person in whom an active synthesis, based on an analysis with much attention to re-education, is essential. In feebleminded patients, only a moderate understanding of the dynamic factors can be obtained. Suggestion, hypnosis, and re-education are most useful here. In the rigid personality, desensitization and socialization are important.

In some cases, there is utilization of an organic basis in the symptom-formation. Some physicians advise tackling this problem frankly, while others shrink from it. It depends on the physician's skill as to how he can draw the patient's attention to this factor and utilize it therapeutically. Considerable danger exists, however, that physician and patient may become attracted primarily to a physical treatment. The psychiatrist will usually proceed with psychotherapy whereas the internist tries to utilize symptomatic medication in addition to psychotherapy.

Among the various psychotherapeutic procedures, analysis has to be considered the choice. One should guard against doing this without attention to the personality setting and synthesis. In using analysis one must realize the limitations which the individual case imposes and evaluate carefully the amount of time and the expense involved. It happens too frequently that, perfect results being sought, analytic investigations are still pushed when active termination through a personality synthesis and re-education had long been indicated. This is always an important consideration in the treatment of psychopathic personalities or when hysterical manifestations have been present through a long period of adult life.

Distributive analysis and active synthesis (see Chapter VI) is the most desirable therapeutic procedure for the average type of hysterical reaction. It can be adjusted to the personality setting and well combined with other psychotherapy, especially re-education, suggestion, and hypnosis. A far-reaching analysis, revealing the psychogenic factors and leading to their adjustment, may be indicated. In a feebleminded person, questioning the patient and relatives in a few consultations will reveal the essential facts, and the main effort then has to be directed at leading the patient to make necessary corrections. Brief analysis will also be sufficient in most traumatic hysterical reactions. To investigate too thoroughly, believing that all the intricate workings of the integrated personality need to be understood by the patient to prevent recurrences, is unnecessary and frequently undesirable. Every case must be studied from an individual point of view and indications and contraindications carefully evaluated before one decides on a course of treatment. Even then, the physician should be willing to turn to other therapeutic means if he changes his formulation of the case. In using active analysis, a frequent mistake is made by trying to push the patient too fast. The resistance of the patient to verbalize material which he begins to remember or to bring in correct correlation is marked in hysterical patients. Poor understanding is indicated if the physician speaks of dishonesty or accuses the patient of an insufficient desire to get well. Even if this charge were so, it would have to be made a therapeutic problem and not a topic for accusation. The inability to discuss problems or the avoidance of discussion because of the rationalization that a certain experience has really no bearing on the illness is striking in hysterical reactions. With treatment, the patient's formulations of his illness becomes in succession more inclusive. Case 4 in Chapter VI is a good illustration of this.

The psychoanalytic procedure is indicated in patients of a sufficiently stable make-up who are able to reach a synthesis without the active assistance of the physician. Freud's dynamic conception stresses that unsatisfactory repression leads to expression in symptoms (conversion), which are primarily of the somatic type. The central problem is the repression of infantile genital strivings in the parent-child relationship (Oedipus complex). The outstanding feature in the hysterical development is the child's fixation on the Oedipus situation. These strivings are repressed. With disappointment through events in later life, a regression to the Oedipus complex and a reactivation of the desires connected with it occur. This results in a renewed struggle for their repression and expression in hysterical symptoms. Somatic tendencies are frequently utilized in the formation of the symptoms. Identification with others and imitation may play a role (e.g., in hysterical group reactions in boarding schools). The primary gain from the illness is the evasion of settling the Oedipus complex satisfactorily. The secondary gain is the material gain (evasion of actual difficulties in life). Nothing essentially new needs to be added to the general principles of psychoanalytic therapy which has originally been developed for the treatment of these reactions. Transference was discovered in the treatment of hysterical patients. It is most obvious in these cases and can be brought to the patient's understanding relatively easily after the resistances have been worked through. The unconscious content usually directly determines the form of transference. The progress of treatment is satisfactory because the physician has a safe criterion of the analytic progress in the patient's reaction to the interpretations which the physician offers and in the changes in transference and the symptoms. In general, hysterical reactions are considered an indication for psychoanalytic treatment. The contraindications are the general contraindications mentioned in Chapter IV. One also needs to turn to different methods (e.g., hypnosis), when immediate help is necessary (Fenichel).

The psychoanalytic goal is to find the forces which cause the repression. The first goals of treatment were catharsis of the dammed-up emotions linked to certain life experiences, later the unearthing of a repressed trauma which was supposed to be of a sexual nature, and still later, the analysis of various complexes which exerted a disturbing dynamic influence. In the treatment of hysteria, psychoanalysis investigates the whole personality and its development as well as the dynamic factors of repression. One can therefore readily understand the long duration of treatment which is justified when the involved nature of the dynamic factors and the possibility of a far-reaching adjustment of the personality demands an intensive investigation. In the average case of one's daily practice, psychoanalytic treatment is neither desirable nor practical.

Suggestion will always play an important role. The suggestibility of these patients, however, has been greatly overemphasized. Hypnosis is indicated in a small group of monosymptomatic reactions and should always be combined with distributive analysis if one wishes to go beyond symptomatic cures.

Re-education has been used a great deal. Some physicians use analysis merely as a means for re-education. This procedure is no doubt a neglect of its therapeutic value. Re-education is especially indicated in psychopathic and feebleminded persons and as a valuable symptomatic aid in patients who have developed hypochondriacal and anxiety reactions and habit-formations. One of the outstanding proponents of analytic re-education was Adler. The training of will power, which some German authors advocated, can never be more than a help to the essential analytic therapy. The attempt to effect a cure by stirring up reactions of fear by painful stimuli, cannot be considered a scientific or humane treatment and is not advocated any longer.

I shall omit a case presentation. Cases 3 and 4, Chapter VI, are sufficient illustrations. The treatment of psychic impotency (Cases 33, 34 and 35, Chapter XVII) also demonstrates the main therapeutic points. Most cases can be treated in one's office without interrupting the patient's routine of work. Hospital treatment is indicated when the patient should be removed from an undesirable environment, or when a state of invalidism has developed. Many of these patients become easily dependent on hospital life. An interesting case was that of a 21-year-old girl who was admitted to the hospital for hysterical stupor attacks. After several months in which little material was obtained, the patient began to talk, and in a few weeks the essential psychogenic material was discussed.

There was, however, little symptomatic improvement. Two months later, she was transferred to a state hospital where she recovered completely in a week. In this feebleminded girl, the hospital was an attractive haven and there was no urge to leave. The desire to stay was a sufficient factor to produce symptoms which had been due originally to quite different dynamic factors. These had been adjusted through distributive analysis and synthesis. It was wise advice of Freud never to treat a psychoneurotic patient without demanding his share from him, financially and otherwise.

Hysterical reactions in children occur frequently in relatively uncomplicated situations and strain. It is therefore usually unnecessary to go into far-reaching analysis. Direct questioning is usually successful. Correction of the disturbing situation is always desirable. Children are highly suggestible and the physician should make free use of this tendency psychotherapeutically. Hypnosis is rarely necessary. M. Klein has urged far-reaching psychoanalytic investigations, whereas, A. Freud opposes this and uses a conservative and cautious procedure. From the material presented by these two authors and from my own experience and that of others in childhood neuroses, I would be inclined to consider A. Freud's procedure preferable.

OBSESSIVE-COMPULSIVE NEUROSES

Usually manifesting themselves in early adolescence and progressing during adult life, obsessive-compulsive-ruminative tension states (A. Meyer) are serious reactions which frequently incapacitate the patient. As in every other illness, the therapeutic possibilities are greatest at the beginning. Patients and physicians alike, however, are inclined to consider the early manifestations as character traits which the patient or the environment should be able to adjust without medical help. In making this strong statement, I am fully aware that many compulsive traits are lost with further development and that no full-fledged neurosis develops. Even persons with such traits would have been greatly benefited by a psychiatric interview, which should have been indicated to determine whether definite treatment was necessary.

The diagnosis usually presents little difficulty. Special attention needs to be paid to possible depressive features. Obsessions and compulsions may be the main complaints in an unclearly recognizable depression and may clear up entirely when the patient recovers from this illness. The treatment is then primarily guided by the depth of the depressive setting (see Case 12, Chapter IX). The claim of some authors that all recovering obsessive-compulsive states belong to the group of depressions is an exaggeration. Even if so, it would not affect the treatment as outlined below. It is not unusual that obsessions and compulsions occur in a schizophrenic reaction. Their treatment usually has to be limited to re-education based on an understanding of the personality. Insulin and convulsive therapy, which have been recommended by others, have not been beneficial in our cases. Obsessions and compulsions occurring for the first time in later life should be considered symptoms of an organic change in the brain (presenile and cerebral arteriosclerotic changes) and their symptomatic treatment would depend on the setting.

The present-day dynamic formulation of these reactions directs the therapeutic approach, which consists of analysis of the dynamic factors, study and readjustment of the personality, and re-education. Most prevalent is the opinion that more or less specific personality make-ups are the necessary soil for these reactions. In contrast to this, Freud believed that the outstanding personality traits are already neurotic manifestations. He therefore wished to achieve their correction primarily through analysis.

Analysis should always be combined with active interference with the patient's activities. At the beginning of treatment, the physician should work out a plan of living based on minimal requirements to which the patient is expected to adhere. It is not always feasible to prohibit all compulsive activities from the start and to expect a normal and active life. A great deal, however, can be expected from the patient if one offers through discussions an outlet for the tension which results from the suppression of the compulsions. This tension is used as a therapeutic stimulant for the analysis. Like a whip, it drives the patient through his resistance. Mere suppression of the compulsions without utilizing the resulting tension and offering it an outlet in discussion is a mistake. Considering the ruminative tendencies of these patients, one should warn against self-analysis, and when this occurs notwithstanding, the constructive aspect of the treatment must be stressed and made the therapeutic issue. Hypnosis is rarely helpful in breaking tendencies to rumination and self-analysis.

The personality setting needs to be determined early. In well-organized personalities, more constructive results can be expected through an analysis than in psychopathic persons. The latter form a large contingent of these cases. Feeblemindedness limits the utilization of analytic investigation. Rigid and aggressive persons are frequently unable to work constructively with the material which was obtained through analysis. In all these cases, re-education leading to modification and reformation of faulty habits will assume a correspondingly more important place in treatment.

Re-education must be adjusted to the individual case. It is never merely a request to suppress compulsions and to complete the various tasks of daily life in a reasonably short time. Faulty thinking habits (rumination and scruples) demand attention. Concrete advice can be offered only if one understands the individual personality. Interests, of which the patient has been barely aware, can be utilized, and he can be guided to cultivate them instead of indulging in unhealthy thinking. His tendency to overconscientiousness and to perfectionism should be corrected by urging him to be satisfied with results as they are obtained with reasonable effort and within a reasonable time. The patient should learn to take a broad point of view and to recognize the relative importance of the place he is taking in life's activities. He must be willing to leave tasks unfinished, if necessary, and avoid indecision, even at the risk of making a mistake. He needs encouragement to develop spontaneity in his actions, to let impulses come to the fore, and to feel responsible for their management. It is necessary to distinguish between this wholesome dealing with spontaneous desires which involves self-control and the insufficiently controlled emotional outbursts which the patient has developed during his illness.

Adler emphasized the personality factors and the need for re-education. He stressed the unfortunate influence of too critical an education, which attempts to make the child perfect. To this influence, the child reacts either by identifying himself with the person who exerts the authority and develops the same attitude, or with spite. Compulsions at first are the striving for perfection and are utilized to prove the patient's superiority over others with less high standards. In addition, compulsions are symbolic expressions of self-punishment to having these ethically undesirable tendencies. A mystical component (superstition) also plays a role in the symptom formation. The illness leads to increasing separation from life and to a domination of the environment. Treatment consists of making the patient aware of these dynamic factors and utilizing them for re-education. Attention also needs to be paid to expressions of gastrointestinal inferiority (e.g., constipation), which are frequently found together with compulsive neurosis.

Some writers have advocated urging the patient to indulge in his compulsions so that these acts wear themselves out. The results are a marked increase in compulsive needs and tension. Compulsions are not meaningless activities which can be dealt with like reflex phenomena, but are of ritualistic significance, offering protection and satisfaction to the patient.

Distributive analysis and synthesis makes use of all the previously discussed tendencies and is adjustable according to the personality setting and opportunities. Its results depend on the physician's knowledge. The most frequent mistake is the analysis of symptoms, thereby becoming distracted from more fundamental investigations which should furnish material for readjustment. The analysis of symptoms is frequently destructive because it increases fruitless self-analysis. Incorrect evaluation of the possible significance and importance of various features may cause the physician to be satisfied with an insufficient analysis and to lay too much stress on a superficial study of the personality and a more or less rigid re-education.

The psychoanalytic approach has the great advantages and disadvantages of a strictly-outlined technique with definite goals. The psychoanalytic theory stresses as outstanding the dynamic factors of regression to the anal-erotic and sadistic childhood level. Compulsions are a defense to, and gratification of, anal-sadistic strivings. Through his symptoms the patient achieves a distorted satisfaction, punishment and atonement. The therapeutic analysis turns to an investigation of early childhood and of the factors which played a role in character formation. Anal-erotic personality features and sadistic needs and gratifications demand special attention in the setting of the general psychoanalytic procedure. The physician should urge the active suppression of symptoms. The resulting tension is used therapeutically. Fenichel points out the following difficulties in contrast to hysterical reactions. The regression to the anal-sadistic stage leads to increased ambivalence and to bisexuality. These features become obvious in the transference situation; the patient asserts himself against the physician and tries at the same time to submit, thus gaining sexual satisfaction. Because of the patient's ambivalent attitude, there are greater difficulties in offering interpretations and they are less readily utilized than by hysterical patients. The compulsive patient has a two-fold attitude to his symptoms. To some extent, he is anxious to cooperate but then again prefers to make use of magical superstition instead of logical thinking. His constant critical attitude to himself makes it difficult for him to adhere to the rules of free association. Speech and thinking have a sexual symbolic meaning and, affected by the illness, are therefore imperfect tools which he must use in the analysis. The secondary gain from the illness is narcissistic. The patient has formed reactions which lead to exaggerated standards. The patient is afraid to lower them and their adjustment presents marked difficulties. All these obstacles necessitate an analysis of long duration with frequently unsatisfactory results. The person who is not well-trained psychiatrically may overlook these obstacles and try to reach unattainable goals by prolonging the treatment beyond practically justified limits. A psychopathic or early schizophrenic setting, unalterable rigidity of the personality and its habits, and a lack of sufficiently usable assets are the frequently overlooked factors which necessitate active synthesis and re-education.

It is unwise to try to prove the superiority of any one therapeutic approach. The results will always depend on the physician's knowledge and skill, and his ability and willingness to see indications and contraindications. The passive psychoanalytic technique, which involves considerable active interference with the compulsions, frequently achieves surprising results in stubborn, self-assertive patients, who have great difficulty in discussing problems even if they are aware of the need. Indirect methods should be utilized in the distributive analysis and synthesis of these patients. There is still too great a tendency to dispose of such cases as "hopeless" because they are "dishonest."

In the average type of compulsive disorder which has lasted for a considerable time, therapeutic possibilities can always be found, but the results are usually limited. Personality investigations along distributive lines are most promising. Even with considerable improvement, marked compulsive tendencies may remain and frank symptoms may recur frequently when the patient is put under strain.

Case 27:

A 32 year old engineer was admitted to the Payne Whitney Clinic on August 26, 1946 because he suffered from obsessions of hetero-homosexual content. He was a pleasant man who talked freely but with obvious underlying anxiety. In the first two interviews the development of his obsessions was obtained. Since January 1944, he had felt restless sexually and dwelled upon phantasies of promiscuity to which he reacted with guilt. In the spring of 1946 he developed obsessions of exhibiting his sexual organ before colleagues, of having anal intercourse with male and female children, and finally with his 6 and 3 year old sons. Fear of insanity began to trouble him. From May until August he saw a psychiatrist once a week. He expressed his obsessions and anxieties to him and became temporarily reassured. A review of his life history revealed he was an only child of a rigid, devoted father and an emotionally very unstable, anxious mother. The mother had taken over the whole education of the son who felt insecure and suffered from childhood nightmares. He did excellent work in school, was active in sports, and was well liked. At 20 he graduated from college and secured a position in a large firm in which he has progressed steadily. At 21 he married his childhood sweetheart, who was a cheerful, outgoing, capable woman. Sexual life in marriage was unsatisfactory because of the wife's frigidity. The patient resorted to masturbation, resenting bitterly that his wife's behavior forced him to resume this habit which he had hoped to control with marriage. Since 12, frequent masturbation with phantasies of exposing himself before a woman had caused much guilt.

In the beginning of September, the patient's personality development was reviewed in some detail. An ambitious, hard-working student and later engineer, he developed an increasing need for perfection in his performance and since adolescence manifested minor compulsive activities, e.g., rechecking lights and locked doors. He became procrastinating and worked best under pressure. He was proud of his self-control and refrained from any marked emotional display. He was shy, although fond of people, and depended on his wife in social contact. Interest in maintaining a good physique and in regular bowel habits was considerable. He rarely gave himself full credit for his achievements and depended greatly on praise and admiration from others.

It was recognized that the patient suffered from marked obsessions and anxiety which made him self-conscious and caused him to stay by himself. He was urged to participate fully in all activities and not permit himself to withdraw from the group, even if this routine should increase his symptoms. His wife was advised not to visit him because her presence increased his tension and his resentment to her. Interviews of an hour's duration were given three times a week. He was eager to talk about his sexual thoughts. To him insanity meant loss of sexual control. His resentment to his wife was based entirely on her frigidity. During the second week his attitude of admiration, and fear, of his domineering father was traced to childhood. He discussed the strict toilet training carried out by his father and how he had been dependent on and afraid of him. He felt keenly the lack of affection from his overanxious, self-centered mother. His choice of engineering had been influenced by his father's profession and his excellency of performance. These discussions were followed by considerable symptomatic improvement. When, at the end of September, homosexual desires were brought up by the patient the frequency of obsessions increased. He remembered that nightmares and nail-biting had occurred between 5 and 8 and that during that period he had engaged in frequent sexual play with boys and girls. At 9 he began to masturbate. He reviewed his unsuccessful struggle at control and insisted that he did not want to recover unless it would mean elimination of masturbation. He was disturbed by a physical attraction to his physician. Transference relationship was explained to him on the broader interpersonal relationship than as an exclusively sexual problem. Decentralization of the sexual topic was considered desirable and various emotional reactions to his physician were analyzed. It became obvious to him that he experienced a mixture of a need for dependence and hostility, as well as of resentment and gratitude. In October symptoms decreased. A renewed analysis of his fear of insanity brought out his fear of permanent dependence on masturbation which he was now urged to control. He felt tense and angry with his frustration. Exhibitionistic desires were now considered a desire for admiration, a need to prove his masculinity, and to deny his passive dependence. In studying his attitude to women, he recognized a general resentment to all women and not only to his wife. However, not until December was this reaction related to his overprotective, domineering, self-centered mother. He viewed his masturbation activities as compulsive and not entirely due to unsatisfied sexual demands. His childhood fears were spontaneously connected with masturbation guilt and castration fears, related to his rigid, disciplinarian father. In response to a dream he discussed the possible existence of guilt in his marital sexual relations and early sexual desires directed to his mother. This discussion, as was pointed out to him, was on an intellectual level and devoid of an emotional working-through of the problem. The patient reacted with a brief period of resentment for being forced to assume the burden of solving his own problems. He reviewed his need for praise which he had missed in his work. Fear of discovering something intolerable through the analysis was finally allayed in several interviews. At the end of October, his obsessions had become infrequent.

In November, the relationship to his children was studied, his need to repeat his own father-child relationship, obtaining satisfaction from the obedience of his children but wanting at the same time their admiration and affection. He resented their claim on his wife's affection. His work was interesting and he liked it, but he was constantly afraid of competition and dreaded failure. Authority was resented and feared, emotions which linked to his own father relationship. Visits to his family brought forth anxiety and a return of the subsiding obsessions but to a less degree than previously. These visits were followed by increasingly productive discussions which now took place four to five times a week.

In December his father's attitude to his early childhood up-bringing and the stress on control of bowel functions brought up a need to analyze his body overconcern and self-admiration. His rigid standards and his overemphasis on attention to detail were related to genetic factors. His resentment to his mother in early childhood and to his wife became understandable, both representing protection and rejection, physical attraction and frustration. In his marital life he had frequently attempted to live out his masturbation phantasies, obtaining exhibitionistic satisfaction instead of sharing with his wife. A self-centered and selfish attitude had developed since childhood and explained his wife's resentment to him which was now obvious to him during his visits. He was urged to apply this increased knowledge to his dealings with his wife and children. A discussion of patient-physician relationship now proved to be fruitful. The homosexual tendencies were accepted without further disturbance, and more emphasis was laid on the physician's representing feared authority, affection, and protection. This analysis led in January and February to a freeing of himself considerably from his father's influence and resulted in increased self-reliance and security.

In January the patient resumed part-time work and spent every weekend at home; in February he did full-time work on a special project assigned to him by his firm. The parental influence was recognized in his dependence on older men and in his rigidity of standards. This rigidity and his procrastination also served as a protection against possible failure and related anxiety which the patient was unable to tolerate. Fear of his own aggressive impulses had been present since childhood and had become intense during recent years. These fears had been expressed in his fear of insanity. During January and February it was possible to discuss the sensitive material without a return of obsessions. Their nature had become clear to the patient and the emotional factors involved worked through satisfactorily. He was able to tolerate homosexual incestuous strivings within himself and his anal eroticism. Through the treatment, his sexual life became integrated in a heterosexual direction. It became possible for him to replace his pleasure in imaginations by that of achievement in reality. His narcissistic self-centeredness and insecurity expended into a sharing with others when he became free of his parental influences. This enabled him to assume the role of father and husband which gave more security to his wife and children than previously.

Advanced cases with marked disorder of behavior should be treated in a hospital where suppression of the compulsions and re-education can be carried out in the setting of routine and group activities. Even in cases which have to be hospitalized for years, the physician should constantly keep in mind that the accumulating tension needs relief through discussion and that he has to use the patient's emotional reaction therapeutically. The pulse curve is usually a correct objective indicator of this tension. As in every psychoneurosis, the danger of finding a refuge in the hospital is great. There is therefore a constant need to utilize situations which might make outside life attractive.

Early compulsive tendencies in children yield well to modified education and environmental and situational factors. In some children intensive treatment by means of play analysis may lead to complete recovery. When marked compulsions have developed early, treatment in a psychiatric hospital offers good opportunity for adjustment. It is frequently surprising how easily dynamic factors can be obtained from the child and utilized constructively if explanations suitable to his intelligence and state of development are offered.

PHOBIAS

Fears which a person cannot throw off no doubt resemble obsessions. They are nevertheless, discussed separately because there are definite differences which are therapeutically important. Phobias occur in a personality which shows few of the features predisposing to obsessive-compulsive neurosis. There are conscientiousness and the need to live up to high standards, but they are not accompanied by the tendency to rumination and exaggerated scruples. Phobias are of relatively simple protective character and lack the essential ritualistic features. The prognosis is therefore much better than in obsessive-compulsive reactions, especially as they occur frequently in well-organized personalities with utilizable assets.

Freud's placing of phobias between hysterical and compulsive states is not only attractive from a dynamic point of view but is also stimulating to one's therapeutic planning of these reactions, which are frequently seen by the practitioner and form an especially large group in late adolescence.

It is not always easy to distinguish between phobias and anxiety reactions. The distinction is important because phobias are always due to definite psychodynamic factors deeply linked with the personality. A thorough investigation is therefore indicated. Anxiety states occur as a reaction to strain and are frequently determined less by factors in the personality than in the environment. In both, the tendency to react with hypochondriacal concern and a resulting hypochondriacal invalidism is considerable and demands therapeutic attention.

Treatment utilizes analysis with active interference, a study of the personality setting, and re-education, especially of tendencies to anticipation and bodily overconcern.

Analysis should be primarily guided by general psychobiologic principles. An investigation into the meaning of the phobias will not lead far in the beginning but offers good results in a short time, after the patient has gained a satisfactory understanding of himself. The patient is urged to carry out activities, disregarding his phobias. With improvement, he is even urged to seek situations which had produced fear. This is desirable as a stimulative therapy, the resulting tension leading to better progress in the analysis and serving as re-education.

The personality of these patients is frequently well organized and fast progress may therefore be made in gaining a general understanding and synthesis of the personality. In a psychopathic setting, active synthesis and advice for the correction and working out of a suitable plan for life plays a more important role than far-reaching analysis. When phobias occur in a schizophrenic or depressive illness, their treatment will naturally be guided by the general setting.

Re-education tries to increase self-confidence and self-reliance by use of what has been obtained through the analysis, stressing the need for a healthy routine and modification of unhealthy habits of thinking and attitude. For the treatment of the hypochondriacal reaction, refer to page 374 and for that of anticipation to page 381. One has to consider the fixity of habit formations of fear, realizing that such a habit may persist as an attitude even when the causative dynamic factors have been corrected. Re-education is important therefore and should be freely combined with suggestive therapy. In one of my patients, hypnosis was found useful in overcoming an attitude of anticipation and fear. This case also illustrates that hysterical and compulsive reactions may appear in the same person. Such cases probably cause various authors to disregard the useful distinction of sub-groups and to claim that all psychoneurotic reactions should be treated essentially alike.

The psychoanalytic school formulates phobias as the expression of an instinctive conflict. It is a projection of inner dangers into the outer world. Anxiety is produced by situations which either offer an inducement to satisfy the strivings of which the patient is afraid or hint at the danger which would threaten if the patient gave in to his desires. Substitution and displacement are considered the essential mechanisms; the Oedipus complex and castration fear, the important dynamic factors. Psychoanalytic treatment is carried out with modifications — after the structure of the neurosis has been loosened and a good transference established, an active interference by the physician is indicated. (He urges the patient to overcome his phobias actively and to expose himself to anxiety.)

Distributive analysis and synthesis is usually the psychotherapeutic approach indicated. Its directness shortens the treatment and allows the free use of re-educational therapy. Psychoanalysis takes longer and is therefore best reserved for cases in which a deeper involvement of the personality seems to have occurred, or in patients who have considerable difficulty in discussion. In these persons, distributive analysis with utilization of indirect means is also indicated, as Case 4 in Chapter VI demonstrates.

BIBLIOGRAPHY

Pertinent literature is found listed under Chapters III, IV, V, and VI.

Chapter XVI

STUTTERING, TICS, OCCUPATIONAL NEUROSES, COMPENSATION REACTIONS, PSYCHOPATHIC PERSONALITIES

IN ALL THESE reactions one seems to deal with handicaps and disturbances in the constitutional endowment and more incidentally with psychogenic and psychoneurotic reactions. The treatment is a more or less far-reaching study of the personality with emphasis on individualized re-educational procedures. The most serious therapeutic fallacy in these reactions has been to mistake the ease of neurogenic malfunctioning for conversion symptoms and to overlook the factors of conditioning and habit-formation. However, the neurogenic aspect has been made the main issue by many neurologists and treatment is limited to specific training, with neglect of the personality setting.

STUTTERING

This speech disorder is of functional origin and in contrast to the structurally determined disorders of articulation. The symptoms are due to the interference of emotions with the free flow of speech. The patient therefore does not have the same difficulty with the same consonants and vowels all the time. He talks well when feeling at ease, i.e., in most persons when they are alone or talking to animals, or singing. Stuttering has therefore been called a disorder in conversation. The outstanding personality features of stutterers are their tendency to be too much aware of the impression they make on others combined with a sense of inadequacy. This leads not merely to a varying degree of self-consciousness but also to a defense reaction of stubbornness, an unwillingness to admit mistakes and to face defeat. Their feelings which are related to self-esteem are easily hurt. Their group adjustment is therefore faulty — they are self-centered and frequently aggressive. As children they are usually poor playmates and do not fit in well with other children. Not only in talk and gesture but also in their emotions they are hasty, some lacking emotional control, others hiding their feelings which are easily aroused and frequently lead to emotional short circuit. They are unable to throw off experiences which are laden with emotions and they harbor resentment. In children this is frequently expressed by sulking. There is a strong tendency to anticipation which, when the situation arises, has already undermined the patient's ease. Some persons are sensitive to situations in which they are exposed to a large group; others are sensitive to definite personalities or to forming initial contacts. While it is most difficult for one stutterer to meet strangers, another can do this well but is most disturbed with his own family or with friends. They are ambitious, but frequently have general and ill-defined goals which make their realization difficult or impossible. They are reserved and lack the ability to discuss their problems with ease. On the whole these personalities are not fully organized and develop with increasing rigidity and, when adult, lack sufficient plasticity. In self-assertive make-ups this may lead to an aggressive self-assertive attitude to life, in submissive persons to passive resistance and inability to adjust. Many stutterers show traits which are found in the group of immature personalities. They are characterized by a lack of consistent activity and of expression of genuine individuality. These persons have insufficient control of emotional display, are easily thrilled and enthusiastic, but also easily discouraged. They have a need for affection which is frequently not connected with real sympathy for others, and they react with antagonism toward some people and their ideas, without sufficient sympathy. A constant craving for something new and a desire for change, a liking for romantic stories and adventures, imaginations of being a hero, revolt against things as they are, and superficial cynicism are frequently observed. Their emancipation is insufficient. They are resentful to criticism and react with sulky and surly behavior, combined with a tendency to be revengeful and a desire for retaliation. Many have a marked fear of the dark and childish fears of robbers. Such fears are not necessarily on a sexual basis but can be due to immaturity of imagination and habit-formation. Occasionally, immature thinking is characterized by lack of constructive discrimination. Physical immaturity frequently accompanies immaturity of the personality, but not always.

Stuttering starts in the years of greatest plasticity of early childhood, at a time when functions are not yet well developed. The development of this malfunctioning becomes part of the general development of the personality. It is therefore not surprising that it becomes a set part of the personality which can only be modified slightly if a person with full-fledged stuttering comes for help after maturity has been reached. Conditioning to more or less specific situations and increasingly rigid habit-formation greatly handicap our therapeutic attempts at modification and correction. The prognosis is usually better when stuttering develops in later phases of childhood, i.e., at around six when the child has to make the adjustment to the larger group and its demands in school, or at a time when there is a subsequent need for life adjustments.

Treatment attempts to modify the personality and to use available means at correction of the personality and speech habits. The personality at the time of study and the various phases of its development should be carefully studied and formulated to the patient in language which he can grasp, pointing out the most striking features which need to be modified and how this can be achieved. Outstanding life situations and environmental influences need to be analyzed constructively. These latter features are of predominant importance in small children and form the basis for a suitable direct and indirect education. In small children, as well as those of school age, psychotherapy by means of play analysis and environmental and educational changes are indicated. In older children and adolescents, a discussion of the personality is desirable. A far-reaching analysis is, however, rarely justified and only if definite psychogenic factors which the child will be able to grasp are at work. Habit training and correction of the formed undesirable habit takes into consideration the child's personality and the points of best modifiability in the patient and in the environment. It should utilize direct and indirect re-education with attention to the individual's suggestibility. In a self-assertive child discipline and authority may provoke an attitude of opposition and resentment which disturbs his ease continually. In a submissive, suggestible child authoritative suggestions may lead to symptomatic improvement. Indirect and direct suggestive influences should be used freely in re-education but merely as a part of all other measures which lead to a correction of the undesirable personality traits. Hypnosis is frequently of great help in breaking already well-established faulty habits of speech and attitudes in children and adults. Speech-training on the other hand is contraindicated, as one does not deal with a disorder of articulation which needs to be corrected systematically, and for the reason that it attracts the patient's attention to the speech. The goal should be to make the patient speak without being constantly aware of it. Speech should flow freely and rhythmically. Attention and effort interfere. The good results which have been obtained occasionally through speech-training are due to indirect suggestive influences and lead only to a symptomatic improvement.

A certain amount of direct speech correction on a modified basis may be helpful. The stutterer usually talks hastily and too loud and even with definite cluttering. These patients should be urged to talk slowly, breathing deeply and regularly. In others it is necessary to point out to them that they slur and speak indistinctly. The same corrections should be applied to the general behavior, to actions, and decisions.

The older theories of stuttering presented it as primarily a neurogenic, organic, or functional disorder and neglected the personality setting. This led to an entirely symptomatic treatment. The observation that the correction of educationally poorly managed left-handedness led to improvement of stutterers should urge us to consider the factor of handedness carefully. It should, however, be considered as an aggravating, but not fundamental, factor, and not prevent us from studying and modifying the personality factors. In recent years attention has been directed to personality factors. Anticipation and anxiety have been emphasized. It has been stressed that timidity and marked sensitiveness are the outstanding predisposing constitutional tendencies which cause the child to begin to stutter when experiencing a fright. This development is certainly rare and cannot be made the general basis for treatment. Stekel groups anxiety under phobias (anxiety hysteria), believing that a sexual trauma causes the reaction in a neuropathic constitution. Stuttering is frequently claimed to be some kind of sexual symbol. His case material shows that such cases exist but they form a small group. Adler stresses inferiority, which uses the stuttering as an excuse for avoiding decisions and a protest against being neglected. Psychoanalytic literature offers much case material. The outstanding

dynamic factors found are anal-erotic, sadistic, and narcissistic strivings, and of somewhat less importance, the factors which result
from the Oedipus and castration complex. Stuttering seems to be
therefore similar to compulsive neurosis. Coriat stresses, in addition, fixation of oral-erotic tendencies and mentions as oral-erotic
character traits omnipotence, overevaluation of intellectual attainment, and envy. For treatment, one should not analyze fear and
anxiety but the underlying psychodynamic factors and these outstanding personality features. A physician who wishes to treat stutterers
should be acquainted with the observations of the various investigators. He should consider these findings as possibilities and deal
with them constructively when found, but not use one or the other
as the general therapeutic principle. Not infrequently, stuttering
occurs with sexual maladjustment, e.g., psychic impotency. A constructive analysis is then necessary to achieve more than symptomatic
improvement and one should not be satisfied by merely explaining
both reactions by lack of self-confidence and the tendency to anticipation.

The discussion of a case will demonstrate the treatment of
stuttering, outlining the personality analysis and adjustment and the
re-educational procedure. In the latter are included the specific
speech correction as well as general habit education. A formulation of ease and tension and the factors which cause both is essential. In correcting speech one needs to stress the advisability of slow
and distinct talk with sufficient breathing pauses. This should not
lead to excessive slowness of speech. Instead of the previously
advised monotony of talk to enforce relaxation, one should try to
establish a rhythm of speech. The danger of symptomatic overattention must be kept in mind. Reading aloud, in the office and at
home, may be helpful in marked stuttering but should not be carried on over too long a period of time and should be limited to
the beginning of the treatment. Talking with others and in an increasingly larger group is more helpful if it can be carried on under
supervision and with analysis of the disturbing factors. There is no
need to be afraid of infectious stuttering. When it occurs, one deals
with a suggestible person who is predisposed to stuttering through
his constitutional make-up. Such induced stuttering is easily corrected by suggestion and hypnosis if attended to promptly. In stut-

tering in various members of a family these same factors play a role. The constitutional tendencies which form the basis for stuttering may be inherited, but not stuttering itself. Relaxation in stutterers can be enforced through Frank's psychocathartic method (see p. 108), which at the same time will re-activate emotionally disturbing situations and memories. Hypnosis helps in the same way. Detailed speech re-education can be carried out under hypnosis. This is not used frequently as it is too time-consuming and forces one to spend too much effort on the merely symptomatic aspect. Recreation, especially in athletics if competition is not stressed, helps to increase ease in dealing with the group and to establish healthy self-confidence. Although some patients succeed in losing stuttering by overcompensation, this tendency should not be fostered as it does not lead to a healthy personality adjustment. In children one should be aware of the tendency of the patient and persons in the environment to use stuttering as an excuse for failures based on other inadequacies. It is therefore essential that one always determine the intellectual endowment and whether too much is expected from the child. It is best to inform child, parents, and teachers that a normal education should be carried out and the child encouraged but not excused, e.g., from reciting. Treatment needs to be carried out over a long period of time with consultations once a week, and later every two to three weeks. Where psychogenic factors play a role more intensive treatment is indicated in the beginning.

Case 28:

A 21 year old girl was referred to me in 1927 because of stuttering which started at the age of 5, and had such a marked increase since about 16 that she was now unable to carry on a conversation. She was a milliner and had to be satisfied with work and an income which she felt was by no means adequate to her abilities. At first, one was unable to obtain a satisfactory history because she stuttered so badly that one could barely understand her. After about an hour she began to feel more at ease and some idea of the development of her illness was gained. Hypnosis was started in the hope of being able to relieve her of some of her symptoms. She first came for three hypnotic treatments a week of ten to fifteen minutes' duration. After the second session a middle deep hypnosis was obtained. No deeper hypnosis was attempted as this stage had a sufficiently suggestive influence. After about two weeks she began to improve somewhat so that one was able to get a better history. Consultations were spaced to only once a week. Until then, suggestions had been offered that her muscles, especially the muscles of her throat and neck, were relaxing and that she would be able to use them without much difficulty. The fact was impressed on her that while talking to somebody her attention would be drawn to what she wanted to say and not to the speech mechanism.

The patient had shown difficulties in her speech since early childhood but they grew markedly worse when she went to school. She had always been very sensitive and timid and afraid of talking because others laughed at her. Her difficulties increased according to the environment and circumstances. The teacher paid much attention to her speech difficulty and it was not necessary for her to recite or to answer questions when her stuttering was marked. Nevertheless, this speech difficulty became so interfering that she had to stop high school in the second year. This was also necessary because of financial reasons. It was a severe disappointment to her because she had expected to go into nurses' training. All her wishes were still centered around this goal. She was turned down in one hospital because of her speech difficulty and she had to take a position as maid to children. Finally she obtained her present position in a department store and her main reason for requesting treatment was the hope of entering training when her speech improved.

After four weeks, the psychocathartic procedure of Frank was utilized in addition to the hypnotic suggestions. She began to become more relaxed and often experienced pictures of situations which were of importance to her. We always discussed them afterwards and this allowed us to get a better understanding of her personality and to achieve some readjustment. She was also advised to begin to read to a friend, but was told that this training was usually overvalued because after a short time the patient gets accustomed to that person and further reading will then be a waste of time and distract the attention from the more important problem of getting an understanding of the personality. The patient began to see that her family situation was a rather unhealthy one. She was the older of two girls and since her parents' death when she was 15 had felt that she ought to take the responsibility of her sister who was three years younger. The patient had little confidence in her ability in general and had always been dependent upon others. Her standards and ideals were always high but rather vague. There was always a desire to devote herself to others, and her most happy year was when she took care of a small child. Because of financial reasons she was forced to take a position where she could earn more money. The patient had then reacted with some sleep difficulties, felt nervous, and her speech had become much worse (at 18, in 1924). An aunt invited her to live with her but she never felt happy there. She began to react with nausea, abdominal pain, and extreme fatigue to any difficulties in her family and also to difficult decisions. Her attitude to her family was one of devotion and resentment. She felt that her aunt and grandparents, who had never been interested in her, were friendly then because she was financially independent. She also was unable to forget that they were unfair to her in childhood. She was devoted to her sister, but quite worried about her because she married when she was 16. She worried that her sister was living with people who were vulgar and coarse. She wanted to reform her sister and give her higher ideals in life. Her whole attitude was immature. She never tried to face a situation as it really was. Her sexual development and present interests were not outstanding factors, as became evident during the discussions.

The patient was advised to give up her home with her aunt and to stay at the Y.W.C.A., and she was urged to mix with people. This was a marked difficulty for her. She had overcome her shyness and her concern about her speech difficulty. Being a likeable girl, she soon made friends but till the end of treatment had to be urged to be with others. She usually reacted with more stuttering to discussions of these difficulties, but I was able to diminish the symptoms with hypnotic suggestions, which were carried out over a period of three months. After two and a half months the patient was able to talk fairly well except if something unexpected happened or when she had to make an important decision. Attention was directed toward educating her to form her own ambitions. She obtained an understanding of the underlying factors which caused her to have the wish to take up nursing, i.e., her wish for social standing and a desire to take care of others, and to overcompensate her own feeling of insecurity. She had a marked tendency to daydreaming. She often criticized others without a clear understanding of the situation and was impatient in dealing with people, unwilling to change her ideas. She had always become emotionally upset and easily discouraged by minor obstacles. During her treatment she took up work at night school. She began to observe her lack of ease and her hastiness. She was advised to talk slowly and to fight her impatience, restlessness, and hastiness. Her description was the characteristic one of a stutterer: "It seems I just don't have the time — it seems to me I am always in a hurry."

The treatment lasted six months, with an occasional consultation during the following two years. This did not involve much time as the consultations had been spaced to once in two weeks after the first two months. The patient matured greatly, understanding herself better and knowing how to deal with her interests and desires. She worked as a milliner for four more years and then entered nurses' training. Her speech difficulty is now only present when her ease is considerably disturbed and she takes it as an indication for the need to find the disturbing factors. Plasticity, which, however, was not very marked, and suggestibility at the period of late adolescence were the prognostically favorable factors. In a rigid development less favorable results would have to be expected with regard to symptomatic improvement. The patient has continued in good social adjustment with little speech disorder when disturbed. She is now married, and is taking care of her family which includes two children.

Accessory movements are frequent in stutterers. Some patients used them originally for enforcing relaxation or to force words out. In others there is a combination of tics and stuttering. The prognosis is less favorable in these cases. The advice to use accessory movements to get distracted from the speech difficulty is most unfortunate. Rare types of stuttering affect playing the piano, trumpet, etc. They seem to be related to various cramps. Other speech disorders, e.g., baby talk, delayed speech, excessive rapidity and cluttering, lisping, etc., are primarily educational and behavior problems with which the practitioner needs to be acquainted, and which should be referred to a psychiatrist if personality factors prevent the correction. In all these cases the determination of the intellectual level is important.

Stuttering always starts in childhood. The patient frequently loses it spontaneously in adolescence and with maturity but a physician should not delay treatment because of this possibility. In such favorable cases a few therapeutic suggestions will hasten the improvement and make a good personality adjustment more likely. Hysterical stuttering may start in adult life and should be treated accordingly. Some observations point also to a possible compulsive nature. In these reactions sexual factors seem to play an important role. With disturbance of the organization of the personality, childhood stuttering may reappear. I have seen this in schizophrenic illnesses and especially in pre-senile and arteriosclerotic cerebral changes. It then requires symptomatic attention.

TICS AND OCCUPATIONAL NEUROSES

Tics originate from coordinated and purposeful movements which served as reflex, defense, or expressional movements. A psychogenic as well as a neurogenic basis of tics should therefore always be considered. They rarely develop before the age of seven and frequently show a marked increase in puberty. The personality is similar to that of stutterers, and habit-formation is an important factor. Abortive forms of tics occur occasionally and can be easily corrected. In a 5 year old boy a slight coughing tic had developed as an attempt to attract attention from his parents who, because of recent tuberculosis in the family, were greatly distressed by it. Intelligent educational handling made it disappear after a year but later, even in the early twenties, this patient still showed a tendency to it when feeling self-conscious. A brief personality discussion made the symptom disappear completely. Such cases demonstrate that habit formation depends largely on the personality setting.

Many tics have a definite sexual origin. To this belong many scratching tics. The nature of the tic is frequently difficult to recognize because the originally clear and full movement becomes abbreviated. It is therefore always necessary to study carefully the setting in which the tic started. Afterwards less and less important factors may reproduce it. There is always a danger that, in the analysis of such conditions, the physician may try to find constant recurring factors and lose himself frequently in the study of minor situations. This, however, does not mean that there are not many cases where recurrent situations must be considered.

Tics of the eyelids are frequent. They may originate in a merely incidental scratching caused by a foreign body, and develop into a habit. In some this may lead to a blepharospasm which in others is on an entirely psychogenic basis, usually expressing the unwillingness of the patient to see certain life situations. The prognosis and therapy depend on the personality setting. In well-organized persons a brief study of the factors involved and a constructive formulation make the symptoms disappear in a short time. In psychopathic personalities re-educational procedures are of importance.

Speech tics are not frequent. They are usually on a compulsive basis and express coprolalia in a clear or abbreviated form. As they usually occur in seriously psychopathic personalities the prognosis is not very good. The treatment should be directed to an analysis of the personality and to re-education. Hypnosis, which in other tics is occasionally successful, leads to only temporary improvement in coprolalia, if any. Minor speech tics, especially with involvement of the throat, are frequently habits which develop easily in self-conscious persons.

Spastic torticollis is usually on a psychogenic basis. It expresses the unwillingness of the patient to accept certain difficulties, a turning away from them. The prognosis is usually not good for permanent recovery because these patients are unwilling to make the adjustment. In two cases I saw good improvement after removal to the neutral hospital atmosphere and treatment by distributive analysis. However, both patients had an immediate recurrence when returning home. It is hard to say in such cases to what extent voluntary factors can utilize the psychogenically established habit. In early torticollis the possibilities for psychotherapy are much better. It is essential that physicians recognize these cases as psychogenic and do not waste time and money on orthopedic and surgical treatment except where definite organogenic or neurogenic factors cause it. Bandages and operations cannot be justified in psychogenic torticollis and tics. In both conditions occupational habits may have been utilized.

Occasionally these reactions occur in a schizophrenic setting. They may also develop in a presenile illness or in a depression. Torticollis, for example, may be the expression of aversion to accepting the depression or the underlying dynamic factors. The treatment is then that of the whole psychopathologic reaction and not merely of the symptom.

The therapeutic approach is constructive distributive analysis and re-education of the personality. The symptomatic treatment has to make use of suggestion or hypnosis and advice to suppress the tic. When done systematically (Meige and Feindel) this education to inhibition and suppression can have very satisfactory results. Exercises of immobilization and of movement are utilized. The patients are taught to keep still for two to three minutes in the posture in which the tic occurs least frequently. This is done three to five times daily, at regular times and at least once daily under the physician's supervision. The patient is advised to carry out slowly and correctly certain movements, first at the command of the physician and later spontaneously. It seems best to use restrained rest and inhibited movements from the beginning and to let the patient carry them out in front of a mirror so that he becomes aware of the movements in detail. With improvement the duration is prolonged to a maximum of about five minutes and the interviews are spaced. The patient is always carefully informed of his progress and failures. He must be told in the beginning that all depends on his persistence in carrying out the exercises carefully for months or even years, even after the symptoms have temporarily disappeared. The physician should find various exercises according to the tic and also the personality involved. In some cases relaxation exercises are advised in addition. In exercises of the hands both hands should be used simultaneously. There are many variations of the procedure of Meige and Feindel to make it more suitable to special tics. The principle is, however, always the same. Such a treatment should be combined with regular routine which fills the patient's whole day. It is obvious that education of the whole personality and suggestive influences play a considerable role in this procedure. Many times the breaking away from environmental or other undesirable association is necessary.

Occupational neuroses, among the wide variety of which writers' cramp serves as prototype, are of functional origin. Some cases belong to phobias; in others one deals with a symptom in another personality disorder, e.g., schizophrenia. Usually one deals with constitutionally poorly organized and unstable persons of the type which has been described above. Fatigue, undernutrition, and toxic factors precipitate the disorder. Anxiety and anticipation are the disturbing emotions. Every case deserves individual attention, an analysis of the whole setting, and of the patient's personality development.

Case 29:

A 28 year old stenographer, who had been in her present position seven years had during all this time noticed a tendency for her hands to jerk when taking dictation. In the last three months she noticed increasing cramps which forced her to take a vacation. A brief study revealed that she was a shy, not very sociable person who had always paid much attention to her health and reacted with gastric complaints to minor strain. After a disappointment in love two years before, she developed slight depressive moods. Previously she had always felt depressed before and during menses. In the last six months she had reacted with vomiting and belching to increase of work and changes in the office. Her writer's cramp was due to these life difficulties and emotional factors. In the office where she now had to work for a driving and abrupt man she felt ill at ease, anxious to do her work fast and well, but unable to do so. Her feelings were easily hurt, and she was unable to throw it off. In her depressed mood she began to stay at home and omit all recreation. Going to the office became a dread to her while previously she had enjoyed her work. In a few consultations (over a period of two weeks) the patient learned to understand herself better. She reorganized her life, including social and physical recreation. Returning to her work she was able to make a satisfactory adjustment. An opportunity for ventilation, encouragement, and strong suggestive reassurance with regard to the use of her hands were of considerable therapeutic importance. (No follow-up note was obtained.)

In advanced cases the treatment will take several months. Patients should be urged to return to work as early as possible or to enter a hospital where intensive psychotherapy with occupations without disturbing environmental influences can be carried out. Hypnotic suggestions are helpful, especially in anxious persons who anticipate the immediate return of the symptoms when starting their occupation.

COMPENSATION REACTIONS
(Compensation Neuroses)

With the development of insurance to accidents and illnesses and the possibility of gaining compensation from injuries, psychogenic and psychoneurotic reactions in relation to injuries and illnesses have become frequent. Until recently the general tendency has been to consider the desire for adequate compensation as the leading factor and to arrange for some kind of final settlement. Little hope was held for influencing the reaction psychotherapeutically until the financial attraction had been removed. In recent years, because of a closer study of the patient's personality and of the factors which caused him to refuse a medically reasonable settlement, a more dynamic understanding and treatment of compensation neuroses has begun to be accepted.

Even when the financial factor is of leading importance and makes the patient unwilling to accept the psychogenic or emotional basis of his illness, the physician still needs to analyze why the patient has such a set attitude. In some patients it is the desire for getting as much as possible. In many others, however, it is not primarily the materialistic aspect but the feeling that they have the right to expect the desired compensation. In still others there is a marked need for full justice, frequently even with a desire for revenge against the person who carelessly, whether or not this be actually correct, has caused the accident. To this group belong paranoid make-ups and the querulous paranoics. Then again fear of insecurity may be the deterrent factor, doubts that one will really be able to work as satisfactorily as the physician assures him or that the symptoms will actually clear up. Environmental factors or the dealings with representatives of the insurance company may influence the patient unfavorably. It also happens, unfortunately, that physicians aggravate the patient's attitude.

Case 30:

 A 55 year old railroad engineer, when convalescing from a prolonged grippe which worried him considerably, developed a depression to his son's sudden death. After six months he improved, but since then (for four years) had been in a depressive rut, feeling slightly depressed in the morning, irritable and apathetic during the day, unable to work, and constantly talking about headaches and feeling weak. The physicians who treated him felt that the compensation from his health insurance played the main role and the insurance company therefore tried to discontinue the compensation. The then 60 year old patient demanded new examinations and was referred to me. At the first consultation I was impressed with the fact that the patient was able to accept the formulation of rut-formation and that he was in need of definite routine and occupation. He was urged to enter the hospital, as such a well-planned treatment would be impossible at home and also to remove him from his over-concerned and worrying wife. To this he agreed. The physical examination revealed chronic otitis media with discharge which had lasted for six years, a few carious teeth, and slight inflammation of some finger joints. We reassured him as to his general health and advised him to enter into full routine and to associate with the other patients. He began to improve steadily and learned to disregard his complaints. His wife was also encouraged and urged not to discuss his illness during her weekly visits.

 We dealt with an unintelligent, sociable man with very few interests, always economical and since his present illness greatly concerned about their meager income. He was in constant fear that the physician would declare him well before he was fully recovered and that, being unable to work, he could not support his family. He had always been set and unforgiving if hurt. The statement from the physician and insurance company that he ought to be able to work had hurt his pride considerably and he developed resentment. Our own attitude and formulation offered the basis for healthy rapport. The hospital atmosphere created a wholesome, suggestive, and distracting influence. Our reassurance was always strongly suggestive and this and the improvement of his ear condition under conservative treatment counteracted his hypochondriacal concerns. He learned to overlook the slight pain in his fingers and was willing to resume work. He was not intelligent enough to understand fully the personality factors which are mentioned above. They were, however, taken into consideration in our formulations to him. After two months he was ready for discharge. He had learned to accept that there was at present no possibility of returning to his previous position and was willing to accept work as a fireman. On our recommendation he started to work immediately and has been doing well since (three years). A lapse of a week between discharge and resuming work, that is a week of insufficient routine and time for anticipation, might have undone a great deal. (No follow-up note on the patient was obtained.)

A careful study of the accident and illness and its actual and possible results, of the attitiude of the patient and of those in the environment to it and of the personality setting are necessary for successful treatment. Psychogenic reactions are of importance; i.e., psychobiologic disorders which are caused by the patient's expectation that he might develop certain mental or somatic symptoms. The factors in psychogenic reactions are suggestibility which also leads to induced symptoms and imitation, the formation of overvalued ideas, catathymic influences, and repression. One should consider the immediate emotional reactions to the accident and the physiologic features which accompanied them. Strong emotions of fear, especially fright, affect one's ability to grasp a situation and lead to a narrowing of consciousness. Hysterical reactions occur when, besides expectancy, a definite wish or desire for gain enters. It does not merely need to be material gain but may be a desire for retaliation or resentment and many other motives, according to the personality at the time of the accident and its sequellae. The formation of the symptoms depends on the type of the experience and how it affects the body. An injury to the head easily causes various types of headaches and head sensations, and injuries to other parts of the body corresponding symptoms and complaints. Formation of symptoms further utilizes organic inferiorities and the individual possibilities for somatic reactions. Well known, for example, is the utilization of an occult spina bifida. One should therefore always study carefully the physiologic reactions of the past, especially vasomotor and gastrointestinal reactions, the possibilities of endocrine disorders, and interrelations of these reaction tendencies and emotions.

The attitude of the patient and of the persons in his environment vary greatly according to what is valuable to them and what they fear they might lose. This attitude may refer to financial factors and their direct and indirect influence. It is possible that the money means a great deal because of greed or because it would permit the patient to start on some important venture such as marriage or business improvement, or because the resulting illness will lead to economic difficulties or ruin. In others, the interest in one's body has always been marked. An injury may stir up hypochondriacal overconcern and anticipation. A scar has often a definite meaning to the patient. Surgeons easily overlook this and may not use as careful plastic surgery as is desirable in such a make-up. The personality reaction to the loss of an eye or a limb should be carefully studied. Impediment of hearing leads to grave social implications, especially in persons who have tendencies to a paranoic constitution (see Chapter XI). The attitude to the group and to the family may enter considerably; separation from them and possible prolonged hospitalization may mean a great deal to certain persons. Environmental concern, resentment, and greed affect the patient and may induce various reactions and symptoms. Many sensory disturbances, paresthesias, and anesthesia are produced by too obvious and repeated physical and neurologic examinations and questions referring to such symptoms in suggestible, anxious, hypochondriacal, and hysterical personalities. A complete and careful study is important and repetitions may be necessary. These repeated studies and observations should not be carried out in too obvious a form and should be accompanied by reassurance which counteracts undesirable suggestive influences. The constitutional possibilities of emotional reactions, especially depression, should be studied and prevented by careful psychotherapy. Formulation and advice should be offered according to the patient's intellectual equipment and according to his ideas about injuries.

The physician ought to base his reassuring formulation on a careful physical examination. Any physical complication should be treated with due consideration of the person's reaction and tendencies.

Replacement of spinal fluid by air has been recommended. Penfield advocates air injection for the treatment of chronic meningeal headaches, trying to break down old pia-arachnoid adhesions. The cardinal symptoms are localized pain in the head and transient vertigo. The headache is localized near the site of the blow and, in some cases, on the opposite side of the head. There are many other surgical procedures which are advocated for various posttraumatic complaints. On the whole it will be advisable to be conservative and be guided by a critical evaluation of actual findings.

Treatment of compensation reactions should always be individually adjusted, taking into consideration all the factors which have been mentioned and dealing with the whole, integrated personality. Prolonged psychogenic reactions with inability to work occur primarily in poorly organized psychopathic and immature personalities, in feebleminded people and in persons who suffer from brain defects caused by trauma or organic psychoses. The setting of a psychoneurosis or psychosis and defects of various organs also aggravates the condition. Psychogenic and hysterical reactions are frequent in children, expressing a desire for punishment of the person who has caused the injury or for affection and care from the environment, the desire to be the center of attention, or the utilization of the illness as an excuse. These reactions clear up soon if they are not kept alive by adults (family, nurses, and other patients). In any compensation neurosis which does not yield to treatment in a reasonably short time or where personality or environmental factors make it desirable, removal to a neutral environment is indicated. Hospitalization and psychiatric treatment should be the usual choice. It is essential that psychotherapy, i.e., reassurance through careful examination, discussion of the insurance problem, distributive analysis of all the factors involved, and a gradually more inclusive formulation, direct and indirect suggestion, be combined with active routine and occupation. Such a patient should live in the group and participate in its activities. Isolation is only justified in dramatic hysterical display and only for a short time. Occupational therapy, in accordingly adjusted form, which utilizes the patient's interests, is also indicated in patients who have to stay in bed for physical complications. Hysterical and psychogenic manifestations should never lead to bed treatment. Hypnosis may occasionally be desirable, but one can usually dispense with it. The treatment can be carried out in a general hospital but in most patients, especially in persistent or symptomatically involved cases, a psychiatric hospital is indicated. Some authors urge the establishment of special hospitals for such patients in order not to overcrowd the psychiatric hospitals and because of the prejudice of the public. This would seem to me therapeutically undesirable. It is necessary that physicians and the public understand the realm of psychiatric treatment and hospitalization and that a broader attitude be developed.

Many times such a patient feels incapable of returning to his accustomed work or the physician considers him more suitable for different work. It is advisable not to spend too much effort and time on a vocational re-education and training, which is indicated and offers good results in non-neurotic crippled patients. Placement in other work or on a farm should be advised instead. Psychiatric re-education, however, with well-planned occupational therapy and routine, is always indicated whenever a patient is unable to resume work. The various procedures which have been advocated during the war cannot be considered valid at a time when one should be able to offer sufficient therapeutic attention to the individual case.

The early recognition of a beginning compensation neurosis and determination of the patient's attitude to accidents and to the factor of compensation is important. Many physicians are lenient, feeling that the impersonal insurance company is well in a position to help the patient although the illness is not directly caused by the accident. The public in general has this same attitude. In addition, there is a general tendency to overevaluate accidents and their possible implications. Other physicians feel unable to decide whether there could not be some organic factors involved. The presence of psychogenic factors does not exclude an organic basis. Only careful observation, which, however, must be combined with the above-outlined psychotherapeutic approach, will answer these questions. One should keep in mind that there is always the possibility of fixation on originally organic pains. A serious mistake is made if physicians do not take the patient's complaints seriously or jump to the conclusion of malingering.

There occur different emotional reactions to an accident, especially fright (suddenness of the experience), fear of recurrence (e.g., in explosions and earthquakes), anxiety (resulting from the possibility of death or suffocation), and horror (seeing others killed). Correct treatment by the first attending physician will decrease these emotions and the accompanying physiologic symptoms in a short time. In constitutionally predisposed persons they may, however, persist and form the nucleus of the neurosis. The physician should be careful not to speak immediately of shock reactions. Among outstanding symptoms are cardiovascular and sleep disturbances and loss of weight. In asthenic persons between forty and fifty, slight physiologic changes, which have preceded the accident for years, increase and convalescence will then take a longer time. In some cases it may lead to marked aging. These symptoms are sequellae of the accident and not neuroses.

Case 31:

After collision with another automobile in which his car turned over, but without injuring him, a 27 year old man developed marked headaches and vomited frequently during the first two days, was tearful and tremulous. He was greatly upset because the other driver refused to pay damages, blaming the patient for reckless driving. He was admitted to a general hospital where he was at first apathetic and sleepy, then (after five days) became irritable and easily upset by noises, shaking and quivering. This lasted five days. He then improved gradually and was discharged to home care with a special nurse after three weeks' hospitalization. He now changed little, was easily irritated and frightened and upset by noises, frequently stuttering. After two months he was admitted to another general hospital, remaining in about the same condition except that the stuttering decreased. Some half-hearted attempts at occupational therapy were undertaken but the patient did really what pleased him. He received considerable amounts of barbiturates for broken sleep and much orthopedic attention to pains in his lumbar region. Slightly unequal pupils and his complaints led to the diagnosis of an old fracture of the skull and shell shock. After five weeks he was transferred to our psychiatric clinic.

On admission the patient was in good physical condition and neurologic examination was entirely negative. He was easily frightened by noises. When light was flashed into his eyes he pressed the lids together tightly and showed a marked tremor. The pulse was around 96 and he had frequent bowel movements. The thyroid gland was somewhat enlarged and soft. There was occasional stuttering when he became excited especially when discussing his accident and the resulting complaints. During the whole examination, and later on the ward, he showed marked craving for sympathy and attention, trying to impress others with his high abilities. He was cheerful and self-assertive, assuring others that he understood his condition well and that it was shell shock. To any fast movement or noise he reacted with slight fright, trembling and grimacing.

A brief study revealed that this patient was immature in thinking and action, sociable but unable to make close and lasting friends because he always wanted to be in the center of everything and tried to impress others with vague talk about philosophy, his self-esteem easily hurt, and sulking about various injustices. He was interested in athletics and proud of his physique. His ambitions were not well defined. He wanted to make much money to be able to educate himself better and to have a home and family. His intelligence was about average. After several years' steady work as a salesman he had become dissatisfied and considered changing in the last year. His sexual life had never been active. Until the age of 23 he had idealized a girl and began to have intercourse only after she had become engaged to another man. After his first sexual intercourse with a friend he felt disgusted, worried over the possibility of venereal infection, asked for several blood tests, and had pains in his penis for two years. The diagnosis of possible posterior urethritis was made and the pain disappeared under massage. The patient had a congenital urethral malformation and lower right testicle which worried him considerably. During his few experiences in intercourse his erection had never been satisfactory, but he obtained an ejaculation. Every few months he had spontaneous ejaculation with dreams which he did not remember. In the last year he had no sexual experiences, thinking a great deal about the girl he had loved for years, trying to convince himself that she would be happy with the other man. The girl married four weeks after the accident and he had been informed of it only a few days before the wedding. His father was a hypochondriacal person who had been constantly afraid that something might happen to his children on their way to school and had spoiled the patient greatly. The mother was a stable person. Two sisters and a brother were in good health. They always considered the patient an immature person who had never been emancipated from home.

Discussing the accident, he expressed resentment to the insurance company's unwillingness to pay him $50,000 and to the other man's aggressive and unyielding behavior. He wanted to have him punished. The police, however, decided that it was entirely his own fault. He had lost his position a week after the accident when his firm failed, and he had expected to gain enough compensation to lead a carefree life until he found something suitable. His outstanding reaction to the accident had been evasion of his responsibilities, followed by fear of serious injury, and finally anger about the ensuing difficulty, and his inability to throw off his fear. The development of his symptoms worried him greatly. When the headaches began to decrease with sedatives he began to worry over taking so much medicine and because a physician had told him his back pain might be due to an injury to his kidney. He also resented a physician's statement that he had always led a sheltered life and had been emotionally poorly controlled. His demand for compensation had been supported by his physicians and by his father, who expressed frequently his satisfaction that the patient was so highly insured through an accident policy that he could receive more money than he had earned previously. In the hospital he had always received much sympathy and attention from the nurses. The physicians had expressed their concern and puzzlement freely. When hearing the news of the wedding he had become greatly upset and discouraged over his life and future.

After a brief careful examination and observation of a few days we felt certain that organic factors did not enter, discontinued all sedatives at once and urged him to enter into a full routine. The patient was cooperative but resented that he did not receive more attention than others. His behavior to nurses was erotic but he was unable to recognize these strivings. I offered him a careful formulation of the factors involved. He learned to accept it after a few days but insisted that he was justified in receiving a large compensation. With all the facts as mentioned above, I doubted that it was primarily a financial factor and therefore stressed the other points and his whole personality. He improved rapidly and was discharged symptomatically well after two and a half months. A tendency to slight stuttering when excited had apparently existed previously, and the patient was again no longer aware of it. Little was obtained with regard to a more thorough personality understanding. Discharge was urged because he seemed to accept the hospital as a convenient shelter. The insurance company had declared its willingness to pay the hospital expenses as long as we felt it was necessary. The patient, who had developed confidence in the hospital, accepted this when he was approached after six weeks' treatment. Before discharge he also withdrew his suit, recognizing that there was little chance for success and that he had been primarily guided by motives of revenge and an immature attitude. (No follow-up note was obtained.)

In many patients a psychotherapeutic approach alone does not lead to recovery. This happens especially in cases where the financial factor is of essential importance and the patient intellectually or constitutionally is unable or unwilling to analyze this attitude constructively. It is then wise to urge a definite settlement which should be large enough to be attractive. The settlement should be carried out without delay and psychotherapy directed to this new situation and the future. Many patients hesitate to accept the settlement because they are anxious and uneasy about the possibility of getting worse in the future. In others the relatives need to be led to modify their attitudes. A physician should not feel that with settlement all the symptoms will disappear at once. This may happen, but more frequently the patient needs brief psychotherapeutic consultation for a more or less long period of time.

The role of the practitioner has been discussed in various places.

He should try to prevent the development of a compensation neurosis and correct the tendency to overevaluate the accident as a frightening and horrible experience, that of having gone through the danger of death. In all cases where compensation may enter he must be guided by his medical ethics and not by sympathy. He should always ask to see the insurance policy and advise the patient whether he is justified in expecting any compensation, and discuss it frankly with the patient's lawyer. When noticing the beginning of a compensation neurosis he should turn to intensive psychotherapy and treat all the factors involved, formulating the problem to patient and relatives. The insurance companies should have psychiatrically trained physicians on their staff with sufficient authority to enable prompt and individually adjusted cooperation. Lawyers and courts need to learn to appreciate these problems and avoid undue delay. The numerous possibilities for appeal and delay over months and years are especially undesirable. Huddleson's criticism is that the actual verdicts are too tardy in time and too liberal in amount. He therefore urges legal reforms and better public education. The establishment of special insurance courts with special courts of appeal has proved to be very satisfactory in some European countries and will be a need in the future with the increase of compensation insurance. Physicians who testify must realize that they have to offer an unbiased opinion. This is not possible if one's sympathies are involved and certainly not if the fee depends on the outcome of the trial.

The same psychodynamic and therapeutic principles which were discussed in this chapter exist in patients whose psychopathologic reactions are related to combat experience.

PSYCHOPATHIC PERSONALITIES

The treatment of psychopathic personalities depends on the characteristics which lead to difficulties. Re-education based on a constructive analysis of the personality is the main procedure. One should be guided by the fact that every person has features with which we can work and that a more or less suitable situation should be created. Perfect results cannot be expected and relapses should not discourage. The physician should be guided by what he considers essential and give in only on non-essential points. The patient should understand that certain undesirable reactions on his part will produce reactions from his environment which are undesirable to him and that sympathy and pity will not modify the attitude of others. He has to become self-dependent and recognize the need to adapt to life. His constitutional deficiency is not an excuse but a handicap.

Many attempts have been made to group psychopathic personalities. This is practically important because it allows more systematic and planned treatment, but it is artificial. An exaggeration or deficit of any of the features which were described in Chapter I can lead to psychopathic maladjustment. One should be careful not to use the term too broadly. Many patients need adjustment along various lines. It is then wiser to speak of personality difficulties and undesirable features. In these cases a distributive analysis leads to more or less good results, dependent on the general stability and plasticity of the personality. In psychopathic personalities, one deals with a far-reaching difficulty. The person is usually loosely organized and there is little need for, and possibility of, spontaneous adjustment of contradictory strivings. There is a disturbance in the synthesis of the personality. Another group is characterized by a rigidity and lack of plasticity. These patients must learn to become more plastic. Their treatment is therefore essentially the same as in the paranoic constitutions. One also includes in psychopathic personalities patients who show reactions which, if they were present in full-fledged form, would present well known clinical pictures, e.g., the cyclothymic and schizoid reactions. For their adjustment the principles of the treatment of mood disorders and schizophrenic illnesses have to be considered.

Many psychopathic persons who come to the physician are characterized by insufficient control of excessive emotional reactions, cravings, and desires. To the first group belong the excitable persons who often react to despair with outbursts of anger, with suicide, or with stupor and psychogenic deliria. A brief period of hospitalization is always indicated if previous attempts at adjustment have failed or if the patient might be dangerous to himself or others. The latter should be considered especially when alcoholism or jealousy plays a role. The treatment consists of determining what factors or situations precipitate and aggravate the outbursts and what can be modified in the patient and in the environment. In these, as in other psychopathic reactions, much attention should be paid to a healthy life routine with desirable recreation. In patients with marked resentment to life and in the discontented person the task is to look for interests which might offer satisfaction, perhaps in different work or in a hobby or social interests. In these cases and in those who suffer from their inadequacy an analysis of the factors which may have prevented a satisfactory attainment is indicated. One needs to investigate the relationship of their ambition and the content of their imaginations to their actual abilities and opportunities. A more relative and constructive conception of success and failure is necessary and a clearer understanding of what they wish from life.

The vacillating and suggestible person who lacks persistence and gives up easily or changes according to other interests in himself or to factors in the environment needs somebody to lean on and to help him actively. This does not mean that he should become dependent on others. The goal is an increase of self-reliance and reliability. In many cases, especially in the immature group, insufficient emancipation from their family is a factor.

In others the attitude to the group needs correction. Opportunities for social contact will increase social ease and develop interests in common with others. In some, athletic recreation, in others groups with cultural, political, or religious interests can be utilized. Control of imagination is necessary in persons who are unable to find this ease with the group, because they are constantly concerned about the impression they make on others or look for indications of slights or of disparaging expressions.

The need to correct one's imagination and to test it on reality is important in autistic and schizoid persons. This is also important in those who are given to fantasy and can no longer see spontaneously and clearly the border between fantasies and true memories and therefore fall into lying and pretense. This becomes especially difficult when it occurs in persons with insufficiently developed standards.

The anti- and asocial groups embrace a wide variety of cases. Normal personalities, and especially any of the previously mentioned psychopathic personalities, may become involved in criminal acts. In a relatively small group we deal with an actual ethical deficit, the origin of which seems to be in the earliest phase of infancy or possibly in the constitutional make-up. Such patients are most trying and even prolonged treatment over years in a psychiatric hospital may prove to be futile. Hospital treatment, however, should always be tried with the frank understanding that readmission would be immediately resorted to if any misdemeanors occur. It is important, then, for the physician not to have too set an attitude, avoiding, however, a leniency which the patient will abuse. Removal from the home environment and attempts at reconstruction in a suitable setting may often help considerably. Re-educational attempts in a group of other such psychopathic personalities, and especially with other criminals, cannot be successful. The place for such patients is in a psychiatric hospital rather than reformatories and similar institutions.

It would lead to mere repetition if I attempted to outline the treatment of psychopathic personalities in detail. Every patient must be studied individually to determine what personality and somatic factors can be modified and what is available for an individualized re-education. This may be attempted outside the hospital, in the usual, or in an adjusted, environment, or in the neutral setting of a psychiatric hospital. Minor psychoneurotic complaints or more or less marked psychoneurotic reactions need to be treated by distributive analysis combined with constant synthesis and re-education. In many psychopathic personalities one deals with a neurotic personality development which, however, may have started so early in life that it has become ingrained and is part of the whole personality, no longer reducible, and only modifiable to some extent. In few cases does a prolonged and far-reaching analysis of the personality help to an extent which justifies the amount of time and energy spent on it. One still must admit that this group of personality disorders has not received sufficient therapeutic interest, and that better procedures may result from a more intensive study.

BIBLIOGRAPHY

1. GREENE, J. S., and WELLS, E. J.: *The Cause and the Cure of Speech Disorders*. The Macmillan Company, New York, 1927. (A practical outline of the treatment of stuttering, stammering and voice disorders.)

2. CORIAT, I. H.: Active Therapy in the Analysis of Stammering. *The Psychoanalytic Review*, 17, 1930. (A discussion of literature is found in Coriat's monograph on *Stammering*, Nervous and Mental Disease Monograph, Series 47, 1928.)
3. DESPERT, J. L.: Psychopathology of Stuttering. *American Journal of Psychiatry*, 99, 1943. (Review of current theories.)
4. MEIGE, H., and FEINDEL, E.: *Tics and Their Treatment*. William Wood and Company, New York, 1907.
5. HOPPE, H. H.: The Treatment of Spasmodic Disorders. White and Jelliffe, *The Modern Treatment of Nervous and Mental Diseases*, Vol. 2. Lea & Febiger, Philadelphia, 1913. (Presentation of the re-educational methods of Meige and Feindel, Oppenheim, Pitres for the treatment of tics and torticollis.)
6. HUDDLESON, J. H.: *Accidents, Neuroses and Compensation*. The Williams & Wilkins Company, Baltimore, 1932.
7. REICHARDT, M.: *Die psychogenen Reaktionen einschliesslich der sogenannten Entschädigungsneurosen*. J. Springer, Berlin, 1932. (Study of psychogenic reactions and compensation neuroses.)
8. LINDNER, R. M., and SELIGER, R. V. (ed.): *Handbook of Correctional Psychology*. Philosophical Library, New York, 1947. (Includes a discussion of the concepts and theory of psychopathic personalities.)

Chapter XVII

SEXUAL DIFFICULTIES

A CLEAR understanding of normal sexual life, its development, and the factors which play a role at various phases is essential for an individualized treatment of the various kinds of sexual difficulties. Most of these patients with such difficulties do not come to the psychiatrist but ask their family physician, the gynecologist, or urologist for help for various physical manifestations which are the expression of their sexual maladjustment. The psychiatrically trained physician is frequently not only able to give advice for general sexual hygiene but also to treat minor disorders successfully. When one finds a more ingrained difficulty or marked personality involvement, referral to a psychiatrist is necessary.

There is a marked tendency among physicians and lay persons to overemphasize the role of sexual desires and gratifications in one's life. It is necessary that we be willing to recognize these functions whenever they are of actual importance but in the setting of the psychobiologically integrated personality. The development of sexual life and the dynamic factors involved have been studied to a far-reaching extent by the psychoanalytic school. I shall merely refer to what has been discussed in more detail in Chapter IV. These findings have greatly influenced the dynamic therapeutic approach to sexual difficulties. A physician should consider them even if their expansion into a general system and the theories which have arisen from these observations are unacceptable to him. They offer guidance in a pluralistic and distributive treatment of the individual patient.

SEXUAL REGULATION AND CONTROL

Sexual functions need to be investigated as a part of a broader personality study. Attention must be directed to present needs as well as to the development of the habits and attitudes which have been formed in the patient. Sexual control, which is as necessary as control of all our other psychobiologic activities, can only be carried out successfully if one is aware of one's own peculiarities, i.e., the amount and type of passion and the factors which stimulate it. In order to gain such an understanding, a patient should be urged to accept a period (on the average of two to three weeks) of complete sexual abstinence. Otherwise, stimulation blurs the actual facts. Many patients who believe that they are highly passionate will find out that they are in reality not very passionate, but keep themselves constantly stirred up through various factors. Most frequent is indulging in stimulating imaginations or dwelling on physical attractions. Everyone should recognize which parts of the human body are especially attractive to him and learn to avoid dwelling upon them in social or business life or when walking on the street, and refrain from indulging in such preoccupations. Specific situations which create desires depend on the individual attraction to certain partners. To this belong the attraction to prostitutes, to persons who are generally admired and who have glamour (e.g., actresses), and to situations which involve danger or romantic possibilities. Dancing, movies, books, and conversations therefore have a different influence on different personalities.

Physiologic cycles are characteristic of the individual. They may be more or less marked and circumscribed and lead to sexual tension, a term which is used freely but has not yet been sufficiently investigated. In women, these cycles are in connection with menstruation (premenstrual or postmenstrual, less frequently intermenstrual or intramenstrual). Seasonal changes have a definite influence. Frequently these physiologic cycles are accompanied by depressive features. In some, mood cycles dominate the physiologic and psychobiologic changes. Toxic factors, especially alcohol, stimulate sexual desires but decrease potency. The effect of certain foods, in contrast to lay opinion, is of minor importance. It is quite likely that the frequent involutional increase is on a physiologic basis, while the increase of sexual desires and activities in the beginning or organic psychoses is due to diminished inhibition and self-restraint. Unrecognized physical symptoms may accompany these sexual cycles. The physiologic relief in men occurs in night emissions, with or without dreams. In women, the various spontaneous relief factors are less obvious.

Education and environmental influences form our sexual control.

The physician therefore needs to be prepared to offer individually adjusted advice. In infants, unnecessary handling of the genitalia, frequently with the excuse of cleaning, should be avoided. Parents should not become alarmed by the infant's or child's interest in his genitalia, but should distract the child. In childhood, one should always offer enough information to satisfy questions and apparent needs but not more than the child can understand at the time, and one should be careful not to increase his curiosity. In adolescence, a complete sexual formulation — physiologic, psychobiologic, and social — is indicated. Incidental homosexuality should not be stressed unduly. One can prevent a youngster from being induced into undesirable sexual practices if the sexual activities are formulated as something essentially private. This does not lead to a need for secrecy or undue modesty if one realizes the importance of privacy in general in our physiologic and psychobiologic activities. A physician should be willing to accept broad limits of normality. Instead of preaching, he should outline the possibilities and dangers which are involved in the individual case and discuss them not merely with the patient but also with the relatives concerned. In adult sexual activities, a partner is always involved who also needs consideration and may need help. Codes which are necessary should not be fixed and rigid but used as guiding principles. In one's sexual life, one should be guided by the attitude of the group, in the sense which has been outlined in the introductory chapters, i.e., with a preservation of one's individuality. Reactions of spite should be prevented or adjusted. Marriage is not merely a sexual union but includes companionship and the principle of family formation. It should therefore always be on a permanent basis and not as a trial or gamble. When the latter tendencies exist, a thorough discussion or even prolonged analysis is necessary to obtain clarified ideas. The same applies to the unwillingness or inability to accept monogamy as the guiding principle.

In sexual life the physiologic and psychobiologic factors need to be integrated. This occurs with puberty and during adolescence. The separation of sexual and love factors is undesirable and, if this becomes a fixed principle, pathologic. Our whole sexual control should be based on the principle of sexual integration in the setting of the psychobiologically integrated personality, with special attention to the needs of individual and group adjustment. This problem is therefore merely one of the many problems with which everybody is confronted. Most people, and unfortunately most physicians, are at present inclined to make it a central or exclusive and separate problem. Therefore the first therapeutic task frequently is its decentralization and making the patient willing to accept as broad an attitude to it as to other complaints.

Sexual control considers and utilizes the quantitative and qualitative sexual factors, the physiologic and psychobiologic potentialities, strivings, interests, emotional and situational influences, and imaginations. Everybody's sense of responsibility should extend to all these factors. It is frequently overlooked that by indulging in certain imaginations one increases associative facilities and that, on the other hand, by control of voluntary imaginations, spontaneous imaginations decrease. Thus a person can learn to strengthen desirable thoughts and their associative links and to loosen and diminish undesirable associative connections. This leads to a healthy repression. In relations with others, interests which leave out the sexual factors can be cultivated. Dangerous situations should be avoided and substituted by others. Athletic outlets not only help to diminish sexual needs physiologically, and should therefore be resorted to at times of increased sexual cycle, but also helps to cultivate other interests and a healthy type of socialization. A well-regulated life with balanced work and recreation is necessary.

In the individual sexual development, many variations which demand medical advice occur. Relatively rare is precocious sexual development which is frequently combined with sexual overactivity. In certain races, for instance the Southern European race, early puberty is frequent and should not be considered pathologic. Early puberty, however, may present a difficult problem if it is combined with sexual push. Early sexual push occurs in psychopathic and schizophrenic children. In the latter group, however, I frequently found precocious sexual desires combined with delayed puberty. In these fortunately rare cases, education in a guarded environment, if necessary in a psychiatric hospital, is necessary to protect the child and achieve sexual control with increasing general stability of the personality. These reactions are seldom entirely due to a psychoneurosis. If they are, an analytic procedure should be combined with placement and educational influences.

Boys may become markedly upset by their first erections and emissions. A physician should discuss this carefully and alleviate resulting anxiety and panic reactions. In girls, similar reactions occur to the onset of menstruation. Disgust reactions, if not corrected, may lead to a wrong attitude to sexual life and result in frigidity.

Sexual hyperesthesia is rarely on a definitely constitutional basis but is more often the expression of an hysterical reaction and occurs especially in psychopathic and feebleminded settings. Such hyperesthesia may be a general ease of sexual stimulation or limited to various body zones [not necessarily to the usual erogenous zones (see Case 4 in Chapter VI)]. In these cases, as well as in the cases of excessive sexual desires which occur in psychopathic individuals and also in old age, a careful personality analysis during a period of abstinence is necessary to determine the actual degree of sexual abnormality, the dynamic factors involved, and the available possibilities for an adjustment of various factors of the personality, including the sexual. Castration is not desirable because it does not always lead to diminution of sexual desires except if performed in early childhood (before eight). Sterilization prevents pregnancy but offers an undesirable and even less controlled freedom. Intercourse or marriage, for therapeutic reasons, can never be defended. In women, there is usually a marked decrease of sexual desire after menopause. In men, fertility usually ceases around sixty but intercourse with slight impotency is possible much later. With senile changes, increase of sexual desire may occur in both sexes, but more frequently in men. These desires lead to increased adult sexual relations, but a greater danger is their tendency to lead to sexual play and talk with children and to exhibitionism. In these senile cases permanent hospitalization is indicated.

Case 32:

A 40 year old woman asked help for her uncontrollable sexual desires which drove her into increasing promiscuity, and for fearful dreams and nightmares about her divorced husband's maltreating her physically. All these symptoms had started with his remarriage two years previously. The patient's sexual desires had become stirred with her marriage to a passionate man at 19 with whom she lived monogamously until 24. During his absence in war, after a few months of abstinence, she began to have regular sexual relations with a lover. These relations she continued after her husband's return. Both began to take alcohol freely and smoke incessantly. She obtained a divorce because of his brutal behavior at 32, but kept up irregular sexual relations with him. Promiscuity increased, leading finally to almost daily intercourse with different men. When drinking, she carried alcohol well but lost some of her inhibitions and invited sexual intimacies which were followed by remorse. In about six consultations over a period of several weeks, the patient learned to recognize herself as a person who had always been self-willed, never willing to modify her expectations, and lacking control of her desires and emotions, inclined to be impulsive, going to extremes, and never obtaining full satisfaction from anything for any length of time. Men had always been mere sexual objects to her because she was selfish and unwilling to offer herself. When she recognized her dreams as sexual wish fulfillments and a desire to still possess her husband, they disappeared entirely. She began to understand her reactions of spite and resentment to life but was unwilling to adjust them. When she stopped smoking and drinking entirely, she became aware of increased sexual desires when waking up. During two months she adhered to strict sexual continence and found to her surprise that her desires were diminishing considerably with the avoidance of stimulating factors and increasing control of her imaginations, which was facilitated by taking up regular occupation. The patient left town after three months. It is unlikely that she will be able to make a permanent adjustment and her prognosis is considered poor because she has not been able to reach a constructive and practical synthesis of her personality. She was frankly unwilling to accept self-control as necessary in her life. Her resentment that her husband's second wife succeeded in making him stop drinking and work regularly has not been corrected. Because of this and her persisting love for him, she has periods of moodiness during which she feels the need of, and the right for, alcoholic stimulation.

This case illustrates well that the persistence of an unattainable love object may lead to increased sexual desire and promiscuity. Other factors causing sexual instability in some women are insufficient decrease of the sexual tension with orgasm or the possibility of several orgasms in one intercourse. In others it may be based on vaginal hyperesthesia or on too easily and too frequently produced orgasms. In these cases, cold sitz baths in the morning and evening, physical outlets, and the understanding of the need for the spacing of the fulfillment of desires in general lead to a satisfactory control. Promiscuity is frequently founded on the basis of these above-mentioned causes. It is more often due to having never been able to find a real love object, leading to a lack of integration of love and genital desires. Prostitutes frequently belong to this group. They obtain pleasure only from sexual relations with the person they really love. Most prostitutes are usually anesthetic and not hyperesthetic. The same factors usually explain male sexual promiscuity.

MASTURBATION

Masturbation should be considered normal if it occurs as a phase in a person's development. It occurs in practically every man; it is less frequent in women for anatomic and physiologic reasons. In trying to gain an understanding of this problem, the physician must know the frequency of its occurrence, what time of the twenty-four hours it occurs, the type of procedure, and the choice of the part of the body. The content reveals the underlying dynamic factors. Contentless masturbation is more difficult to correct because it is either more or less automatic, frequently symptomatic of a schizophrenic reaction, or due to marked dissociation, or the expression of narcissism. An example of lack of content caused by dissociation is Case 33 (page 441), and that caused by narcissism is Case 38 (page 461). It is essential that the situations which create the urge be studied. A study of the whole personality and the sexual life as outlined previously will allow us to relate desires to definite psychobiologic or physiologic factors. A full bladder, for example, may cause a desire to masturbate which can be corrected by urinating immediately. Physical stimulation may be caused by horseback riding, or tight clothes; in small girls it may be due to unrecognized physiologic itching because of eczema or oxyuris and infections, and in small boys occasionally to phimosis.

Masturbation usually starts with puberty, in boys frequently as a spontaneous reaction to erections. Its being induced by others is less frequent than has been believed previously. If this is the origin, it is important that one analyze carefully the original situation, determining whether the persons involved played more than an incidental role in the patient's later sexual life. Frequently associative links or definitely homosexual factors persist. In some it starts with local irritation. In this connection it is necessary to warn against too careful cleaning in small children and to emphasize the danger of douches and enemas. The latter often cause marked anal-erotic pleasure and takes the place of genital masturbation.

Masturbation leads to relaxation and sleep. In states of anxiety and tension and occasionally in agitated and tense depressions, patients therefore may resort to it.

The patient has to understand the need for the control of masturbation as of any other sexual activity. This does not necessarily mean continence, but spacing, and the acceptance of it as a needed although adequate outlet. The dangers are not important from the point of view of physical or mental damage, but considerable for sexual maladjustment. Not being dependent on a partner, masturbation becomes more readily excessive than other sexual activities. In women, it may lead to frigidity because the erotic pleasure becomes fixed on the clitoris and is not transferable to the vagina with intercourse. Therefore such women obtain orgasm in intercourse only if certain postures or manipulations lead at the same time to stimulation of the clitoris. Further, it permits psychic promiscuity and intensification of the dynamic factors connected with it. This may lead to psychic impotency, especially frigidity. Masturbation as a habit merely develops the sexual sensations with orgasm as the goal and neglects or omits entirely the desire for, and pleasure in, having some one else participate in the sexual act. It is therefore frequently difficult in persons with marked habit-formation to experience sexual intercourse as a physically and psychobiologically intimate union of two persons.

Therapeutically important is the correction of the patient's attitude to masturbation and the formulation of it to him in the light of general sexual hygiene. According to his physiologic cycle, he needs physical recreation. In women, sitz baths morning and evening help promptly. Although bromide (1 to 2 gm. — 15 to 30 gr.) decreases sexual desires temporarily, it should not be used freely.

The patient should learn to understand his own possibilities of sexual control. He should be urged not to struggle constantly against it, but to accept the fact that relapses may occur and that only a gradual education is possible. He is usually inclined to make it a problem of ethics or will power, instead of the general personality. In children, if no physical factors cause it, educational means are usually successful, i.e., teaching the child to sleep with his hands outside the covers and to distract it with playthings, etc., when it occurs in the daytime. Only if this fails is more thorough psychiatric investigation indicated.

PSYCHIC IMPOTENCY

This frequent disturbance may affect erection, ejaculation, or orgasm. Various forms and degrees can be distinguished clinically. In the beginning, premature discharge (ejaculatio praecox) caused by anxiety and infrequently by hyperesthesia, may occur only occasionally, then increase in frequency, and finally lead to total impotency. In some, it is so marked that it prevents intromission. Other patients first notice merely a weak erection, which makes intromission possible but diminishes the pleasure and prolongs the time for discharge. The next step is increasing lack of satisfaction to the gradually diminishing pleasure, and then weak discharge with little orgasm. In this stage, the man usually feels the completion of intercourse a duty to his partner and begins to stop during the sexual act. The final outcome is usually lack of sexual relations, forced prolonged intercourse without ability to obtain orgasm and discharge, or shortened duration with or without discharge. All these developments lead to an increasing feeling of inadequacy and disappointment.

Psychic impotency may be purely symptomatic, or it may be the essential difficulty. In all cases one must study the physical condition, ruling out an organic or neurogenic disorder, and exclude toxic factors (alcohol, drugs, excessive nicotine), depression, and early schizophrenic reactions or illnesses due to cerebral involvements, especially general paresis. In real psychic impotency, the difficulties are usually primarily in the sexual field. Various dynamic factors may then play a role — dissociation of physical (genital) and love factors, fixation of the sexual desires on certain persons, homosexual factors, or various sexual perversions. In many cases, however, we find a more or less marked personality maladjustment or a well-defined psychoneurosis. It is also important that one consider the reaction and influence of the partner. Lack of response or remarks during intercourse, both of which occur in frigid women, may disturb the man and the emotional interference may check the discharge. Disappointment about his apparent inability to stir his partner may lead to similar reactions. Other patients have the habit of watching the partner or themselves closely during intercourse and cannot give themselves completely. Many men expect too much pleasure from intercourse and orgasm and are disappointed.

Freud has analyzed the dynamic factors of sexual life carefully. He points out two possibilities in the failure of sexual integration. It is possible that a man has developed a love object which is formed by his mother as the ideal partner. To him the physical aspect of the relationship is therefore a degradation of the object of his love which he cannot tolerate. Such a man will be impotent with the woman he admires and loves. On the other hand, he may be sexually successful with a woman who merely attracts him physically. This explains why a man who is impotent with his bride may be potent with a prostitute and had always been so before his marriage. The other group is formed by men for whom the personality aspect is essential in their sexual life. The purely physical aspect is merely incidental. Their high ethical ideals condemn intercourse except in marital bonds or at least with someone whom they esteem. Such men are impotent with prostitutes and in extramarital relations, but able to have satisfactory intercourse after marriage. These men frequently explain their failure by fear of venereal infection. This fear is usually the expression of guilt and the impending self-punishment for desiring something unethical, i.e., intercourse with a promiscuous woman. When attempting intercourse, nevertheless, they have an ejaculation before intromission is possible or are entirely impotent.

Freud's formulation demonstrates clearly why it would be useless to advise a person who is impotent with his bride to find assurance in intercourse with an experienced woman or to urge a young man who is afraid he might be impotent in a planned marriage to try himself out. In addition, such advice could not be justified from ethical and medical points of view. It exposes a patient to danger of venereal infection and may cause serious guilt reactions in him. The physician does not have the right to force his own standards on a patient.

Other psychoanalytic investigators stress the importance of anal-erotic, sadistic, and narcissistic features. The inability to have erections is considered the expression of inhibition of the patient's love for his mother and of an identification with the feminine sexual role. In premature ejaculation, the same feminine attitude may be important, or a sadistic attitude to the woman may be hidden behind the apparent passivity, or an erotic fixation on urination. Impotency, vaginismus, and frigidity are conversion symptoms of motility and sensibility to prevent sexual pleasure but these sexual disorders are caused by a deeper personality involvement than in hysteria. The factor of guilt in connection with the infantile castration fear is especially stressed. The fear that the genitalia may be injured in the vagina may cause impotency. An underlying masochistic attitude is considered especially poor prognostically.

A careful history of the patient's sexual development and general sexual life and a brief personality understanding should be obtained in the first consultation. Of special interest in the sexual history are the occurrence of the first intercourse and of the beginning of the impotency, the type of partners involved, the specific situations, whether sexual relations and desires correspond to sexual pace, attitude to sexual life, masturbation, and early childhood experiences. Dreams may reveal the goal of the sexual desires and latent homosexuality. Repressed perversions should be considered. Coitus interruptus or birth control may be a disturbing factor. A brief orientation is important with regard to the attitude to mother and ideal wife and the choice of partners, to marriage, companionship, and family formation. General hygiene, work strain, and suitable recreation should be discussed. With these facts the physician should be in a position to formulate his patient's case dynamically and decide on the most suitable therapeutic procedure — persuasion and suggestion, hypnosis, or analysis.

In any therapeutic approach, however, a thorough explanation of the obvious intelligible factors is necessary, e.g., an alleviation of unfounded fears, corrective advice in an unhygienic sexual life, formulation to the wife, adjustment of the patient's routine and general hygiene (including use of alcohol and nicotine). In the treatment the patient's attitude to the sexual question, his desires, wishes, and ethical standards should guide us. In unmarried people the choice of the object needs to be carefully investigated; in married men we should try to correct the exaggerated attitude to the wife by clearing up the dissociated factors which influence the patient. If a patient cannot gain sufficient self-confidence through treatment to decide on an impending marriage, the analysis should turn to an investigation of the preventive factors. In milder cases, however, according to Stekel, the physician is justified in taking the responsibility for sexual success if he is convinced that the patient made the correct choice. I would hesitate to do this if I had not obtained in addition definite proof of improvement, e.g., in dream content.

"Persuasion" (Dubois) and suggestion are successful in mild cases of psychic impotency, especially in unintelligent, suggestible patients or in cases where misinformation and wrong sexual hygiene, faulty general hygiene, or faulty attitude of the wife are of importance. To this group belong men who are insecure in general and have marked body concern.

Hypnosis is indicated in patients in whom the dynamic factors are less important than lack of self-confidence based on feelings of general inadequacy or body overconcern, or where the patient would be unable to deal constructively with the dynamic factors. Through hypnosis, one is able to change the dream content and to establish self-confidence. I usually suggest dreams of the desired heterosexual content and, at the time when a spontaneous emission should be expected, intercourse dreams with emission. Through hypnotic suggestions, the sexual desires are stimulated and directed to a definite love object. Time determination, i.e., that the urge for sexual intercourse will occur spontaneously at a certain time and lead to successful intercourse, should only be given if one is certain of an hypnotic amnesia. Otherwise, anticipation and resulting doubts and anxiety will interfere. Hypnosis frequently leads to satisfactory sexual relations within two to three weeks. However, it achieves merely a symptomatic cure. The therapeutic choice is an analytic procedure which acquaints the patient with all the dynamic factors and allows a thorough adjustment.

Case 33:

A 31 year old man complained of moderate impotency (weak erection, discharge after a minute with little pleasure and without relaxation) and slight anxiety attacks. At 21 the anxiety symptoms started, increasing with a love disappointment at 24, and again at 28. In recent years he had developed dull headaches, constipation, and fatigue. The patient had been stimulated sexually by his nursemaid at 4, had intercourse with colored maids at 10, later with a neighbor girl at 12, masturbated from 12 to 19, and again had successful intercourse with college girls from 19 to 23. At that age he fell in love and was continent for nine months. Then, having read that masturbation and excessive sexual activities might lead to impotency, he began to worry over his past. At that time he noticed a varicocele (which disappeared after two years) and a decrease of morning erections with increase of dreams with emission. When fondling the girl he loved he noticed lack of erection and worried about marrying her. In order to reassure himself he picked up a prostitute after having taken a few drinks and experienced his first impotency. He failed to find reassurance with another prostitute and broke his engagement. At 29 he had normal intercourse several times with a girl of his own set but again failed afterwards with a prostitute.

This man had always been shy, self-conscious, and easily discouraged. Since puberty he had developed high ethical standards, especially in sexual matters, and was ashamed of his childhood experiences feeling that one should have intercourse only with women for whom one really cared. He had always been considerably concerned about his physical health and his personal appearance. His woman ideal was a person who resembled his mother and idealistic personalities which appeared in stories read in adolescence. His fiancé had corresponded to this physically and as a personality. Important to him was a proud, old family background, similar to his own. He had a disgust for prostitutes and girls whom he considered cheap. The last two years he had been treated for verumontanitis and had tried to understand his problem by reading much sexual literature which increased his hypochondriasis.

The factors in this case were sexual maladjustment (unable to emancipate himself from his mother who formed his woman ideal, and guilt to masturbation in adolescence), tendency to discouragement and reactions of inadequacy which have led to failure in his life ambitions, procrastination, and marked hypochondriasis. His anxiety symptoms and their increase were reactions to corresponding sexual problems and difficulties in life. This patient, who was seen for two days only, was urged to adjust his life in general, lead an active and healthy routine, and to guard against hypochondriacal concern. Sexual hygiene in general and with regard to his own problems was discussed. The patient has made a better adjustment since. His sexual life is satisfactory, with occasional successful intercourse with friends. This patient ought to be able to adjust his sexual problems in married life if he can adjust his personality problems. (It has not been possible to obtain recent follow-up data on this patient.)

Many cases are treated for verumontanitis, which is an expression of sexual malfunctioning and not its cause. It is essential that a urologist have psychotherapeutic knowledge and be able to treat cases of psychic impotency correctly.

Case 34:

Treatment with hypnosis was necessary in the following 29 year old patient who refused any lengthy analysis. This set, aggressive, successful man came half a year after his marriage because he was unable to obtain pleasure from intercourse, orgasm, and emission, although he was able to penetrate. Twice weekly he had intercourse which was frequently prolonged to half an hour and longer. He stated, however, that penetration had been impossible until the hymen had been removed. In the last four weeks erections had been lacking completely.

A brief study revealed a rigid, self-centered and egotistical person, highly ambitious, proud, and guided by set ethical standards. His mother, who was of a similar make-up, was his ideal. His wife was a pleasant, rather submissive person whom he loved and idealized. From the beginning, it was apparent that we dealt with a personality problem rather than a mere sexual one. The patient accepted this to some extent, but was not able to apply our formulation constructively with regard to his general as well as sexual life. His wife was instructed in sexual hygiene.

The patient was easily hypnotized. The need for temporary continence was explained to him. In the first hypnosis the patient was led to re-experience his last intercourse in order to obtain a clear picture of his attitude during the act, which was one of constant observation of himself and of his sensations. Sexual dreams, which previously had been rare and always dealing with impotency, were then suggested and were changed gradually — dreams with erections being first produced, and then with successful intercourse but without discharge. Next, through post-hypnotic suggestion, erections were obtained when he was with his wife. Intercourse was again attempted and lasted two to five minutes, but without relaxation and pleasure. It was not suggested that this occur in dreams, but he soon had intercourse dreams with discharge, pleasure, and full relaxation. Because of his constant self-observation he was, however, never able to relax in real intercourse or to reach orgasm and emission although the whole act gave definite pleasure. A few brief discussions of selected dreams made it clear to him that he expected excessive pleasure from intercourse and especially from orgasm, which he had never experienced (this is my only patient who, I am sure, had never masturbated). Through hypnosis he was made conscious of the sensation of orgasm and it was stressed that his orgastic pleasure would correspond to his desires. He was warned against distracting imaginations in daily life and during intercourse which would diminish his sexual tension. His dreams about circus girls and adventurous women led me to make these suggestions and to reformulate the concept of integrated sexual life. Rediscussions of personality stressed his tendency to cruelty and his unwillingness to give, his need for constant self-assertion, and fear of letting himself go because of underlying lack of self-confidence. After one year of treatment, which for three months had been two to three times weekly, afterwards once in two to three weeks, the treatment was stopped. For half a year the patient had been able to have pleasant intercourse of five minutes' duration but never reaching orgasm and emission. He was then not seen for over a year. During this time his sexual life had become entirely normal. He explained at a later visit that he finally began to apply better hygienic rules to himself, avoiding indulging in adventurous sexual preoccupations which had always been denied. He began to watch his wife instead of himself and received pleasure from noting her pleasure, and to think more of what he could offer her than the gain for himself in his sexual as well as general life. He adjusted his ambitions more to reality, was more willing to see his shortcomings and limitations, and with this developed more self-confidence and ease. This patient has remained sexually well-adjusted during the last twelve years.

This patient is mentioned as an illustration of treatment with hypnosis as well as one of the few cases where the impotency is primarily characterized by inability to experience orgasm with emission. Abraham's theory that narcissism is of primary importance in delayed or impossible ejaculation can be applied to this case. In this and other cases the tendency to be close with money is a striking personality feature. This tendency is an expression of anal-erotic factors often found in psychic impotency.

In some cases circumcision, phimosis, varicocele, unequal testicles, etc., are the basis for concern, leading to feelings of inadequacy. One of my patients overcompensated with desires for extraordinary potency and being admired for it like Casanova.

However, he had no intercourse before he married. As a student he visited a prostitute but was afraid of having intercourse and merely watched her undressing. The fear of intercourse and of infection was on the basis of fear of castration. In such cases, when a patient learns to control his imaginations and receives hypnotic suggestions to increase self-confidence, a lasting and good adjustment is possible with brief treatment. Poor results are usually predicted in latent homosexuality or perversion. This prognosis is frequently unfounded, as many cases can be cured through a careful analysis. It depends on the stability of the personality involved. In less stable patients, hypnosis and careful discussions may lead to a satisfactory adjustment.

Instead of discussing in detail all the possible factors in psychic impotency, the following case is presented for illustration of an analytic-synthetic approach in which free associations were used to some extent. The patient was seen three to four hours a week over a period of two months. In the presentation, dream analysis is emphasized particularly. This is done because the patient's dreams are unusually telling and offer good illustrations of the value of dream analysis. In order to save space, only the therapeutically most important features of a few dreams are discussed. The reader should keep in mind that these dreams were only one of the means to get closer to an understanding of the factors involved.

Case 35:

A successful 39 year old lawyer, married a year and a half, had never been able to give his wife full sexual satisfaction, as his erections were always brief or faded away during the love play. His wife was slightly frigid and had a prolonged orgasm. The patient stated that he had had four sexual affairs before marriage, all with women ten to fifteen years his senior. He was pursued by these women and never actively sought them. His wife was the first woman he had pursued, except for a girl (A), whom he had loved at 25. That courtship was terminated by her engagement to someone else. In the beginning, the patient considered his whole difficulty mainly sexual, but he gradually learned to consider it a personality problem.

He was a cheerful, optimistic, idealistic person, although well adjusted to reality. He was socially successful, a tall and attractive man, expecting a great deal of himself, ethically very strict, and in general perfectionistic. Since adolescence there had been a certain body-concern, characterized by a desire to build up his body. However, during a two-year physical invalidism (chronic nephritis) from 22 to 24 he was not given to hypochondriasis. His wife represented his ideal physically and as a personality, but her self-assertion frightened him to some extent.

The patient's high standards in performance along ethical and intellectual but not social lines had been fostered by his successful father, who died when the patient was 30. His mother still played an important role in his life. He had always felt close to her and at 13, when disturbed by the beginning of dreams with ejaculation, he went to her for help. He had a sister who was five years his senior and who was, to some extent, emotionally dependent on him.

The patient's courtship had lasted three years. In the second year some physical intimacies had occurred, but no intercourse had been attempted until a year before marriage. This had been a complete failure. His wife had told him before marriage that she hesitated to marry him because he probably would be a poor lover. Since their marriage, she tried to manage sexual life according to her ideas, which she had obtained from books. The patient expected a great deal from intercourse. It means to him losing himself, and he felt that children should only be conceived in a state of mutual orgasm. During the act he constantly wondered whether he would be good enough to give his wife orgasm.

The patient felt that his sexual life was clear and did not consider himself passionate. When smoking was stopped, there was a marked increase in sexual desire, and dreams, which had been scarce before, became frequent. Some of these dreams proved to be exceedingly helpful and their analysis shortened the treatment considerably. One of his dreams, occurring in the fourth week of treatment, woke him up at the stage of emission. He was having intercourse in a little park with the first woman (B) with whom he had indulged in sexual relations, and he experienced great joy. She suddenly laughed sarcastically and said, "I got you after all and I'm sick." This shocked him, but he decided to forget it and get full pleasure out of the experience. He finished the intercourse, but his discharge occurred before her orgasm. He then lifted her head. She looked hurt and her face changed into that of his wife, then changed back to the previous face. She again stated, "You are mine and you are sick and you can't have me." He got up and she ran after him. They raced along a dock. He dived into the water between two steamers and the dock, but while diving he thought it was a mistake. He grabbed the cable of an anchor and slipped down into the water. He then swam downstream — a narrow stream through a pleasant landscape — and thought, "It is not right that this is so pleasant and calm. I have been infected and need to do something." The next scene was in his home city, in which a dinner was given in his honor. A neighbor showed him a mark on his wrist, saying, "I am sick." (The patient has in reality such a mark on his wrist.) He said to himself, "Why am I not sick? Dr. D. has cured me." Then he woke up, but went back to sleep soon and had a second dream in which he told his physician the first dream. The physician said, "Now we are getting somewhere," and the patient thought that he would now be able to talk more freely about the ideal of his own personality. He was irritated because the physician did not understand that an ideal is always made up of the qualities which we do not possess, i.e., in his case, to be stong, powerful, and have will power. This thought changed then to the thought, "Now my ideal is to be a perfect lover."

The analysis of the first dream brought up clearly the conflict which he had experienced during the first sexual relationship. The woman (B), who had seduced him, was the wife of a man whom he liked very much. He therefore felt guilty of a breach of friendship and broke the relationship off after a few weeks. She had wanted him to marry her 17 year old daughter. The girl pursued him later, desiring to become his mistress. For ethical reasons and because the girl was not attractive enough, he did not give in. The patient has never experienced as much joy in sexual relations as with the first person (B). Fear of venereal disease, induced by his father when he was about 16, had played a certain role in his life. This fear was really protection from intercourse, which he did not want for ethical reasons, and especially because he was afraid of being shown up as inadequate. The dream revealed to the patient that it was his feeling inadequate as a personality and not a mere sexual disturbance which was a basic factor in his illness. It revealed also an ambivalent attitude to treatment and the development of a new attitude. He later realized that the statement, "You are sick," meant his impotency and that he was impotent because his first intercourse occurred in a situation of which his personality did not approve. He wondered whether there was any definite relation between that first love affair and his married life, as was indicated by the woman's face changing into his wife's face. However, he was not able to get very far during this dream analysis, although the statement, "You are mine and you are sick," indicated to him that he had not been able to get away from this woman and that she was still pursuing him. The thought that it was a mistake to dive into the water indicated that it might be a mistake to try to get away from her as he was able to enjoy life and women although he was sick.

The second dream referred to discussions of his personality, which he had resented as he was not able to answer the question of the ideal for which he was striving. In the dream, not being able to find the answer, he again thought, "The important problem is really to be a perfect lover." In the discussion of the ideal of his own personality, the patient began to see the need for integration of divers elements — intellectual, artistic, and cultural. In recent years his development had become more and more intellectual to the exclusion of other personality needs.

In another dream he saw himself go upstairs in an opera house accompanied by two women, the older a voluptuous brunette and the younger a blonde. He saw their bodies through their dresses and he awakened with an erection saying, "Mother and daughter." This dream referred again to the mother-daughter relationship in his first love affair. Its importance was explained by the background of his relationship to his own mother and his sister. Sexual factors played a less important role than the desire to protect his mother and sister and take the role of his father in their lives. This he had practically done since his father's death.

A few nights later he dreamed that his wife was away and that he met another woman with whom he "played around." During dinner they decided to run off with the thought of spending the night together, which caused him great anticipation of sexual pleasure. He felt in the dream that he did not want this out of spite because his wife had left him, but to show his independence. He went to a drugstore to look up the name of a hotel and wondered how he could satisfy her desire for a marriage ceremony that would not be a fake and yet not make him lose his wife. He decided that the best solution was not to go back to the woman, and he left through another door and took the train home.

This dream was quite important. The woman of the dream was a girl (C) with whom he had had a love affair, but had never mentioned her to me because he had not treated her fairly. She was also the only girl in his life who had been a virgin. He had never been able to free himself from her. The last intercourse occurred about the time he met his wife. She wished to marry him and he had left her in a way which was not quite honorable according to his rigid ethical concepts. His own standards demanded that a man who seduces a virgin should marry her. The dream also brought to discussion his attitude to marriage. He had always believed that he had adjusted very easily, but saw now that he resented deeply having to give up certain personal habits and not having the feeling of complete personal freedom any longer. Whenever his wife was away, he was able to do many things which he had had to delay because of social obligations. He saw from this dream analysis the need for a new orientation of his life. He resented his own weakness, i.e., inability to say, "No." The patient mentioned briefly that his wife had not been a virgin when they married, having had a lover a few years previously.

The question of why these women in his past interfered with his relations to his wife could not be answered satisfactorily. He wondered whether he had married his wife because he loved her, or to escape from difficulties which he had created in his past and with which he did not feel capable of dealing.

In another dream, the patient was dining with his mother at a seaside hotel when the woman (B) of the previous dream and a young man entered. His mother greeted this obviously bridal couple very haughtily, saying that it was an outrage for an old woman of 70 to marry a young man. He corrected her by saying that she was not 70 but only 60. This dream led to further discussion of the same woman (B), who in a dream the following night appeared again. His wife was running away from him (the patient said, "from her," meaning the woman of the previous dreams). He pursued her with the desire and a determination to catch her. This chase led first through the streets of a city, then the yards of the Phipps Clinic, some more streets, and finally to a summer place in the country near a lake. All along the way, people had been interfering with his progress, trying to grab him, but mostly throwing obstacles in the way, such as barrels and pieces of furniture. The patient reached his wife in the little house on the lake, had intercourse, and remembered that she looked up at him with a happy smile on her face, apparently completely satisfied. He had a great feeling of relief and pride.

These two dreams led to a final understanding of the woman (B) who had been interfering in the working of his personality. Through his dream, the patient reached an understanding of the importance of the age factor in all his premarital sexual relations. It clarified his emotional dependence on his mother, although this had never reached a full sexual meaning. In selecting his paramours he was attracted to women who took the mother's place. Because of this, he had a feeling of immorality in his sexual relations. He also had never cared for these women and had given in to their pursuing. Their satisfaction therefore had not meant anything to him and he probably had never been able to give orgasm to any of them. His mother had actually objected to his relationship with older women, probably to a large extent on a jealousy basis. The first dream demonstrates how he deceived himself successfully about the age and mother relationships of these women, although he had to admit to himself that they were really rather old for him.

The second dream showed progress in the treatment and gave a picture of his actual relationship with his wife. Many obstacles had been thrown in their way, some of them by his previous sexual relations, some of them by other personality features. Through the help of psychiatric treatment, he finally would reach the point where he would be able to have satisfactory sexual relations. His slip of the tongue indicated that he felt his wife was running away from him because he had not been able to settle his previous love affairs. He still had a feeling of guilt with regard to the woman (C) and wondered whether he should not help her financially as she had developed tuberculosis and was in a distressing financial situation. She had been a virgin and he had always felt guilty about seducing her. His high ethical sense made him feel responsible for her later sexual life. His wife and this girl were in many ways similar, whereas the other women of his past life had only age and their mature attitude in common.

In one of the last dreams the girl (A), whom he had loved as a young man, reappeared. Analysis of that dream showed that he had primarily loved her for her personality and, to a less extent, for her physical attractions. The same night he had another dream in which he was a boy playing with another boy in a freight yard. They played in and out, all over the engine, and in a little cab. He looked out through the open door and saw an official moving back and forth. He was dressed in a very imposing uniform. On a stand hung a white dress that had just come back from the cleaner. He said to his friend, "We must be careful lest he see us." They then indulged in mutual masturbation, accompanied by erection and ejaculation. He was surprised to notice that his semen was mixed with urine. This dream took him back to his childhood when he had played around freight yards, and to the only boy with whom he had practiced mutual masturbation. He saw that there were still some homosexual interests which played a role and interfered with a satisfactory sexual adjustment. The white dress coming back from the cleaner indicated his ability to get well (cleaned). The official represented partly his father and partly his own conscience. Erection and discharge showed that there were still some desires for a repetition of the childhood experience, but mixed with the feeling that it could not be satisfactory (semen mixed with urine).

After this the patient had many more dreams but they all dealt frankly with intercourse with his wife and the ability to satisfy her, or with more general personality problems. There was a definite desire for promiscuity. Jealousy based on his insufficiency, and resentment against his athletic wife appeared in several dreams. He also envied the large penis which he had seen on other men.

When talking of perfectionism, the patient used the word, "protectionism," several times. The analysis of his perfectionistic attitude showed that he used it to protect himself. It allowed him to put off certain work which would expose him to public criticism and which would not allow him to change (fear of finality). "Perfect protection is the end of perfectionism." This same attitude with regard to sexual life prevented him from having children. His concept was to try to achieve pregnancy only from a state of mutual orgasm. He was afraid of having children because they would make his marriage still more lasting, as a divorce would then be impossible for him. Through these discussions, he learned to see the necessity for adjustment of these strivings in sexual life. This meant a willingness to accept his own and his partner's satisfaction in a more relative and not exclusive way. In a few consultations, his wife's sexual attitude was also investigated and modified. The treatment lasted about two months and has led to a good sexual adjustment (for four years) and to a change in his personality which, I feel, will make the sexual adjustment permanent. From information received in 1947, this patient's sexual adjustment has remained good.

FRIGIDITY

Frigidity is the counterpart of psychic impotency in women. It is frequent, but more apt to escape medical attention because it interferes less or little with marital relations and is frequently accepted by the patient as a normal expression of a non-passionate make-up. In many patients, adolescent masturbation has caused it. In others, ethical difficulties may be the essential factors, e.g., in unmarried girls who try intercourse out of curiosity or because they feel under obligation to live up to the codes of their friends. In women who are primarily mother and only secondarily wife, frigidity develops occasionally after they have become mothers. Latent homosexuality may be a factor, as may be hysterical reactions in which early disgust played a role. Usually such patients also suffer from dysmenorrhea. More important may be emotional dependence on the father and lack of emancipation from him, or fixation on another man. A crude husband may offend a bride, and, through disgust, cause frigidity.

Vaginismus, with or without painful sensation to intercourse, is due to fear and disgust. Some psychoanalysts found it related to the female castration complex (an inhibition of the desire to destroy the male genitalia of which they are envious). In brides, and in women indulging in premarital experiences, it is usually the fear of defloration which is not only caused by hearsay but based on deeper dynamic factors which are related to the first intercourse and the loss of virginity. Disgust is frequently the reaction to marital conflicts, e.g., to an alcoholic or unfaithful husband. In some, vaginismus is due to the fear of detection of previous masturbation. Impotency of the husband or his brutal or obscene approach may lead to it. Psychotherapy with reassurance and suggestions, together with practical advice for quiet and deep abdominal breathing, are sufficient help in some of these minor fears. In others, a more thorough investigation is indicated. The physician should always discuss their sexual life with the husband and influence his attitude. Therapeutic operations, e.g., removal of the hymen, are rarely necessary. If there are definite physical indications for such an operation, a brief therapeutic discussion should always precede it.

Patients with frigidity after operations, or as a result of early involutional changes, need psychotherapeutic help. They should understand that the inability to experience pleasure in intercourse does not mean diminished love for their husbands. Although their own pleasure is lacking, they should be willing to offer pleasure to the husband. This does not mean acting, to which so many frigid women resort.

In some patients delayed orgasm, caused by a prolonged sexual curve of the woman or short duration of the intercourse, is mistaken for frigidity. The advice to the husband to attempt to prolong intercourse is not always wise. In certain men it may lead to sexual dissatisfaction and anxiety symptoms. Increased attention to sexual play as a prelude is usually more satisfactory. Disturbance of the female orgasm may be caused by an erection of too short duration or the fear of orgasm. It may be fear of losing sphincter control, which is usually an expression of fear of losing oneself in orgasm, which is found in self-assertive and hysterical patients. In some women it is caused by the fear that the penis might be too small, a fear which is usually based on the fear of losing it.

In most cases of frigidity, a thorough study and adjustment is not possible because of the patient's unwillingness to spend sufficient time on treatment. This is the more regrettable as the treatment of frigidity and psychic impotency is not only interesting, but leads to good results. Hypnosis can be used successfully in suggestible patients and also changes their attitude to intercourse and sexual activities in general. In the majority of cases, however, one needs to be content with offering constructive advice through a discussion of normal sexual life, stressing the psychobiologic aspect and the needs of the partner. Many women have difficulty in accepting the passive role in intercourse and maximal submission in orgasm.

VARIOUS COMPLAINTS TO SEXUAL MALADJUSTMENTS

In the discussion of psychoneurotic and also of depressive and schizophrenic reactions, I discussed complaints which are due to sexual maladjustment. They consist of backache, ache in the neck, and fatigue in regions of the body which show relation to normal sexual fatigue. In such cases, whenever an orthopedic examination is negative, a study of the patient's sexual life is indicated. Anxiety symptoms and genito-urinary complaints are frequent and cause the patient to seek help from the internist or urologist. A brief study of all the factors involved usually allows a constructive adjustment.

Case 36:

A young priest who was a cheerful, active, and determined person, but who lacked confidence in himself and had a marked tendency to anticipate difficulties, always had to push himself in his preaching. When ordained, he was concerned about his health because of a serious physical illness, and was disturbed by ethical conflicts. At that time he had his first ejaculation while preparing his sermon and noticed a twitching of his face and neck, and hot flushes. From then on emissions occurred usually on Saturday nights when he was unable to sleep, thinking of the sermon the following day. Later he also noticed a pain in his lumbar region. As these ejaculations increased, he was treated for a prostatic condition. When the patient was seen in consultation, the ejaculations were formulated to him as being largely due to hypochondriacal overconcern, lack of confidence in himself, conscientiousness, and ethical conflicts (he had marked guilt feelings to his ejaculations because they indicated sexual desires which he felt he should be able to control). Although verumontanitis was present, local treatment was considered inadvisable because the local condition was of secondary nature and his physician was urged to attempt a personality adjustment. (The further development in this patient is unknown.)

Pains in the right lower quadrant, in the right leg, and frequently referred to the right ovary cause such patients to seek help from the gynecologist. Others complain of hyperesthesia in the lateral epigastrium, or during the examination, of hyperesthesia of the cervix or endometrium. Menstrual disorders (amenorrhea and dysmenorrhea), pruritus of the vulva, anesthesia of the vaginal entrance, lack of secretion or hypersecretion of the Bartholin glands, ful feeling in the vagina suggesting a prolapse, are frequently on the basis of sexual dissatisfaction or disturbances in sexual development. These complaints are mentioned in detail because not enough attention is paid to them and usually, instead of appropriate psychotherapy, some kind of surgical treatment is offered or merely the statement that there is nothing wrong physically.

Menstrual disorders deserve a detailed discussion because of their frequency and the satisfactory results of a psychotherapeutic attack. The influence of emotions and suggestions on menstruation is well known and explains the fact that unpleasant or highly disturbing life experiences which are not necessarily of a sexual character easily affect the menstrual flow, e.g., accidents, fright, disgusting experiences. Too early menstruation, too long or too marked bleeding, irregular intervals, or cessation of menstruation may result. Such experiences easily cause menstrual disturbances if they happen to occur around the time of menstruation or when predisposing factors play a role, such as asthenic make-up, vagotonia, and Graves' disease. Besides local organic endocrinologic causes, depressions and other personality disorders have to be ruled out. The treatment consists of analysis of the factors involved, explanation of the working out of these factors, and suggestion. In most cases a brief analysis is satisfactory; in others, however, a more thorough study is necessary, e.g., when homosexual factors play a role. Amenorrhea, caused by fear of pregnancy, which in a depression may develop into catathymic delusions, occurs frequently. In some cases it has been found to be a wish-fulfillment of the desire to be a man.

In dysmenorrhea, situational and sexual factors need to be considered. In adolescents, an insufficient hygienic understanding with shame or guilt reactions or the environmental overemphasis on pain are frequent causes. When sexual desires precede the onset of menstruation, the girl reacts easily with menstrual disorders. Late dysmenorrhea, e.g., the onset after a few years of normal menstruation, is caused by sexual upheavals, concern about masturbation, and fear of intercourse. Dysmenorrhea frequently starts during the engagement period when a girl struggles against sexual desires, and indulges in frustraneous activities or intercourse. Fear of intercourse, marriage, and childbirth may be of importance in some; in others, conflicts because of breaking away from parents and home or fear of impending responsibilities. Sexual or situational difficulties may cause the disorder to start with or after marriage. In some patients anal-erotic factors are of importance. The personality setting should always be studied and the possibility of marked body overconcern or hysterical factors taken into consideration.

Case 37:

A 26 year old woman complained of pruritus of the vulva and marked dysmenorrhea, for which codein was offered freely. When she asked for help because of excessive sexual desires, marriage had been advised by the gynecologist. She was treated in weekly consultations, and was helped to readjust her personality and to find interests and recreation as a balance to the work routine, to establish better socialization, and to learn to take her sexual problem as part of her general personality difficulties. She decided against indulging in promiscuity, which she had considered for several years, because her ethical standards did not allow it, and learned sexual control. After half a year, all her symptoms had cleared up.

In most of these cases, we deal with sexual maladjustment as part of a general personality problem and not as an hysterical or compulsive reaction, although both are possible. The localization of the complaints utilizes physiologic and psychobiologic sexual functions. Our sensory organs play a considerable role in sexual selection and may therefore be affected as an expression of sexual maladjustment. Sexual upheavals frequently lead to sensitiveness to certain odors. Masturbation, cunnilingus, and anal-erotic interests can lead to specific preoccupations and sensitiveness. In many cases, there is a definite connection with the nose, indicated by itching, picking, burning, sneezing, and congestion. Another frequent expression is found in itching of the skin and in various skin disorders. A brief analysis of sex life and hygiene and, in women, cold sitz baths, usually clear up these symptoms in a short time.

HOMOSEXUALITY

Homosexuality is the sexual attraction, in overt or more unrecognized strivings and acts, to members of one's own sex. Previously it had been explained on a constitutional, and most frequently on a somatic, basis with the claim that we always find precocious sexual development, sentimental and immature rather than frank love expression, and signs of physical degeneracy. Accordingly, several descriptive groups were distinguished. As a result of Freud's influence, the psychologic factors have been more stressed in recent years, leading to either an exclusive stress on psychodynamic and developmental factors or to a more pluralistic atttitude in which these as well as constitutional and endocrinologic factors were evaluated and treated according to the individual case.

Probably every modern formulation now stresses the undifferentiated sexuality of the infant. Most investigators agree that bisexual factors are active in every adolescent and adult, and that their predominance depends much on developmental and situational factors. The developmental factors and various phases of sexual development with the possibility of fixation in infancy and childhood and the corresponding dominance of various unusual sexual strivings and satisfactions have been made the basis for treatment by Freud and his school. Intensive investigations have shown that homosexuality is of equal importance in men and women. The previous impression that homosexuality was relatively frequent in men and rather rare in women was caused by the attitude of our civilization, which willingly tolerates the expression of affection among women and prosecutes by law only male homosexuality. The latter factor also explains the impression that homosexuality occurs only in inferior personalities and psychopathic patients who were unable to adjust in general. In the pre-psychotherapeutic era, homosexual patients came to the physician's attention only because of actual or threatening legal involvements.

It is essential in treatment that one study the personality setting and modify the factors which are open to therapeutic influence. This implies that primary attention is paid not only to psychobiologic factors, developmental and situational influences and their modifiability, but also to the personality organization and somatic features. In this way, we are able to distinguish three large groups which demand different prognoses and therapeutic approach — homosexuality in the stable person, in the unstable and loosely organized psychopathic personality, and homosexuality which is linked with definite persons. These homosexual attractions and fixations occur especially in adolescence and early adult life. In stable personalities, a far-reaching investigation of the dynamic factors and the personality development is indicated. In the unstable group we deal primarily with a personality problem. Stress must then be placed on the general personality adjustment through a distributive analysis and individualized re-education. When definite attraction to, and dependence on, certain persons develop in stable individuals, the patient's personality determines whether or not a more or less thorough investigation should be undertaken. It is frequently possible for some patients to obtain a thorough understanding of the dynamic factors, while for others, e.g., adolescents and feebleminded persons, a situational adjustment is of primary importance. We should realize further that homosexuality may be symptomatic in schizophrenic and paranoid reactions, in panics, and in early organic (paretic and senile) disorders.

It seems to me that Freud's conception is correct — that the most important psychodynamic factors are formed in the parent-child relationship and through early environmental influences. Freud arrived at the formulation that male homosexuality develops because the boy is unduly influenced by his mother or by women who take her place; he admires them and identifies himself with them through his ideals. This can be intensified by antagonism to, or hate of, his father, who represents his own sex. Educational factors (being kept from healthy contact with boys and urged into girls' play and activities) emphasize these tendencies. In girls, we deal with corresponding factors and development. In male homosexuality which is caused by identification with the mother, three further developments exist. A strong narcissistic tendency leads to the aggressive type in whom narcissism is more important than the desire for femininity. These homosexuals turn to men of a similar age in whom they can see themselves. Fixation on the anal-erotic stage of sexual development causes the passive type. These men want to be taken by a man like a woman. A third type, which Freud considers prognostically more favorable than the other two, is due to hate of a brother overcompensating into love. In female homosexuality, the same factors play a role, i.e., identification with the father which, because of narcissism, develops into the aggressive, and because of anal-eroticism into the passive homosexual type. A third type of homosexuality is that in which hate of a sister, later overcompensated in love, plays a role. In most homosexuals, several of these factors are present and are of varying importance. The psychoanalytic formulation does not overlook later situational factors but considers them merely precipitating. Homosexuality which is caused by the occasion of being in a group of one's own sex with no possibility of heterosexual contact (e.g., in prison) has to be viewed in such a way. In many who indulge in a transient homosexual episode, this remains a mere incident in their lives. In those, however, who are developmentally predisposed, it leads to permanent homosexuality. Disappointment in heterosexual love may cause such predisposed persons to turn to their own sex.

I do not wish to convey the impression that Freud's formulation takes care of all the possibilities of homosexual development. Publications of thoroughly investigated homosexuality in stable persons are not frequent, but with more case material, additional psychodynamic factors will no doubt be found. Adler points to more general personality factors which are occasionally of importance, but not exclusively, as he claims. He found that these patients have an inordinate ambition together with an extraordinarily pronounced caution or fear of life. In homosexual men, the fear of women cannot be conquered by the patient. In women, the refusal to accept the female role (masculine protest) is essential. In psychopathic personalities, besides those above-mentioned factors, many others are usually significant. The investigation of somatic factors has thus far not been productive. The general somatic make-up often impresses one with the possibility of constitutional predisposition. These somatic factors, however, cannot be influenced — endocrinologic treatment, including implantation of testicles or ovaries, for example, has been a failure. The presence of somatic features of the opposite sex causes most physicians to anticipate a poor prognosis. This, however, is not always justified. We do not know much about the importance of such body features on the psychobiologically integrated sexual life. Many men with a feminine pelvis or with feminine gestures and gait, and many women with masculine features or behavior are sexually well adjusted. I stress this because many physicians are too much influenced by such features and seek to find homosexual factors as an explanation for the personality difficulties for which the patient consults them.

It is undesirable to expand the term, "latent homosexuality," which should only be used when definite homosexual strivings and desires are active in the person who is not aware of them. It then will depend on the whole setting whether we shall guide the patient to recognize these strivings in order to be able to correct them or deal with them constructively, or whether it is wiser to neglect them by steering the patient in another direction therapeutically. Not every homosexual trend in a disorganizing personality disorder or in adolescence indicates latent homosexuality. With the concept of bisexual strivings and interests in the incompletely organized and immature personality, one should be willing to accept these features as part of normal development. In the well-organized adult, these tendencies exist to a more or less marked degree. Even in a homosexual person, heterosexual interests exist in varying degrees.

The older treatment has tried to suppress homosexual, and to stimulate heterosexual, strivings through suggestion and hypnosis. I never saw good results from treatment with hypnosis. In some cases where homosexual and heterosexual strivings keep more or less in balance, heterosexual interests and fancies may be cultivated and homosexual strivings repressed. This symptomatic success is dangerous, however, if it is not accompanied by a thorough personality understanding and insight. In such cases, marriage cannot be advised. A physician should not make the decision of marriage for the patient. If successful treatment has led not only to a heterosexual adjustment, recognizable in day fancies and night dreams, but also to an understanding of the dynamic factors and their adjustment, the physician may acquiesce to the marriage plans. If either one or both of these requirements have only been partly achieved, he should advise against it.

The choice in modern treatment is a thorough analytic investigation in which the physician should be guided by the principles of sexual development and environmental influences which seem to be most common. However, he should not believe that this is the necessary or only key for therapeutic success, but should follow any other leads which present themselves. In some cases psychoanalysis may be indicated, or a free association procedure with dream analysis and careful study and use of the therapeutic situation may be most successful. In other cases, a more analytic-synthetic procedure along distributive lines is more desirable. I personally feel that in the treatment of all sexual difficulties the physician should take an active part and direct the treatment. Otherwise there is the danger that the patient may try to consider it entirely as a sexual problem instead of one of the whole personality. As a result of popularization of our increased knowledge of the dynamic factors in sex life, too many poorly understood ideas have become common knowledge and are used by the sexually maladjusted person for rationalization or short cuts in treatment. A physician should therefore be careful not to offer his own hypothesis as a solution to the patient. During treatment he may offer possible solutions for critical consideration to the patient, but this therapeutic step should be done only after careful consideration of the whole phase of treatment and in a careful form.

In the unstable person, a thoughtfully directed personality study is the first step. It should lead the patient to a realization that he deals with a problem of the general personality and that the sexual problem should be decentralized. General re-education is of importance. Many homosexual patients are, however, unwilling to be cured. They seek help because they are in general difficulties which they try to explain by society's attitude to homosexuality. Usually to this group belong persons who are in legal difficulties. In many of these cases, as well as in the more stable group where a thorough adjustment is impossible because of limitation of time or psychobiologic obstacles (set personalities, lack of sufficient intelligence, possible danger of a disorganizing illness), a re-education along the lines of Moll's association treatment is indicated.

Based on the fact that every homosexual patient has definite heterosexual strivings and interests, Moll urges the patient to cultivate heterosexual preoccupations in the broadest sense as well as definite heterosexual fancies and to guard against indulgence in spontaneous homosexual thoughts. The patient must feel responsible for his imaginations. The physician should find out what heterosexual and homosexual attractions exist for his patient, in acquaintances as well as passing persons, in literature, art, movies, and in the general situations of his life. Then the patient is able to recognize the bridge which leads to a heterosexual life and to avoid dangerous attractions. These patients are in need of a clarification of the term, "sexual," which they usually limit entirely to the genital organs and functions. They should learn to cultivate friendships with persons of the opposite sex and associate with them on the basis of healthy socialization. They need to break away entirely from homosexual groups and learn to see that friendship with members of their own sex does not need to be on a homosexual basis but built on interests they have in common. Athletics are an excellent means for socialization if one keeps in mind that sexual self-exposure and observation of exhibitionist acts by others must be avoided. During the whole treatment, the patient needs to be encouraged and reassured that possibilities for correction exist. The patient should learn to accept the fact that a perfect and automatic adjustment in sexual life rarely exists, and that the average person knows the dangers and how to deal with them. On the other hand, the patient should accept the fact that we deal with an "either-or" situation and that he cannot be both homosexual and heterosexual. This fact is frequently the stumbling block because the average homosexual patient wishes to be heterosexually adjusted but to keep the possibility of homosexual pleasures. In others, an attitude of spite to society as well as to their own lives prevents full cooperation. To re-education belong a well-regulated life and the omission of alcohol which removes the inhibitions that the treatment tries to strengthen.

Castration, for which unhappy patients ask, has been recommended (Thürlimann). Undesirable somatic and psychic eunuchoid symptoms do not seem to occur to any marked extent if castration is performed in patients over 25 years of age. Best results are obtained in patients who have a well organized personality. Poor results were observed in ill-controlled psychopathic personalities. Escape to a country where homosexuality is legally and socially tolerated is most undesirable. It usually causes marked homosexual indulgence with its dangers of venereal disease and involvement with psychopathic and criminal persons, and results in increased difficulties of the personality and life in general. The dangers of homosexual prostitution are especially grave because it can easily lead to legal involvement or blackmail. A physician should always get in touch with legal authorities if one of his homosexual patients is blackmailed. An intelligent prosecutor and judge will be willing to help the blackmailed patient and not urge prosecution for his sexual misdemeanor.

The stable homosexual patient, even if a change to heterosexuality cannot be achieved, must learn to use normal sexual control. The homosexual person should understand that in this way he is not different from the heterosexual and is under the same responsibility to himself and to the group. Many of these patients succeed in leading a life of complete continence, accepting the fact that they are not different from many heterosexual persons whose ethical code does not permit them to seek sexual satisfaction in unmarried life. The cultivation of general and specific interests offers healthy outlets. It is not necessary, and certainly not proved, that this is sublimation in the sense of transformation of sexual into other energy, as has been postulated.

Homosexuality is frequently combined with other sexual perversions, especially sadism, masochism and fetishism. If these additional tendencies are leading factors, the prognosis is worse as it indicates a loosely organized personality which has not been able to develop circumscribed sexual interests. Complete sexual abstinence, which is essential during the treatment of any sexual disorder, is then even more difficult to obtain than in the average homosexual.

The detailed presentation of a case will show many of the possibilities which can occur and the dynamic factors involved. It also illustrates the need of decentralization of the sexual problem and of personality analysis in its broadest sense with attention to a general life, instead of a mere sexual, adjustment.

Case 38:

A 32 year old research worker asked for help for homosexuality, for dissatisfaction with his work, and inability to make a good social adjustment. He had been brought up as an only child by his maternal grandmother after his mother's death when he was four, and his father's remarriage the subsequent year. She demanded a great deal of affection from him and influenced him against his father, whom he began to dislike intensely. His health had always been good and his scholastic achievements excellent. After having obtained his Ph.D. at 24 he worked in a research laboratory. Since early childhood there had been a great interest in bowel movements and at around 11, he experienced orgasm to enemas, which he administered to himself. Masturbation with admiration of his naked body before a mirror started at 12 and has been continued since. In adolescence (at 15), mutual masturbation began. He was usually the aggressor. Physically, he was of the athletic type but with definite feminine features. At 29 he was treated for four months in an orthodox psychoanalysis. He had asked for treatment for his increasing self-consciousness, his inability to adjust his homosexuality, and for increasing sadistic impulses (when whipping a dog cruelly he had experienced orgasm). From this treatment, he obtained a fair understanding of his relationship to his grandmother and father, a vague idea of sadistic tendencies being an ingrained feature of his personality, but little understanding of the general personality setting. He had apparently not been able to utilize what had been revealed by the analysis. During that treatment several heterosexual attempts had resulted in impotency or failure of emission. He had been greatly afraid of pregnancy and being obliged to marry. In the last three years, he had been promiscuously homosexual, and no heterosexual attempts had occurred. Sadistic impulses had not recurred in a frank form.

This history was easily obtained in two hours. It pointed to the need to decentralize the sexual topic and to consider a wholesome personality adjustment of primary therapeutic concern. Stress on the synthesis of what could be obtained through analysis and the obligation to utilize it in re-education was made the basis for treatment. The spacing of therapeutic discussions was therefore considered important. On the average, the patient came for one hour twice a week, with an occasional increase or decrease in frequency if the situation made this seem desirable. Distributive analysis with a modified free association procedure was used throughout. The free associations seemed indicated because of the patient's attitude of formulating his answers carefully and arguing his point. The treatment lasted six months. For the sake of a clear presentation, I shall merely stress the main therapeutic issues and the method of handling them.

The first three consultations in May 1931 were devoted to a review of what had been obtained in the psychoanalysis. Whenever the opportunity arose, the patient's attention was drawn to the fact that he dwelled too much upon sex and omitted the consideration of other factors which were of obvious importance. These first discussions were guided by the need to get a better understanding of the actual sexual status and the patient's knowledge of himself. Complete abstinence from alcohol, nicotine, and sexual activities was urged but after about three weeks, the possible occurrence of masturbation had to be allowed and it was practiced a few times. During the treatment, the patient watched the physician closely for his reactions (he insisted on being allowed to face the analyst during the psychoanalysis, and when this was permitted after about two months, he had a feeling of having gained his point and despised the physician). Dreams were analyzed occasionally. Thorough analysis would probably have led us too far away from the problems which were most necessary to adjust. This case did not offer hope for a complete sexual adjustment, but had to be considered primarily as a personality problem in which sexual difficulties played one of the important roles.

The problems which the patient was able to state were shyness and self-consciousness, constant rebellion to authority and to ideas of the majority, a tendency to procrastination, the inability to form lasting friendships, frequent depressive moods in which he felt the need to resort to alcohol and excessive smoking, and the inability to reach a satisfactory sexual adjustment. He also felt that analysis had not given him a sufficient understanding of his tendency for physical hero-worship, of his inability to expose himself to others, especially intellectually, and his need for self-admiration. To me, an additional important problem was to determine to what extent narcissism was the basis for his homosexuality, and also for his feelings of physical inferiority. The patient was unable to answer questions with regard to his sexual ethics, his type of companionship, and what workable assets he had.

These preliminary discussions revealed a marked tendency to exhibitionism, expressed in naked swimming in mixed crowds, and admiration of his body. Other men were to him a mirror-image of himself. In homosexual, in contrast to heterosexual, activities he would not have to give himself away to somebody strange. Masturbation was never as fully satisfactory as homosexual play. His description of attractive types stressed the athletic make-up of his homosexual friends and personality features similar to his own. In connection with his interest in the rectum, anus, and defecation, the patient mentioned what was known to him as anal-erotic character traits. I was able to utilize this concept for a brief discussion of his selfishness and unwillingness to give affection, and on this basis, his resentment to the expectations of his father.

From June 1st to 16th, the discussions led to an analysis of sexual life in his personality setting. He had always been anxious to keep his body fit and was untiring in his efforts to master athletics. "Overfastidiousness" to body secretions was expressed in disgust at coming in contact with saliva, to touching a vagina, to getting blood on his fingers, but not to his own excreta. He had desires to beat women and to bite their breasts. On the whole, there was a definite streak of cruelty to others and to himself. In dealing with others, he reacted readily with resentment and spite. This, as well as his physical self-admiration, led to an undesirable attitude to others. He was constantly concerned about the impression he made on others, felt easily slighted, and had a marked tendency to suspiciousness. Since his analysis he had been worried about the dangers of narcissism and had tried to change his elaborate masturbation ritual to contentless masturbation. Previously he had touched his buttocks, standing before a mirror, thinking of male friends, then touched his breasts, thinking of women, and thus proceeded to ejaculation. At this stage of treatment, he expressed resentment to homosexual abstinence, which would drive him deeper into narcissism. He considered narcissism the expression of highly developed individuality and insisted that a better group integration would be an inferior adjustment. He felt that alcohol was a desirable help to overcome self-consciousness, and its therapeutic prohibition at this stage undesirable; also, that complete integration of personality strivings would make life uninteresting. Resentment to treatment increased and spite caused him to indulge in drinking one night. He began to feel somewhat depressed because life seemed futile.

The next phase (June 21st to July 4th) was devoted to a study of his resistance to treatment and to the need to achieve a constructive attitude with a feeling of worth-whileness. An analysis of his reaction to co-workers, to superiors, and to his grandmother, when a child and in adolescence, revealed his increasing inability to yield. He had never reached full emancipation and healthy individualization. He had always been afraid of having to offer too much to others and was readily on the defensive. His reaction to the demands of treatment was the same as to any other demands in life. He mentioned (June 24th) that homosexual desires which had disappeared for three weeks, were returning and stated finally, with much expression of shame and anger at himself, that they were now directed to the physician. The analysis made him recognize his tendency to sexualize every intimate relationship with men and allowed him to see that a personality relationship based on mutual interests is possible. In this connection, he remembered a close friendship without physical attraction at the age of 20 to 24. The analysis of this friendship demonstrated clearly the undesirable development of the last ten years in which his sexual desires had become the center of his life and penetrated into all his interpersonal relations. He saw that the treatment was not "anti-homosexual," but that it tried to reduce the all-important sexual factors to a position which did justice to all the personality tendencies, and that self-reliance with willingness to adjust to life, and not submission to medical demands, was the therapeutic goal. A dream in which he had intercourse with the wife of a homosexual friend offered an opportunity to discuss the need for integration of bisexual strivings. He remembered that on an actual previous occasion he had fancied that he had relations with another friend and taken the wife merely as the best means to achieve a homosexual relationship which had been refused. His desire for promiscuity seemed to be more the expression of his unwillingness to become attached to anybody than caused by bisexuality, which had been taken as an insurmountable obstacle. In this connection, he again mentioned analeroticism and wondered to what extent constipation was due to erotic pleasure or to habit-formation. It seemed possible that moving away from his overconcerned grandmother and establishing a healthier hygiene might have had as much to do with the disappearance of constipation when he went to college as the homosexual gratification which started then. In the previous treatment he had gained the impression that the anal-eroticism had been transformed into homosexuality.

The treatment then turned to a study of group adjustment with the purpose of finding constructive possibilities which the patient could put into immediate practice and thus utilize life experiences for active re-education. The need to become part of the group in thinking, feeling, and actions, the urgency to develop interests in common with others, and share with them whatever seemed wise, was evaluated carefully. The patient saw the wisdom of guarding against thinking about the reactions of others and analyzing them. He had, however, marked difficulty in recognizing fully his tendency to perfectionism. Self-assertion and lack of trust, resentment, and discouragement were studied. His frequent feelings of boredom were formulated by him as unwillingness to become integrated socially in general, as well as integrated in the attitude of the group to sexual life. He found that fear of surrendering to women was as great an obstacle to intercourse as his standards relating to an idealized mother and possible castration fears of early childhood. Prostitutes were unacceptable because his body might become marred through venereal illnesses. The influence of alcohol on relieving social and sexual inhibitions was reviewed. Procrastination and vacillation were taken as undesirable means of evasion and protection against carrying out difficult tasks and the necessary suppression of unacceptable desires.

This constructive attempt was followed by a spite phase (July 24th to August 20th) in which the patient felt he should assert himself against threatening dependence on treatment. He had been absent for three weeks on a business trip. Giving in to increasing heterosexual desires, he had approached a girl acquaintance for intercourse. (Heterosexual relations had also been prohibited.) When refused, he had a very satisfactory homosexual experience. This episode was due to his need for the wrong type of self-assertion and to resentment, and was also utilized by him to prove again the inferiority of women and the undesirability of becoming really integrated in group life which included men and women. The concept of integration was again opposed because it prevented freedom, which included the right of satisfying all kinds of strivings. Ambivalence was mistaken for plasticity.

After this, a constructive and more inclusive personality analysis progressed fast. Vanity still found satisfaction in fancies of self-glorification and dramatization which had been important since childhood. His dead mother, whom he had never known, was pictured as beautiful and wealthy and contrasted to his unsuccessful father, who was remarried to an unattractive woman. He hated his stepmother because her appearance made him doubt that his father's first wife (i.e., his mother) had really been so attractive. Day-dreams had been increasingly substituted for actual testing in reality. Enthusiasm in new tasks soon gave way to discouragement when obstacles occurred. Innumerable excuses had always been found for his lack of persistence. In his work he had been more interested in the impression made on others than the actual achievement. The desire to do a perfect task made satisfaction impossible and prevented him from enjoying the performance and progress of work. His personality difficulties served as constant excuse for any failure. The desirability of a general integration was now accepted with a willingness to recognize the need of distinction between leading and incidental strivings. Smooth working of personality features did not predict boredom and "freezing" any longer. Envy and resentment now appeared as unhealthy and undesirable emotional reactions. Interests which could be well utilized in social life were found. However, he was still unwilling to accept the need for wholesome sexual integration and wondered whether homo- and heterosexuality could not be cultivated simultaneously.

The patient now improved fast. His work and social life became satisfactory and depressed moods did not recur. Life seemed stimulating and worth while. The week from August 8th to August 16th was devoted to a review of what had been achieved and why. Self-discipline and willingness to offer himself to others were discussed constructively. The occasion of his stepmother's sudden death and his father's turning to him for sympathy was not merely an opportunity for the study of his reaction, but revealed also that his hatred and resentment had greatly diminished and that he was able to offer sympathy without constant dread of future dependence of his father on him. Sexual strivings and constant activities were viewed in connection with family life and home.

On August 20th, the question of termination of treatment was approached. The patient felt confident that he would be able to utilize in the future the understanding which he had gained, but stated that a solution for his homosexuality had not been found. In the remaining five weeks, the sexual aspect was again investigated. He recognized a wish not to adjust his sexual life in order to prolong the treatment. He then reviewed his anal-erotic interest which had greatly decreased and his masturbation which was now resorted to as a relief from sexual tension with heterosexual preoccupation and narcissism. He was unable to accept the heterosexual relationship exclusively because his ethical standards, as well as the narcissistic fear of venereal disease, did not permit intercourse with prostitutes, and his standards did not allow seduction of a virgin. However, further discussion revealed this as not valid any longer. The main factor was his unwillingness to be tied to a woman for lifetime in marriage and to be responsible for her. A constructive solution was finally worked out in that he could do this if he had interests in common with her, and would base marriage and the formation of a family on a personality relationship in which the sexual factor was only one among many other factors.

Since then (November 1931) the patient has been better adjusted socially, more interested and productive in his work, and rarely given to moodiness. He tries to accept life more as it is and to guard against his still considerable tendency to procrastination. On the whole, he is more tolerant of others. He uses little alcohol and tobacco. He is less self-centered and has formed a few non-sexual friendships. He rarely masturbates and has never relapsed into frank narcissism, and no sadistic desires have occurred. On the other hand, his sexual life has not been entirely satisfactory. There have been two brief homosexual episodes. He planned at the same time to marry a friend with whom he had much in common. Premarital sexual relations were entirely satisfactory for three months. When the time for marriage approached, he lost his libido and became bored with her. After two weeks, both decided against marriage and his old interests and sexual desires for her returned. He realized that he was still unwilling to be satisfied with an exclusive heterosexual life and to take all the responsibilities which marriage involved. He did not blame his constitutional make-up and society any longer but was willing to accept that the whole problem lay with him (The patient married later and had a satisfactory sexual life for about four years. In connection with disappointment in an antici-

pated success many psychoneurotic symptoms developed with a return
of marked homosexual desires but without overt activities. This information was obtained in 1943.)

The influence of definite personalities in life in general as well
as in the limited field of sexual interest always deserves great attention in psychotherapy. It is marked in childhood, but even more
so in adolescence when the emancipating personality gropes for
new guiding principles and ideals. In persons who never develop
sufficient individuation and self-reliance, this need for idealization of
special persons and hero-worship may persist during life. As adolescence is also the time of sexual orientation, it is not surprising that
attachments to persons of one's own sex are readily formed. They
may take definite sexual form and, although frequently recognized
as sexual in character, may be expressed in affectionate friendship.
The adolescent girl's crushes belong to this group. In some, overt
homosexual acts occur either spontaneously or by seduction. They
are usually merely transient episodes in the person's life and of
no dynamic or other significance when maturity has been reached.
On the other hand, in predisposed individuals such experiences may
cause a homosexual orientation for life. It is therefore essential not
to minimize such incidents but to study their significance for the patient and use it for a healthy sexual orientation.

There is a small group of stable adult homosexuals where seduction caused the sexual malorientation on a similar basis. In
others, definite hysterical factors play the decisive role. These patients are usually attracted to one dominant homosexual person and
in contrast to the easily changing homosexual, do not become attracted to others. The prognosis in these cases is good if a thorough
analysis of the factors involved can be carried out, with separation
from the person involved and a corresponding change in environment. It is necessary to secure the other person's cooperation so
that the patient is given a chance to find self-reliance.

Case 39:

A 24 year old girl broke her engagement when she fell under the
influence of a homosexual girl after a brief acquaintanceship. In the
beginning she enjoyed this "beautiful friendship" and accepted expressions of affection. The homosexual girl represented her woman ideal
physically and culturally. Her easily aroused sympathy and affection

made it easy to accept carresses and minor sexual activities which, when she was completely under the friend's influence, led to frank sexual relations. After two years she was persuaded by friends, who were disturbed by this close relationship which led to the exclusion of other friends, to see a psychiatrist. She had become increasingly discontented and restless, often realizing that the relationship was entirely sexual.

In a few consultations, it became clear that her homosexual friend was, from the physical point of view, an identification with the man whom she had loved from 17 to 21 and with whom she had had satisfactory sexual relations. For financial and family reasons, marriage was impossible and the relationship terminated by her lover's leaving town permanently. A year later she became engaged to a well-to-do man who was physically attractive but who had few interests in common with her and whom she did not love, having never freed herself from her previous lover. Unhappy about her life, she appreciated her homosexual friend's offer of sympathy and friendship. She also was a sympathetic listener to her friend's defiance of society's attitude to homosexuality at this time because she herself was in an attitude of spite toward society.

This girl has been primarily heterosexual in her development. Crushes in adolescence were something unintelligible to her and she preferred to indulge in minor petting parties. Even during the homosexual phase her dreams and many of her preoccupations were primarily heterosexual. Without realizing its significance, she had to depend increasingly on alcohol to adjust herself to the homosexual situation. During treatment the patient abstained entirely from alcohol and any kind of sexual indulgence. With this, and the clarification of the factors involved, her heterosexuality again became dominant. She obtained a good understanding of sexual hygiene. When meeting her homosexual friend socially a few months later she was surprised to notice how her whole attitude had changed to one of sympathy, but without any sexual attraction. The treatment lasted three months, with consultations about once a week for six weeks, and later once in three weeks. These intervals between consultations were considered necessary to allow sufficient time for re-education and adjustment of her routine.

Such reactions may easily lead to permanent homosexual orientation. They emphasize the possible dangers of homosexual seduction in childhood and adolescence. On the other hand, the attraction of homosexuals to children has been greatly exaggerated. Danger of homesexual seduction exists also in all places where strict sexual segregation is carried out over any length of time (schools, army camps), especially at the age of sexual upheavals (adolescence), or when spite plays a role (prisoners). Moll urges the need to distinguish such cases as perversity (merely a sexual act without actual perverse orientation) from the perversions.

Other perversions frequently accompany homosexuality, e.g., *masochism* and *sadism*. In pure form these sexual maladjustments are rare and then usually in a psychopathic or early psychotic setting or under the influence of drugs. Masochistic and sadistic features are a part of normal sex life. They are considered perversions only when they are the dominant factors in obtaining sexual satisfaction. Freud feels that we deal with a fixation in the corresponding sexual developmental states in early childhood and a regression to these points when sexual life organizes itself in adolescence and early adult life. The perusal of literature makes one feel doubtful that analysis of these factors alone is sufficient. Most authors stress the need for sexual re-education and life adjustment.

Fetishism is also relatively rare. In one of my cases of shoe fetishism, I found fixation on an early adolescent experience and a habit-formation through indulgence in these fancies. The treatment was partly successful through sexual re-education and general sexual hygiene.

Sexual relations with *animals* occur sporadically in feebleminded persons and psychopaths, usually as the only possible sexual outlet in shy and solitary make-ups. General personality adjustment with stress on socialization is probably most helpful. Similar factors, such as the general make-up of the personality, poor sexual hygiene, and developmental factors, need to be adjusted in *voyeurism*.

Exhibitionism occurs in similar persons, especially under the influence of alcohol, and in senile psychoses. Recurrent cases apparently give good results to castration. On the whole, however, the treatment of personality and not merely of the sexual problem will be indicated.

BIBLIOGRAPHY

1. FREUD, S.: *Three Contributions to the Sexual Theory.* Nervous and Mental Disease Publishing Company, New York, 1910.
2. FREUD, S.: Contributions to the Psychology of Love. *Collected Papers,* Vol. 4. The Hogarth Press, London, 1925. (1. A special type of choice of object made by man. 2. The most prevalent form of degradation in erotic life. 3. The taboo of virginity.)

3. THOMPSON, C.: Changing Concepts of Homosexuality in Psychoanalysis. *Psychiatry: Journal of the Biology and Pathology of Interpersonal Relations*, 10, 1947.

4. KRAFFT-EBING, R. v. (ed. by A. MOLL): *Psychopathia Sexualis*. F. Enke, Stuttgart, 1924.

5. THURLIMANN, R.: Ueber die Indikation und den therapeutischen Erfolg der Kastration bei sexuell Perversen. *Schweizer Archiv für Neurologie und Psychiatrie*, 57, 1946.

Chapter XVIII

ALCOHOLISM; DRUG ADDICTION

IN BOTH alcoholism and drug addiction, the main principles of treatment are alike. Both these reactions are symptomatic of an underlying personality disorder which appears, and must be corrected, after the patient has been freed from the influence of alcohol or drugs. Addiction is a psychobiologic habit-formation, characterized by the features of craving and tolerance and symptoms of withdrawal. The patient does not only develop a desire for the drug and dependence on it, but, as a result of physiologic changes from the prolonged use of the drug, a definite need (craving) for it. Little is known about the physiologic changes which cause this craving. Further, the patient begins to tolerate larger amounts of the drug, amounts which would be lethal in the person who had not acquired this tolerance. Because of the acquired tolerance, the patient needs to increase the drug amount to achieve full satisfaction and again raises his tolerance. A vicious circle, which is limited by the body's reactions to this high chronic intoxication, develops. Sudden withdrawal of the drug therefore usually leads to marked physiologic symptoms. With our present knowledge, however, it is impossible to state to what extent anxiety and other emotions increase or provoke the physiologic symptoms. Considering the factors of craving and tolerance and the accompanying physiologic changes, it is doubtful whether one should speak of alcoholic addiction. In the chronic use of alcohol the patient does not develop the physiologic need. Whether we deal with the same tolerance as in drug addiction is doubtful. It is true that the average alcoholic develops a certain tolerance, but he usually then remains on a certain level and does not react with increased cravings. When the consumption of alcohol increases rapidly the body soon begins to suffer and tolerance begins to decrease in a relatively short time.

ALCOHOLISM

Alcoholism is the most widespread and important of these reactions and will therefore be discussed first. A patient should be considered a chronic alcoholic when he harms himself or his family through the use of alcohol and cannot be made to realize it, or when he no longer has the will or strength to overcome his habit. The diagnosis does not depend on the frequency of acute intoxication, which is merely an indication of his susceptibility to alcohol, but on the development of personality and somatic changes. The first symptoms of alcoholism are on a toxic basis; later structural changes in the brain and in various organs occur. In order to establish the damage which has been caused by the influence of alcohol, a thorough physical examination with due attention to the neurologic status is necessary. Most frequently found are cardiovascular and liver damage (fatty degeneration), chronic gastritis with complaints of nausea and constipation, and renal changes. The general nutritional status frequently suffers. A fine tremor of the fingers is obvious, and occasionally nystagmus, muscle twitching and, in the advanced cases, ataxia. The pupils may react sluggishly to light and accommodation. Alcoholic optic atrophy and paralysis of eye muscles are rare. The deep reflexes are frequently increased, rarely decreased or absent. These neurologic symptoms may present the picture of a tabes or tabo-paralysis. Disturbances of sensibility and neuritis are frequent. Under complete abstinence most of the neurologic symptoms clear up.

An early symptom is difficulty in falling asleep, restless and broken sleep. Potency suffers markedly with advanced alcoholism as a result of neurogenic and organogenic factors. Libido is increased in the beginning and begins to decrease only in advanced stages. Because of degenerative changes in the testicles a definite damage to the spermatozoon may occur. It is claimed that feeble-minded and epileptic children may result from this damage. The use of alcohol during lactation may exert a toxic damaging influence on the infant.

The psychopathologic changes are primarily those resulting from early cortical involvement, expressed in changes in memory function, attention, judgment, and in personality. One should therefore examine carefully for these defects, some of which may be concealed behind more or less marked confabulation. Usually these symptoms clear up under prolonged abstinence. When they persist to a more or less marked degree, they suggest definite cortical changes. Outstanding personality deviations are recognized in impulsiveness, lack of self-control with increased irritability (especially when accused of neglect of duty), euphoric mood with marked lability of affects, lessened perseverance in interests and actions, diminished initiative and ambition. It may be difficult to recognize early changes. In early alcoholism and especially when the patient is well groomed, he is charming to his friends, talks glibly about ambitions and impending successes, and finds plausible excuses for his failures. In his own family the same person may be rude or threatening, even to the point of striking members of his family, showing uncontrolled behavior at the least provocation, and developing marked dislikes and hatred. According to the personality, definite pathologic reaction traits appear, such as jealousy, paranoid tendencies, marked moodiness, and even phantastic-mystical tendencies. These may be forerunners, or a definite part, of the recognized alcoholic illness. There does not seem to be any essential difference between male and female alcoholism.

Alcohol produces a euphoric mood in which the patient pushes away inhibitory factors. He expresses himself more freely and acts with more ease and less self-restraint. Self-consciousness disappears. He feels intellectually stimulated but lacks perseverance in pursuing a goal. There is a definite decrease in efficiency, indicated physically by increase in pulse rate and metabolic changes, and mentally by less agile mental operations. Because of his euphoric mood, the patient deceives himself and believes in his increased efficiency. As a result of a heightening of the sensory thresholds, his sensation of fatigue is diminished, and he therefore erroneously believes in his increased endurance. These pharmacodynamic influences of alcohol explain why certain people turn to alcohol for relief and become dependent on it.

In some persons alcohol primarily intensifies the mood present. Euphoria and its accompanying symptoms result if the person is in a cheerful mood, while depressive features are accentuated if he is is an unhappy mood. To obtain relief the patient may have to resort to alcohol in amounts which will dull him emotionally.

In chronic alcoholism we deal with a habit-formation which is due to various psychobiologic difficulties. The moody person drinks to cheer himself during periods of slight depression and discouragement. He is in the beginning a spree drinker but usually develops later into a steady alcoholic. Alcoholism often starts in the setting of a depression, particularly if considerable situational factors play a role. Shy and self-conscious people drink to attain social ease. Persons with marked feelings of inadequacy drink for self-encouragement, especially when confronted with situations which demand too much of them. The lonely, socially maladjusted person tries in this way to forget his longing for understanding which he cannot achieve. Many solitary drinkers belong to this group. They frequently turn during their alcoholic escape to an inferior environment. Many of them are definitely psychopathic individuals. Not infrequently frank or unrecognized sexual maladjustments are the driving forces. I do not feel, however, that this is a general principle, as Ferenczi has claimed. Latent homosexuality may be a dynamic factor. Frequently indications of homosexual desires are revealed under alcoholic release. A careful study of such patients will then show whether latent homosexuality is a major dynamic factor or merely one of the many inhibited strivings, possibly not even of marked importance. We often find drinking as a direct reaction to disturbing situations in life in order to forget disappointments and failures. Some seek to gain relaxation in states of tension which may be due to the prolonged strain of situational difficulties or to maladjustment in the personality. There are others who rely on alcohol to produce the necessary encouragement and push. These factors explain why a person who suffers from an anxiety neurosis turns so frequently to alcohol. We also must consider social drinking habits which often have a detrimental influence in the case of suggestible persons who are easily influenced by others and lack resistance. To this group belong adolescents and immature psychopathic make-ups. Early alcoholism therefore frequently begins in college and club settings. With chronic alcoholism suggestibility increases and persons who have not been overly suggestible originally may no longer be able to resist the suggestive influence of others. Despite their best resolutions they are easy prey to the invitations or teasing of their alcoholic friends.

Although certain alcoholic beverages are taken primarily because of their taste, this factor plays a minor role in the formation of the habit. More important are social customs and prejudices. The latter are frequently a defense reaction of persons who drink and therefore make every effort to induce others to join their activities. There are, of course, marked individual differences in the reaction to alcohol and many variations of susceptibility and tolerance. It is therefore wrong to claim that a definite percentage of alcohol is non-intoxicating. This holds true only for the average person. We physicians are concerned with the alcohol-sensitive person to whom we have to offer constructive help. Persons who have constitutional tolerance for acute intoxications are naturally more in danger of developing a serious type of chronic alcoholism than the very susceptible person who, because he easily becomes a social nuisance in his frequent acute intoxications, is influenced by his companions to drink less.

Physical factors are etiologically not important except that they may lead to drinking in order to forget pain or to overcome fatigue. While persons with brain lesions have less tolerance, they have no specific craving as a result of the structural change. Attention should be paid, however, to physical changes which have been produced by alcoholic damage and which later may play a contributory role in the need for alcohol. This refers especially to liver and gastrointestinal changes (especially chronic gastritis), and feelings of general malaise.

The treatment of chronic alcoholism has usually been directed along three lines: That of personality analysis, in an endeavor to find strivings which drove the patient into alcoholism, re-education under enforced abstinence, and the use of drugs to change hypothetical chemical processes in the body or to produce a lasting disgust to alcohol through chemical alterations. The attempt to treat with drugs which are supposed to affect chemical etiologic factors cannot be considered scientific. Treatment through so-called reconditioning may offer symptomatic help and must be combined with psychotherapy to be of essential value.

The only treatment which can be effective in all cases and which can be adjusted to the patient's individual needs is treatment which combines personality analysis and adjustment with training of healthier habits over a long period of time and under strict abstinence.

The treatment can be divided into two phases. It should begin with immediate withdrawal from alcohol and be carried out under complete abstinence. Immediate withdrawal is psychologically important. It proves to the patient that there is no medical necessity for the use of alcohol in his case, and this realization is the beginning of his re-education. The patient must break away from many of the ideas, attitudes, and habits of his past life and learn that alcoholic drinks are not necessary for him to be cheerful and happy; that although they may help temporarily, in reality they increase his difficulties. There are no serious symptoms of withdrawal and no danger of the development of delirium tremens. Although the average physician may claim that he has seen delirium tremens caused by the abrupt withdrawal of alcohol, there are no carefully studied cases in literature to substantiate this claim. Other factors (accident, marked loss of blood), and not withdrawal, precipitated the outbreak of the delirium. Most frequently the earliest symptoms of a beginning delirium could have been recognized by a psychiatrically well-trained physician. It is important that the physician use cardiac stimulants for a short time (caffeine) in cases of marked alcoholism, as a substitute for the stimulating influence of alcohol. Attention to the physical condition is important, including correction of the results of faulty dietary habits. In a large number of these patients vitamin deficiency exists. Although vitamin B_1 appears to be the most important in these instances, the deficiency usually is multiple and therefore other members of the B complex will be indicated.

The insight which the patient usually shows at, or shortly after, the beginning of treatment lasts only about one or two weeks. It is not based on real understanding of the danger of his alcoholism, but on alcoholic euphoric optimism. It is followed by a grouchy revolt of two to four weeks, in which the patient insists upon less restriction because he feels he is well and will be able to handle the alcoholic problem in the future or because he does not care for the treatment. Many patients terminate treatment at this point, frequently with the support of members of their family who are optimistically deceived by them. Only after this negative reaction has passed, does real insight develop. This insight makes the patient willing to cooperate and anxious to see how he can develop self-dependence and self-reliance without the aid of alcohol. In any case of marked alcoholism therefore the patient ought to be under close supervision for about two months, preferably in a closed psychiatric institution, with definite restriction of his personal freedom. This period constitutes the first phase of treatment during which a thorough investigation of the personality with due attention to the physical status is carried out. This study reveals the main factors which caused the patient to become dependent on alcohol. In the analysis we should evaluate the patient's shortcomings, his resources, and interests. After real insight has been gained a constructive analysis will show him how his assets can be used to overcome his difficulties.

During the second phase of treatment, which deals primarily with re-education of his habits, our knowledge of his personality should permit us to utilize an individualized approach. It is desirable that this be carried out in an open institution in which the patient can lead a healthy life, with a well-balanced routine which includes work and suitable recreation and a healthy physical regime. Treatment by weekly consultation is sufficient for a brief constructive analysis of recurrent psychobiologic difficulties. The patient will gradually learn to deal with slight depressive moods, to cultivate interests which will allow a better adjustment to the group, and to develop confidence in himself. This self-confidence is the basis for social ease and the ability to face failure and disappointment.

A cure has been achieved when the patient no longer needs alcohol and has confidence in himself because he does not need to drink. Treatment should always lead to total abstinence. Moderate drinking during treatment has been advised by some physicians because many patients develop a spite reaction to the request for complete abstinence. When this occurs, the physician should endeavor to obtain a better understanding of the factors causing this behavior and should not give in to requests for moderate drinking.

The atmosphere of the environment is most important. The patient should not feel that he is inferior to those about him because he cannot drink, but that he has no need to drink. A physician who is a total abstainer will achieve better results than a physician who has one attitude for himself and another for his patients. The totally abstaining physician carries much more conviction in his advice and exerts a strong suggestive influence.

The preparation of the home environment is important. The old associations with alcohol have been destroyed in the hospital and the patient should return to a home atmosphere which supports his new attitude. It is therefore essential that his family be willing to abstain also and that no alcoholic beverages be served in his home. The family physician should understand that no alcohol should be prescribed to former alcoholics, and that a brief interview when the patient is disturbed will make sedatives unnecessary.

It is possible to carry out the first phase of treatment in a modern psychiatric hospital in which the physicians have sufficient time to study the patient carefully, but greater difficulty is encountered in finding institutions in which the re-educational phase can be carried out. On the average, the entire hospital stay should last about a year. The patient should be in a place where he can lead as normal a life as possible and where association with other patients will facilitate adjustment to society. A psychiatric institution cannot fulfill these requirements, and therefore special institutions for alcoholic patients are neecssary. The hospitals abroad which are devoted to this special phase of treatment are, to my mind, not satisfactory. They carry out a summary type of re-education, do not pay enough attention to the patient's individual needs, and omit planned psychotherapy.

In chronic alcoholism, as in the treatment of many other personality problems and faulty habit-formations, physicians and public must realize that we deal with an illness which has developed over a period of years and cannot be treated successfully in a short period of time. As a result of better education, one no longer hesitates to urge a patient to go to a tuberculosis sanitorium for a year without even promising full restoration to health. The same attitude must be taken with regard to advanced alcoholism.

For the largest number of alcoholic patients this type of treatment is not possible because of the lack of adequate medical facilities. It is always possible to offer the first period of treatment in the psychiatric hospital and treat the patient afterwards ambulatorily. In patients treated entirely on an ambulatory basis, the therapeutic principles are the same; namely, immediate withdrawal of alcohol, a study of all the factors responsible for the development of alcoholism, and constructive adjustment of personality difficulties, well-organized activities in the patient's daily life (if possible without interruption of work), avoidance of sedatives, and a prolonged re-educational period, with efforts to induce members of the patient's immediate family to accept abstinence also and to modify their social customs accordingly. If we fail in any of these main points, hospital treatment will be necessary.

Case 40:

A 46 year old college professor came for help after one of his frequent alcoholic excesses. He realized that he would not be able to hide his alcoholism much longer and was in danger of losing his position. For about ten years, feeling lonely and increasingly disappointed in his family life and in his research, he had tried to forget his unhappiness in periodic drinking bouts occurring approximately every two months. In the last two years they had increased to once a month and finally to once in ten days. While drinking in his club he felt more cheerful and at ease with others and was able to become interested in commonplace talk. When sober he was a serious minded man, devoted entirely to teaching and research, talking little, leading a very narrow life and unable to form any friendships. He was very shy and self-conscious, good natured, and with a great yearning to be kind and close to those he liked, but unable to express it. He had married a vivacious woman, five years his junior, who had manifold cultural and social interests but little in common with him. Spoiled and selfish, she was unwilling to yield to him and succeeded in keeping their only child entirely to herself. In the last four years no sexual relations occurred, because of her frigidity. On the other hand, she was jealous of his friendship with a woman of her age. In this relationship sexual factors did not enter, as it was based on mutual interests in his study of modern languages.

In contrast to his previous physicians, I advised immediate and constant abstinence. The main personality features which made adjustment impossible were formulated to him and possible modifications outlined. Although he slept poorly for several nights, no sedatives were given. It was explained to him that poor sleep was one of the frequent symptoms of the withdrawal of alcohol. For one week he was seen daily, in order to encourage him, to restore his shattered self-confidence, and to establish a healthy routine. He was urged to take long walks which he had enjoyed previously and to revive his interest in botany which had given him much pleasure in adolescence. Later he formed a connection with the botanical department in his college and began to participate regularly in their excursions. His wife was unable to see the need for change and has led the same life since. However, he became much more tolerant of her and gradually lost the resentment which had developed in him. His daughter became interested in her father's hobby and accompanied him occasionally on Sunday mornings. Considerable time was spent on investigating his disappointments in teaching and research which resulted in discouragement and feelings of inadequacy. Analyzing the behavior of persons who irritated him and hurt his sensitive nature allowed him to accept others as they were and prevented him from magnifying difficulties.

After the first week the patient came for a consultation once a month for the first year. The second year, consultations were spaced to once in two months. Since then the patient has returned once a year, before the beginning of his vacation, in order to discuss plans for the summer, when he felt lost without his routine. Vacation had usually been the time when he had to resort to escape in alcoholism. The treatment over these eight years during which the patient has never taken any alcohol was primarily planned re-education. This patient has remained in good health since termination of treatment in 1936 and came for only three consultations at times of considerable emotional strain.

The attitude of the patient's wife was unfortunate but not unexpected. In many cases of chronic alcoholism we find a definite indifference in the partner and an unwillingness to change his or her own life for the patient. Another equally distressing type is the wife who sacrifices herself for the patient and believes his constant repentance and promises. Relatives are frequently unable to recognize alcoholism as an illness and consider it as bad behavior or an expression of lack of will power. Not infrequently there are wives who rejoice definitely, although they are not aware of it, in the role of the sufferer and feel that it is their duty to stick to their alcoholic husbands, sacrificing their own life, and the happiness of their children. They do not help the patient and keep him in his alcoholism by their submissive and frequently motherly attitude. They are usually unable to see that it is their duty as well persons to enforce the treatment of a patient who has not enough insight to request the necessary help. It is true that our commitment laws are usually not very adaptable in order to keep an alcoholic patient detained a sufficient length of time. The physicians of each state and county need to recognize this and try to achieve satisfactory changes. This will, however, depend on a change of the attitude of the public as well as of the physicians towards the alcoholic patient, leading to an appreciation of his condition as an illness requiring medical treatment.

It is difficult for a cured alcoholic to resist the influences which attract him to drinking. In order to build up his self-confidence and not to develop reactions of inadequacy because he is singled out as somebody who is sensitive to alcohol, he needs the whole-hearted backing of his family and friends. It is desirable to advise such a patient to join people who do not drink. In many communities there are social and religious groups who cultivate total abstinence. In recent years considerable progress along these lines has been made in this country and abroad. Participation in an active social life will, however, remain exceedingly difficult in a society which does not insist with the same wholeheartedness on the right not to drink as on the right to drink. A psychiatrist who treats alcoholics would no doubt be able to form such groups through former patients. The prevention of alcoholism has attracted so much attention in the last fifteen years that little effort has been spent on the improvement of treatment.

In a brief presentation of this problem in 1933 I urged a practical solution, proposing the establishing of farms for the treatment of alcoholic patients, for carrying out the re-educational phase. The first phase could be carried out in the local psychiatric institutions. It would be essential that such farms be self-supporting. A broad solution of the alcohol problem is medically necessary. In contrast to the treatment of actual drug addicts, there is a definite advantage in treating in groups alcoholics with insight. They exert a healthy suggestive and encouraging influence on each other if treated in the proper environment. One would have to select one's cases carefully and omit destructive psychopathic patients.

The various types of other well-defined alcoholic psychopathologic reactions need little discussion. The most frequent type, delirium tremens, has been discussed in Chapter XII. Delusions of jealousy and full-fledged paranoid reactions were discussed in Chapter XI. Acute hallucinosis is frequent and often combined with delirium tremens. When it occurs in pure form, i.e., primarily auditory hallucinations of threatening content and with delusions of persecution and marked fear without disorientation, hospitalization is urgent. These patients are very suicidal and greatly disturbed. Korsakow's psychosis also necessitates hospitalization, at least until the patient is quiet and well enough oriented to take care of himself. In exceptional cases discharge to the family can be considered later; i.e., after a year or more of hospitalization. There is, however, always danger of relapse into alcoholism and exacerbation of the psychotic picture with more serious deterioration. Alcoholic pseudo-paresis and pseudo-tabes frequently offer a good prognosis with rapid clearing up of the neurologic symptoms under complete abstinence and administration of vitamins. When definite structural cortical damage has occurred the treatment corresponds to that described in Chapter XIII. "Alcohol epilepsy" is not a desirable term. We deal with the occurrence of epileptic convulsions in the setting of chronic alcoholism. These convulsions are merely symptoms; they are either due to definite alcoholic cerebral damage, to special toxic admixtures in the alcoholic beverage, or the precipitation of convulsions through alcohol in the epileptic patients. These cases have not been studied sufficiently and the etiology is still unclear. In all these alcoholic reactions prolonged treatment in a psychiatric hospital is indicated. Careful attention must be given to the physical conditions, (especially to the general nutritional state and the probability of vitamin deficiency), to the cardiac status, and proper gastrointestinal functioning. Hydrotherapy in the form of prolonged warm baths should be offered freely. After recovery from the acute psychopathologic condition the chronic alcoholism needs to be treated.

Cases of acute alcoholic intoxication rarely present a psychiatric problem. The so-called pathologic intoxication is rare, occurring in especially predisposed individuals, e.g., psychopathic personalities, epileptic and schizophrenic patients and after traumatic brain damage. These patients ought to be taken to a psychiatric hospital because they present the picture of an excitement in which they are very destructive and dangerous to others. In the only patient of this type whom I saw, restraint was necessary for the transport because the usual amount of scopolamine-morphine failed to influence the patient. A dry or cold wet pack will be the easiest form of restraint if enough people are available. Otherwise, one may have to resort to definite physical restraint.

Dipsomania comprises a large variety of cases. Most of the patients are psychopathic personalities, frequently with epileptic features. Others suffer from some kind of periodic psychoses. Their prognosis is usually poor. If they are unable to carry on a self-supporting life, permanent hospitalization is necessary. The only hope is hospitalization for a year or longer for treatment of the chronic alcoholism and the underlying personality disorder. If after discharge alcoholic excesses occur, immediate re-hospitalization is indicated.

PARALDEHYDE ADDICTION

Paraldehyde addiction occurs in alcoholic patients. One should therefore never offer paraldehyde freely. Paraldehyde addiction is rare. There was an increase during the prohibition era when people became accustomed to drinking alcoholic beverages notwithstanding their disagreeble smell or taste. The symptoms are those of chronic alcoholism and in addition loss of weight, poor or excessive appetite, constipation, anemia, increased evening temperature, and irregular cardiac action. The paraldehyde breath is always marked. Most of the patients observed are serious psychopathic personalities. It is felt that abrupt withdrawal of paraldehyde leads to a series of epileptic convulsions and a delirium-tremens-like picture, but the same has also been observed with gradual withdrawal.

Case 41:

In a 51 year old man who had been a heavy drinker since college, the physician advised paraldehyde in October 1928, for insomnia, which had been persistent since 1922. He stopped alcohol entirely and for five months depended on a daily amount of 60 cc. of paraldehyde. When admitted to a general hospital (2-19-29) paraldehyde was stopped. The patient became restless, sleepless, and excitable and two days later developed marked delirium with three convulsions, which were relieved by immediate lumbar puncture (the pressure was increased). His delirium was characterized by marked fear, disorientation to time and place; he heard voices talking to him and felt there was something mysterious about it — boats and persons were around him — and he believed that he was taking a lesson in flying. He constantly picked "bugs" out of his hand. He was deeply cyanotic, respiration was shallow and irregular and at times there was definite Cheyne-Stokes breathing.

During the paraldehyde delirium the patient received hydrotherapy (prolonged baths) for five to twelve hours daily with occasionally a cold wet pack and 0.006 gm. ($\frac{1}{100}$ gr.) of scopolamine when excited. The patient was digitalized and diuretin 1.5 gm. (22gr.) three times a day was administered. He was put on increased fluid intake and light diet. After three days he was completely oriented and his physical condition improved greatly. At first he was cooperative in order to obtain a better understanding of the factors which caused his alcoholism, but soon became restless and wanted to leave. During this brief stay in the hospital we were able, however, to get some understanding. The patient, who was an intelligent, highly successful person, had been forced, through his family, into a profession in which he was unhappy. He therefore resorted to alcoholism, which increased whenever he felt discouraged over his work. Insomnia started when he felt that his professional situation became unbearable to him and he resigned from his position. For two years preceding admission he had been drinking very heavily, trying to get sleep also by taking 3.0 gm. barbital daily (45 gr.) and high amounts of bromide. There was a marked tendency to depression on the maternal and paternal sides and the patient has always been moody.

Before discharge we tried to outline a routine which would take care of his spare time and allow him to overcome his moody spells. He did not sleep well yet but felt able to get along without medication. He left for a trip to Europe. When landing, he immediately went on another drinking spree. At that time he was taken to a psychiatrist, who discussed with him briefly his alcoholic cravings and emphasized his advice by hypnotic suggestions. The patient relaxed, but did not develop a deep hypnosis. He stayed with that physician a week, and since that time he has not been drinking at all, although many times there was an urge to return to it. At such times the counter-suggestions which had been offered in hypnosis began to work. The patient has been leading an active and successful life for five years. It is one of the few cases in which I have seen help through hypnosis. One should realize that we dealt with a relatively stable individual who, because of a tendency to moodiness and unfavorable life situations, began to seek relief in alcohol. The suggestions apparently were sufficient to give him the necessary hold when moodiness or discouragement occurred. The paraldehyde addiction was merely a phase in the problem of alcoholism. To date, 1947, this patient has remained a totally abstinent and well adjusted person.

Ether addiction is rare, occasionally occurring in members of the medical group who usually start taking it because of curiosity. Ether causes marked euphoria with slowing of perception and some excitement and resembles much the effect of alcohol, especially when taken chronically. It leads to serious kidney, liver, and heart damage. The prognosis is poor, probably more because of the poorly organized personality make-up involved than resulting from a specific craving for ether. Treatment consists of sudden withdrawal with careful attention to physical involvement, a constructive personality analysis, and re-education in a psychiatric hospital.

Chloroform addiction is rare and apparently limited to the medical group. Sudden withdrawal does not produce any special symptoms.

MORPHINE ADDICTION

Morphine addiction is widespread; its danger and correct treatment, however, are little understood by the average physician and even psychiatrists, because they rarely meet cases which they can study thoroughly. Addiction is frequently induced by physicians who offer morphine freely for pain. It seems to be true that not everybody develops addiction who has to take morphine over any length of time. Cases have been observed in which no withdrawal symptoms were manifest after the withdrawal of morphine which had been given daily in cases of prolonged, painful illnesses. However, these cases are rare and form the exception. On the whole it will be wisest to consider every patient as having a possible constitution for morphine addiction. A large group is formed by persons who have easy access to morphine, i.e., physicians and their wives, druggists, and nurses.

Morphine given by mouth is absorbed from the small intestines. A much faster influence is obtained by hypodermic administration because the liver, which changes the morphine, is excluded. Considering the danger of addiction, we must include morphine derivatives, most frequent of which are dionine, which is part of the frequently administered Schlesinger solution, heroine, peronin and eudokal. The main physiologic results are central analgesia, fatigue, and sleep and, in toxic amounts, respiratory paralysis. In chronic addiction loss of libido, impotency, and sterility result. The psychobiologic features which lead to addiction and which become manifest ten to fifteen minutes after hypodermic administration are marked euphoria with a feeling of contentment and optimism and pleasant day-dreaming but no desire for sleep. The effect lasts from two to four or six hours and is followed by a negative phase, which produces a desire for more morphine.

In very susceptible persons the average amount of morphine produces toxic symptoms in the form of oppression and slight anxiety, dizziness, nausea, and urticaria, increased libido, and in rare cases of idiosyncrasy, collapse which needs to be treated with camphor and caffeine. Usually prompt relief results from a hypodermic injection of 0.0002 to 0.0005 gm. ($\frac{1}{300}$ to $\frac{1}{120}$ gr.) of atropine.

Acute morphine intoxication, with which one is occasionally confronted in suicidal attempts, is characterized by sleep, or somnolence and coma. The pupils are very small, the respiration is shallow, and the temperature low. The treatment is well discussed in textbooks of pharmacology.

In chronic intoxication one can distinguish three definite stages: (1) The euphoric stage, which was mentioned previously, with increase of libido and occasionally also of potency. This is soon followed by (2) adaptation of the body to the toxin. There is reached a definite tolerance to the morphine in which no euphoria is produced any longer but the same amount of morphine enables the patient to work. In order to obtain the desired result, the patient must resort to a higher dosage or more frequent hypodermics. Chronic toxic symptoms now develop — general physical decay with marked diarrhea and constipation, dental caries, degenerative change of skin and nails, and decrease of libido and potency. The pupils react sluggishly to light; pulse is slow, and blood pressure low. The patient feels restless and apathetic. No toxic psychopathologic symptoms seem to develop during this stage of chronic intoxication. (3) A stage of intolerance during which the amount of morphine cannot balance the symptoms of withdrawal any longer.

The withdrawal reaction is greatly feared by the patient and prevents him from turning to the physician for help. Withdrawal symptoms occur at any stage of morphine addiction and in every age but are more marked with the cessation of higher than lower amounts of the drug. Patients usually come for treatment in the second and third stages. When intolerance has started, the patient usually only wishes a reduction to the point of tolerance, and not complete cure. In the second stage, most patients ask for a reduction to the level at which they are able to carry on their work and duties, or which they can afford financially. If the physician accommodates the patient, a reduction on a more satisfactory level will be kept after discharge for a certain length of time and is followed by another increase which brings the patient back to the physician. Such patients may undergo innumerable reduction treatments. There are naturally exceptional patients who are able to keep the amount required within certain practical limits. They are rare, and no physician should be guided by such observations in his therapeutic approach to morphine addicts.

Withdrawal symptoms are general restlessness, yawning, hot and cold flushes, perspiration, increased salivation, combined with anxiety which increases rapidly to a marked extent. The patients are very fatigued but sleep becomes restless and poor. Their mood is usually definitely depressed. There is marked nausea and frequently vomiting and diarrhea. The appetite is usually poor; in some, however, it increases greatly. Very distressing are marked intestinal cramps and pains which may impress the physician as being due to a surgical condition and impede him greatly in his therapeutic decisions. Physicians who are not well experienced in the withdrawal treatment are often afraid to proceed further and resort to morphine again. Many patients complain of neurologic pains and muscle cramps and twitchings. The patients become markedly prostrated. Libido may increase markedly and may be accompanied by painful erections. All these symptoms, and especially the fear of their increase, may provoke a panic.

These symptoms and their duration depend on the amount to which the patient has been addicted, the duration of the addiction, and the individual personality and somatic make-up. They usually reach maximal intensity after twenty-four hours and begin to subside after forty-eight to seventy-two hours. The factors which cause withdrawal symptoms are unknown, and one is not able to say whether they are of a direct or indirect nature. It is certain, however, that fear of withdrawal increases all the symptoms greatly and that psychotherapy, especially suggestion, helps to make them much more tolerable. Morphine addicts are usually well informed of the withdrawal reaction, either from medical literature or contact with former patients. It is important therefore that physicians and public know that the actual withdrawal symptoms in moderate morphine addiction are not very marked and can be well handled medically.

Case 42:

A 51 year old successful business man sought help for morphine addiction which started at 44 when his physician prescribed morphine for relief in attacks of asthma. He obtained from the drug a feeling of well-being and relief from emotional tension when under strain. Several treatments by gradual withdrawal were followed by a relapse after a few weeks. His daily amount was 0.12 gm. (2 gr.), administered intravenously.

On admission he was restless, mildly anxious, and depressed, but in good physical condition. After a period of 12 hours, needed for carrying out the physical and psychiatric studies indicated and during which he received two hypodermic administrations of morphine sulphate .03 gm. (½ gr.), the drug was withdrawn abruptly. Within 24 hours, he became very restless, had marked perspiration, complained of headaches and pains in the calves of his legs, and slept little. The third and fourth night he had nightmares. His most troublesome symptoms were priapism and numerous seminal emissions. To diminish his anxiety he received barbital 0.15 gm. (2½ gr.) four times in 24 hours, and warm baths for 3 hours' duration twice a day. Medication for headaches was given for three days. Massage of his legs was administered twice daily. A mild attack of asthma was terminated by 0.5 cc. of adrenalin (1:1000 solution). He ate a soft diet. Whenever possible, the patient joined in the routine activities. Reassurance was offered by physician and nurses and psychotherapeutic discussions occurred daily. After a week the withdrawal symptoms had disappeared. During four months in the hospital some of the important psychodynamic factors became clear to the patient, including his unsatisfactory sexual and marital life. He recognized the precarious nature of his success which was maintained by excellent intelligence and unusual interest in his work and threatened by his unwillingness to be in full control of his desires. His rebelliousness against conforming to society and against authority was understood dimly only from the point of view of his early childhood development and family setting. He was superficially most cooperative but maintained a defensive attitude and was never able to recognize emotional reactions readily or to express them freely in therapeutic interviews. Since he has left the hospital he has kept free from morphine (6 months), but his prognosis must be considered very guarded.

In exhausted and generally poorly nourished patients, there may occur marked psychopathologic withdrawal reactions, characterized by delirious reactions with marked fear, delusions of persecution, and hallucinations of very small animals (bugs, etc.). These reactions are rare and usually do not occur during treatment if the necessary precautions are taken. More frequent are psychogenic confusional states and deliria. They are the personality reaction to the feared withdrawal and should not be classified with withdrawal deliria. Many so-called withdrawal deliria are due to the free use of atropine or scopolamine which were offered to alleviate the withdrawal symptoms. Collapse is rare and can be helped immediately by the hypodermic administration of 0.03 (½ gr.) of morphine. This danger may exist for a few weeks after sudden withdrawal. If occurring at this late date, morphine administration is contraindicated because it would not only undo the psychotherapeutic results of treatment but also stir up new cravings for morphine because of the resulting euphoria and contentment. Caffeine will then be indicated.

It was mentioned previously that certain constitutions seem to be predisposed to morphine addiction but little is known about this possibility. Some authors claim that a vast majority are persons who like to be in the limelight and demand much attention, the same type which is inclined to hysterical reactions. Many patients are psychopathically unstable persons who are unwilling or incapable of putting up with the struggle of life. If they are of the aggressive type they attempt to overcome their inadequacy to life by seeking a stimulus in the drug and a change of environment through daydreaming and feelings of contentment. If they suffer from a passive inadequacy the addiction may be the expression of flight into an illness. In a large number, sexual maladjustment, especially struggle with homosexuality or even sexual disgust to perverted demands of the partner may be leading factors. In these cases, the increased libido will substitute for the missing biologic craving. Psychoanalytic investigators consider a narcissistic constitution the important factor. The precipitating factors are ill-considered medical administration of morphine for hysterical and hypochondriacal reactions and various complaints in psychopathic individuals. One needs to consider especially the danger of morphine administration for hysterical vomiting and hiccough, intestinal cramps and dysmenorrhea, hypochondriacal pain reactions, especially headaches and anxiety attacks. Seduction by a morphine addict, in contrast to the high frequency in cocaine addiction, plays a minor role. The morphine addict is the solitary type. Imitation is more frequent, e.g., in schools and in criminal environments. Curiosity may lead to morphine addiction, especially in members of the medical group.

As long as a patient does not take more than 0.06 gm. (1gr.) a day we may speak of moderate addiction in which not very distressing direct withdrawal symptoms will occur. From 1 to 2 gm. (15 to 30 gr.) would be considered high amounts. There are even cases mentioned in literature where the patient developed a tolerance to 10 and 15 gm. (150 to 225 gr.)

It is essential that psychotherapeutic rules guide us in the treatment of drug addiction. The patients should be accepted on an honest and frank basis and not with the attitude of dealing with hopeless psychopathic material or with a person with inferior ethical standards. A self-righteous attitude has unfortunately been the rule among most physicians in the past and has kept those drug addicts who offered a good or fair prognosis away from help. It may be that ethical standards suffer with drug addiction and many patients are not able to co-operate honestly in the treatment. This is part of the illness. The establishing of insight, and not condemnation, is the therapeutic goal. Furthermore, most patients are not able to co-operate wholeheartedly because they are torn between their craving for morphine and their desire to get rid of it as well as because of their great fear of withdrawal. Because of these difficulties, hospitalization in a closed institution is the only possible setting for treatment. Treatment without restriction, as is still occasionally promised, is impossible. It overlooks the strength of the biologic craving. One should always ask for voluntary or legal commitment.

In the first consultation the physician needs to determine the amount taken, the duration of the addiction, the physical and mental status, what the dynamic factors are, and in what personality and life setting it occurs. He should be distrustful of the amount mentioned if it is high, but should not show this to the patient. Many patients exaggerate the amount taken and the duration, the seriousness of some of the distressing factors which drove them into addiction, or the grave withdrawal symptoms which they had experienced when trying to reduce the morphine in order to induce the physician to refrain from sudden withdrawal and to choose a slower therapeutic procedure. When the physician has reached an understanding of the case, he should formulate carefully to the patient the need for hospitalization and the possibilities with which modern treatment is able to alleviate the withdrawal symptoms. He should urge and arrange for immediate hospitalization. Otherwise, the patient's doubts and fears will recur and he will lack the courage to enter the hospital at a later date. It is justifiable to administer morphine to such a patient for the trip to the hospital.

If urgent reasons demand a brief postponement, the physician also has the right to offer morphine. He can only do this, however, if he knows the situation well. He has not the right to offer morphine if the patient offers excuses or is undecided for more than twenty-four hours. Every practitioner will be confronted now and then by drug addicts who ask for morphine merely because their supply has stopped. The drug should not be given except when definite physical dangers would occur from even temporary withdrawal.

In the hospital a careful physical and psychiatric examination should be done within the first 24 hours. During this period the patient should receive his usual amount of morphine. The treatment should be started, preferably on the morning of the second day in the hospital, with immediate abrupt withdrawal. This has become increasingly the accepted principle. It has the advantage of shortening the period of somatic and mental re-adjustment and allows more intensive psychotherapy. We need, however, to be able to assure the patient that we are well acquainted with the withdrawal symptoms and know how to modify them, whereas his knowledge is less definite and much influenced by unreliable hearsay, anticipation, and fear. The patient should realize that there are marked individual differences and that withdrawal causes not merely a physical, but a whole personality, reaction in which physical symptoms and emotional reactions influence each other. The alleviation of withdrawal symptoms is therefore possible from both the somatic and psychobiologic aspects.

It will be best to start immediately with prolonged warm baths which may last twelve or more hours. In especially restless, fearful cases, one may change to cold wet packs. No sedatives should be offered during the day but one will rarely be able to omit them at night to procure some sleep in cases where we expect a marked withdrawal reaction. Barbital 0.5 gm. (7½ gr.) with phenobarbital (luminal) 0.2 gm. (3 gr.) are sufficient. High amounts of hypnotics (chloral hydrate, luminal, amytal, scopolamine) have been advised to overcome the withdrawal symptoms. They are not very effective and it will be wise to refrain from their use because these high amounts may add a toxic factor. The patient is put on soft diet including milk with the free use of sodium bicarbonate 2.0 gm. (30 gr.) every four hours to prevent hyperacidity. Carbohydrated water is preferable to plain water in dehydrated, nauseated patients. For nausea and vomiting, ice and iced milk are offered. A craving for sweets should be satisfied. The frequent marked diarrhea is preferably treated with bismuth subcarbonate, never with opiates. Before beginning the withdrawal, mild cathartics are advisable (two compound cathartic pills or ½ oz. of Epsom salts). Massage and alcohol rubs help greatly against the various muscle pains and cramps. Bed rest should not last more than a few days and whenever possible the patient should be in the open. After the withdrawal symptoms have subsided the patients develop a great appetite and gain weight rapidly. In convalescence no special medication is necessary if sufficient hydrotherapy and massage is given and the patients put on active routine as soon as possible.

Choline and ergotamine (gynergen) and endocrine treatment have been advocated in order to influence the sympathicotonia to which the withdrawal symptoms are attributed. Large amounts of antipyretics, especially aspirin, are also suggested. In some of my cases aspirin seemed to offer relief (2.0 gm. — 30 gr. every four hours). It is, however, difficult to evaluate such cases because the intensity of withdrawal varies greatly and is influenced by suggestion and reassurance. If marked anxiety is present the administration of 20 to 30 units of insulin is helpful. Resulting mild hypoglycemic symptoms, e.g., hunger, marked perspiration, or somnolence, are relieved readily by the administration of 50 gm. of glucose by mouth. It will be wise to be ready for any possible emergency reaction (see p. 158). I might add that in my personal experience, it has never been necessary to resort to insulin.

It will always be wise to consider prophylactic digitalization before withdrawal is started. On the other hand, we should be careful not to delay active therapy because of the patient's fears, which are much more marked and distressing than those experienced to an impending operation. Many patients become panicky and are then in an undesirable state for the proposed treatment so that one is forced to use fast or slow withdrawal instead of abrupt. Definite contraindications to sudden withdrawal are cardiac decompensation, nephritis, or generally poor health.

In abrupt withdrawal the symptoms start after a few hours and increase gradually, with marked improvement starting after three to eight days. The physician should always use sudden withdrawal when the amount is less than 0.3 gm. (5 gr.). There is still some discussion with regard to higher amounts. German psychiatrists are still hesitant. The experience in American and British Government hospitals, where sudden withdrawal is the rule, demonstrates, however, that most of the fears, especially of withdrawal, collapse, and excessive physical pain, were grossly exaggerated. With good medical attention and intensive psychotherapy, abrupt withdrawal should be the choice as it leads to far better results. Withdrawal under sleep treatment and anesthesia have not proved to be successful.

Fast withdrawal spreads the gradual reduction of the morphine over a period of not more than one week. The reduction proceeds daily from one-half to one-fourth to one-eighth to total withdrawal. The symptomatic treatment is the same as with abrupt withdrawal. Better results are obtained if one offers codeine and morphine instead of merely morphine during the reduction period. In recent years, there have been increasing warnings against the use of chloral hydrate, atropine, and scopolamine during the withdrawal.

Slow withdrawal takes four weeks. It is psychologically undesirable and frequently does not lead to total freedom from the drug. Its advocates overlook the fact that with slow withdrawal a stage may be reached where the morphine again produces a euphoric reaction and, with this, renewed craving.

Much has been said for individualized withdrawal with a reduction to one-half at the beginning and further reduction according to the withdrawal symptoms. When they become distressing the patient receives a temporary increase of morphine to produce good days during which he is able to regain strength and courage. As in all the slow withdrawals, the patient should never know the dosage which he receives. Individualized withdrawal, which is attractive especially to the physician with little experience in the treatment of drug addiction and which he defends as most humane and psychologically desirable because it appeals to the patient's will to cooperate, is to my mind the least effective. Psychogenically and emotionally determined symptoms dominate the picture and confuse and frighten the physician. It is definitely a symptomatic treatment.

A physician must have the courage to proceed with the treatment correctly and not be swayed by symptoms and complaints. This does not mean that a harsh attitude should be substituted for patience and sympathy. The patient should feel that he can depend on the physician. This same attitude is important for the second phase of treatment, during which the patient's personality is studied closely, the dynamic factors determined, and through a constructive analysis a life adjustment achieved. Through discussions the conflicts which, in the past, caused the patient to take morphine are stirred up. A change of environment should be effected before discharge. Occupational therapy and group activities are highly important. Recreational outlets need to be found and cultivated. The fear that spite reactions may develop to treatment in a closed institution should not prevent such hospitalization. These reactions, especially suspiciousness, which occasionally leads to a definite paranoid picture, need to be analyzed and treated according to the principles which were discussed in the chapter on paranoid reactions. Hypnosis has occasionally been found helpful to change the patient's craving and general attitude. It is of little use in serious withdrawal symptoms. Psychoanalytic treatment, which some consider effective in changing the personality factors which cause the craving, should also be carried out in a closed institution.

Hospitalization should last preferably six months. Afterwards control examinations at least once a year are desirable, combined with urine analysis to determine whether the patient is again under the influence of morphine [the tests are only positive if at least 0.015 gm. (¼ gr.) of morphine has been consumed daily]. Even after years, patients are still susceptible to morphine. It is one of the most serious mistakes to administer morphine to a cured addict. The patients themselves are usually very much afraid of it. When an operation is necessary or a painful illness occurs, the physician in charge of such a case is confronted with a great difficulty. It is usually desirable to consult a psychiatrist who will carry out this aspect of the treatment, trying to alleviate pain with codeine, occasionally pantopon, and psychotherapy. Even with codeine one should be careful and interject one to two codeine-free days after every three to five days of codeine administration. Although very rare, the possibility of codeine addiction exists.

One should never attempt substitution of morphine by opiates or other alkaloids. It leads to addiction and the result is the prognostically very undesirable addiction to more than one drug. One needs to warn against any drugs which are advertised for morphine cures. They usually contain some other alkaloid, if not morphine itself. During the re-educational treatment, nicotine, coffee, and tea should be either eliminated entirely or strictly limited. They often take the place of substitution and prevent the detection of the factors which create craving.

It is difficult to create a desirable hospital setting for drug addicts. In contrast to the treatment of alcoholism, there is a marked danger of the development of an undesirable addiction atmosphere in special sanatoria. Most authors feel therefore that it is best to admit them to psychiatric hospitals where they are not in contact with other addicts. Even then, one must be aware of the constant danger of erotic involvements with nurses and of bribery, even after the withdrawal has been terminated.

Of practical importance among the derivatives of morphine are heroin (diacethyl morphine) and eudokal (dehydro-oxycodeinon). The treatment is essentially the same as in morphine addiction. *Heroin,* which is taken hypodermically and by snuffing, has an especially poor prognosis. It leads to a faster physical and mental decline than morphine. The most experienced physicians urge abrupt withdrawal. There are, however, statements in literature that the withdrawal symptoms may be more marked than in other addictions and occasionally accompanied by several convulsions. It is considered advisable therefore to extend the withdrawal over six or seven days and to offer codeine and phenobarbital during this period, but not morphine and alcohol as has been advised by some authors.

The use of *opium* is rare except in Oriental countries and in the large Oriental colonies in American cities. The present use is smoking. After ten or twenty pipes the smoker experiences great happiness with vivid pleasure and a forgetting of unpleasant experiences with a loss of all disturbing sensations. This lasts several hours and is followed by a few hours' sleep. Awakening, the patient experiences general malaise and therefore looks forward to new relief in opium. The chronic symptoms are emaciation and marked weakness, excessive constipation, apathy, ethical decline, selfishness, and marked sensitiveness to pain. Many opium addicts commit suicide. The withdrawal symptoms are similar to those of morphine withdrawal. In addition to the marked craving for the drug a depressed mood is noticeable. Sudden withdrawal is indicated. Of considerable importance is *paregoric* addiction. It is a combined addiction to opium and alcohol. Sudden withdrawal is advisable.

COCAINE ADDICTION

Cocaine addiction has become of great importance since the first world war. In the beginning the patients administered it hypodermically but in the last thirty years snuffing powdered cocaine has become the exclusive fashion. Most frequently, healthy persons are induced to try it by cocaine addicts. Occasionally it may develop after it has been prescribed by a nose and throat specialist or dentist.

The first effect of cocaine is exciting, leading to marked euphoria, ease of thinking and of associations. All cares disappear and happy imaginations prevail. This is accompanied by a dilatation of the pupils, vasoconstriction, increase of body temperature, and fine tremor. The next stage is paralysis, expressed in vasodilatation, shallow respiration, fainting, decrease of temperature, and finally death. Because of its stimulating and euphoric influence and before the danger of addiction had been recognized, cocaine had been advised for depressions and as a substitute in alcoholism and morphine addiction. The effect of the cocaine starts after ten to thirty minutes and lasts from four to six hours.

Cocaine is frequently used for sexual stimulation. It stimulates women physically and mentally. In men it causes a temporary increase of libido with a decrease in potency. In order to get satisfaction, such patients have to resort to various sexual perversions. Addicts seek stimulation through pornographic literature. In order to produce sexual stimulation in a partner, cocaine addicts occasionally offer the drug in drinks. The result is frequently an acute cocaine intoxication, characterized by a sudden cardiac attack with cold extremities, small and hard pulse, increase of temperature, and dilated pupils.

In acute cocaine intoxication it is best to urge the patient to lie down because of the danger of convulsions. When the patient is excited, dial hypodermically administered or pernocton is indicated (morphine is contraindicated). Cardiac stimulation and artificial respiration are important. Atropine 0.001 gm. ($\frac{1}{60}$ gr.) and adrenalin, which are frequently given, are not effective. Such patients need to be kept in the hospital for two or three days.

The great danger of cocaine addiction is that the addict wishes to take it in company. Every cocaine addict is therefore a source of infection. He usually advises his victim to use repeated small doses in order not to produce too much nausea and anxiety with dyspnea. When taking cocaine together, addicts stimulate each other by indulging in the description of phantastic stories and often suggested hallucinations, sexual perversions, and especially homosexual practices. Addicts frequently assemble in groups for their orgies. Cocaine especially attracts persons in the demi-monde, prostitution, and criminal classes. Most distressing, however, is the high percentage of young people, from sixteen to twenty-two (morphine addiction starts most frequently around thirty to forty-five). Because of their still marked suggestibility, the desire for the new and adventurous, and the sexual push of late adolescence, college students are frequently found in this group.

Because of the disagreeable deprivation symptoms cocaine addicts will try to resort immediately to more cocaine. It is therefore rare that the amount can be held down so that it does not interfere with the patient's obligations in life. On the other hand, this limitation happens occasionally in morphine addiction. One then deals probably with patients who are of a relatively stable make-up and show little constitutional predisposition to morphine. In these cases morphine seems to stimulate intellectually while in cocaine even small amounts decrease the intellectual functioning. Cases of periodic cocaine addiction are very rare. Periodic morphine addiction seems to be more frequent and corresponds to periodic alcoholism. In all these periodic addictions the prognosis is better than in continuous addiction as far as life success is concerned. The possibility for final cure depends on the dynamic factors, the constitutional make-up, the possibility of change of environment and atmosphere, and the duration of the illness and the amount taken.

In predisposed persons acute toxic psychoses occur, frequently as the climax of cocaine abuse, with euphoria, fantastic tales, frightening visual hallucinations with many colors, tactile, and auditory hallucinations. When more cocaine is added these patients frequently have outbursts of rage, directed by jealousy. In chronic cocaine addiction one finds restlessness, intellectual changes (diminished ease of association and grasp; poor memory for recent, and in advanced cases also for remote, events) habit deterioration, and anxiety attacks. When under hunger for the drug, the patients develop a state of fear which may lead to dangerous explosions. Physically they are in generally poor condition and suffer from diarrhea. Subacute deliria of varying duration from a few hours to two weeks are frequent. During these states the patient is either euphoric, has grandiose ideas, and experiences pleasant visual hallucinations; or he is paranoid, hearing threatening voices, being afraid of them and of visual and disagreeable tactile hallucinations, or he is in a dream-like state with vivid cinematographic-like hallucinations, as a passive onlooker. Hallucinosis is characterized by many tactile hallucinations and overactivity with grandiose delusions. A Korsakow's picture, with poor retention and marked confabulation, can occur but may be without polyneuritis and with a good prognosis. The content in all these psychopathologic reactions frequently shows sexual coloring.

The treatment consists of sudden withdrawal in a psychiatric hospital, personality analysis, and re-education. There are no physiologic withdrawal symptoms. The increase of the daily amount of cocaine is due to craving and only slightly to tolerance. No physician therefore should ever give cocaine to an addict who comes for help. He should, however, urge immediate hospitalization, especially as the drug-hungry cocaine addict is fearful and often dangerous in outbursts of panic. Various personality reactions occur in withdrawal but they are psychogenic and not real withdrawal symptoms.

In advanced cases and after long duration of the addiction, these personality reactions are marked and especially dangerous because of the patient's ethical decline. Treatment at home or in a general hospital is therefore contraindicated. The patients need much hydrotherapy for relaxation and for the prevention of excitement, and barbiturates should be given. Sleep and weight usually improve after a few weeks. Because of the type of personality involved as well as the long persistence and easy recurrence of the craving, a long hospitalization (one year) is necessary. Even so, the prognosis is considered poor, definitely worse than in morphine addiction. In a relatively high percentage permanent hospitalization must be considered.

In cocaine psychoses hospitalization is necessary for protection of patient and environment. In a panic outburst such patients may commit suicide. Hallucinations increase fear greatly. Because of their frequent jealousy or definite paranoid delusions, the patients are dangerous to others. On the ward they are difficult to handle and need to be watched carefully. Cocaine gives them a feeling of great physical strength. They are therefore ready for fights or violent outbursts. All these patients need to be treated as excitements, with careful precautions. It is, however, important that nurses and attendants do not develop an attitude of fear. Hydrotherapeutic procedures during the whole day make the management much easier.

Atropine attracts persons to chronic use because it produces a definite euphoria and ease of activity. Addiction occurs. It is therefore important that physicians warn against its use by women who wish to make their eyes attractive at social events. *Scopolamine* addiction has been described in metencephalitic Parkinsonism but not in healthy persons.

Hashish (Marihuana) addiction (eating, smoking, and snuffing) is practically unknown in Europe, but has become more frequent in America. In Mexico and Central America and to some extent in Texas, *mescal* addiction needs attention. The drug is usually offered as a drink, e.g., mescalesos or peyotol. Marihuana, smoked in the form of cigarettes, has an emotionally stimulating effect. It does not produce essential addiction and its dangers have been greatly exaggerated. Its ready availability makes it especially undesirable and often a serious problem among adolescents. In all these drugs immediate withdrawal with total abstinence and a constructive personality analysis and re-education are essential.

Chloral hydrate can lead to addiction in psychopathic individuals, especially in those with depressive mood, anxiety features, and compulsions.

Pervitin, the drug which is closely related to benzedrine, has been found to be habit-forming. This observation should warn one against prescribing benzedrine too readily, especially for prolonged use. The psychiatric usefulness of benzedrine is still disputed.

Barbiturates and bromides are often taken habitually and show damage accordingly but do not seem to result in actual addiction. It is important that one keep a clearly defined concept of addiction and not use this term for any dependence on an habitual use of drugs.

Nicotine, although not belonging to the addiction group, is nevertheless discussed here because it frequently takes a substitutive place in addiction. Nicotine (smoking) may have a marked sexual depressant effect although this feature is not generally known. It acts as a sedative in restlessness and uneasiness and in many persons is stimulating, producing a slightly increased ease in thinking. There is a self-conscious social smoker as well as a social drinker. Many persons are fully aware of their specific reaction. In others, especially in the sexually maladjusted group, smoking helps to conceal the disturbing factors from the patient. It is therefore desirable to demand complete abstinence for a period of two weeks during any thorough personality analysis, to determine the role of smoking, the patient's dependence on it, and his individual abstinence reaction.

Psychopathologic symptoms which occur with chronic nicotine may be the expression of an unrecognized psychoneurosis or the person's reaction to the well-known physical complaints of headache, dizziness, anxiety, and neurologic symptoms. Delirious reactions and excitements which have been described are most likely psychogenic and not toxic reactions. Some claim that difficulty in going to sleep and anxiety dreams may occur. These symptoms are often noticed in the beginning of abstinence in very heavy smokers, together with restlessness, irritability, decreased appetite, and constipation. These personality reactions are not of the withdrawal type but the expression of dependence on the smoking for various reasons which were mentioned, and the inability to use self-control. Smoking is a psychiatric problem in itself if a patient is unable to keep himself within the limits which are necessary to him for his physical welfare or if he constantly struggles against this desire and is unable to adjust to it. Total abstinence will be easier than mere reduction.

A personality analysis will reveal the factors which cause the maladjustment and offer possibilities of control.

Psychopathic personalities form a high percentage of the drug addicts. Therefore, the prognosis is frequently poor as far as freedom from drugs for life is concerned. We may have to be satisfied with achieving freedom for a period of years and help to regain this with repeated withdrawals and attempts at readjustment. On the other hand, one should not be too pessimistic. In the more stable groups, permanent results may be obtained. Statistics are deceiving because their material is drawn from individuals who have been committed for criminal acts or minor offenses. In private practice, one deals with a less unstable group. Separation of cases needs to be considered in hospital treatment and special hospitals for drug addicts should offer possibilities for wholesome group life and individual treatment.

BIBLIOGRAPHY

1. EMERSON, E. H.: *Alcohol and Man*. The Effects of Alcohol on Man in Health and Disease. The Macmillan Company, New York, 1932.
2. JELLINEK, E. M.: *Alcohol Addiction and Chronic Alcoholism*. Yale University Press, New Haven, 1942.
3. KALINOWSKY, L. B.: Convulsions in Nonepileptic Patients on Withdrawal of Barbiturates, Alcohol and Other Drugs. *Archives of Neurology and Psychiatry*, 48, 1942.
4. DIETHELM, O.: The Treatment of Chronic Alcoholism. *The Southern Medical Journal*, 27, 1934.
5. LAMBERT, A. Et Al.: Report of the Mayor's Committee on Drug Addiction (New York City). *American Journal of Psychiatry*, 10, 1930. (This report offers a critical and constructive review of various therapeutic proposals.)
6. MAIER, H. W.: *Der Kokainismus*. G. Thieme, Leipzig, 1926.
7. GASKILL, H. S.: Marihuana, An Intoxicant. *American Journal of Psychiatry*, 102, 1945.
8. BINDER, H.: Kriminalität infolge Pervitinmissbrauchs. *Schweizer Archiv. für Neurologie und Psychiatrie*, 55, 1945.

Chapter XIX

PROBLEMS IN GENERAL PRACTICE

THE PHYSICIAN, the surgeon, and the general practitioner must learn to recognize and treat in every patient emotional factors which influence physiologic functions. Emotional reactions can be understood and influenced only if one can evaluate their significance in the setting of the whole personality. As has been stressed in Chapter I, such an understanding can be obtained if one tries to recognize the influences which have shaped this personality during life. In order to do this, one must review with the patient the persons who have played an important role in his life, the changing social, economic, and housing conditions, the role of work in school and in adult life, his physical development, and his state of health.

Such a review is obtained in every good medical history, but the physician is frequently unable to recognize the significance of the facts which he has obtained. The best way to organize one's material is in the form of a chart of three columns, in which each fact is noted with regard to the time of its occurrence. The column on the left contains the pertinent facts of physical development and somatic illnesses; the column on the right, changes in living conditions, school and work, illnesses, and deaths in the family. The middle column contains personality reactions which have occurred at various times, whether they appear to be normal or pathologic. Looking at these three columns, the physician will observe correlations in time which may appear significant and demand further clarification. This principle of organization of the medical history, which A. Meyer called the "life chart," is the basis of psychotherapy in general medicine. Furthermore, such a chart is essential for all medical treatment if one wishes to treat the patient and not merely a separate physical disorder.

It would be fallacious to believe that the general practitioner can limit his knowledge to an understanding of well-functioning personality, omitting the inclusion of psychopathology. In his ambulatory and hospital practice he will meet all types and degrees of psychopathologic disorders. It is his obligation to recognize and treat them to the best of his ability. In difficult problems he may ask for the advice of a psychiatric consultant. Other types of psycho-pathologic disorders may be treated jointly by him and the psychi-atrist, while still other reactions may be referred to the psychiatrist for ambulatory or hospital treatment.

For ten years, this mode of treatment has been carried out suc-cessfully in the various departments of The New York Hospital. It has resulted in an increased ability of physicians and surgeons to understand and treat their patients as individual personalities, and to recognize and treat various psychopathologic disorders. A review of the case material in the general hospital has revealed a surprisingly high number of marked and involved psychopathologic disorders, e.g., depressive, schizophrenic, and paranoid reactions. Many of these patients came to the hospital because of physical illnesses, while others suffered from somatic symptoms and complaints produced by emotional strain. This fact is not surprising because the same problems are found by physicians working in industry and in public health.

These considerations make it imperative for a physician to learn the methods of study and treatment of the functions of the per-sonality and of psychopathologic disorders. It is not possible to practice medicine without a full understanding of both the well and the sick person.

A broader concept of pathology than has heretofore existed must become the basis of understanding and treatment of the patient. Whether pathology deals with somatic or psychopathologic dis-orders the essential feature is that findings which are unusual in degree, or occurring within the wrong age period, are considered pathologic. In addition, signs of unusual and disturbing behavior in interpersonal relations must also be considered pathologic. The recognition of the factors which play a role in psychopathologic conditions permits the physician to modify them. The role of emo-tions should always be evaluated. Their significance depends on the type of emotion, its strength and duration, and its psychopathologic and general psychobiologic settings. In dealing with the influence of emotions on physiologic functions, the physician is usually con-fronted with a direct influence of recognizable or suppressed emotions. These so-called psychosomatic conditions can be analyzed more directly than the repressed emotions of psychoneurotic reactions which work through dissociation, displacement, and substitution. Every well-trained physician should be able to use well-planned analytic psychotherapy for many psychosomatic disorders. The analysis of the psychoneuroses usually demands the skill of a psychiatrist.

The therapeutic knowledge of a physician should enable him "to study, understand and treat depressive reactions in his patients, whether these reactions belong to the group of psychiatric disorders called depressions or are a mild depressive mood reactive to personal problems or to physical illness with its many possible implications. Among these may be included the meaning of the illness, its economic complications, and its interference with carrying one's responsibility. The period of convalescence as well as changes caused by aging give rise to disturbing emotional reactions. Personal difficulties of adaptation may be expressed in queer or suspicious behavior, in paranoic delusions, in antagonism to or overdependence on the physician, in jealousy reactions, or in schizophrenic withdrawal. The sexual life of most patients presents either some aspects which are unclear to them or definite difficulties which might be discussed to the patient's advantage. There is no patient who will not benefit greatly by a review of his mode of living and an investigation of whether, according to his individual needs, he balances work and recreation and pays adequate attention to his physical needs, especially food intake, activity, rest, sleep, and sexual satisfaction."*

This general discussion demonstrates the necessity of basing the treatment of problems in medical practice on an understanding of the personality as outlined in Chapter I, and of utilizing the broad principles of psychotherapy which have been presented in previous chapters. It would be futile and wrong to present prescriptions for various specific conditions, basing these prescriptions on current psychopathologic hypotheses. Our knowledge of the influence of emotions on physical functions, in health and illness, is limited as has been mentioned above. It is, however, recognized that the emo-

* Diethelm, O.: *Psychiatry and the War,* ed. by Frank J. Sladen. Charles C Thomas • Publisher, Springfield, Illinois.

tions of anxiety, tension, and resentment are especially important. In some conditions one or the other of these emotions is considered especially important but one should not be biased, seeking only the expected emotion. In cardiac conditions, e.g., one frequently finds resentment to be of especial significance. On the other hand, anxiety and tension may be of equal or at least aggravating importance. The following case may serve as illustration:

Case 43:

A 45 year old successful business executive who had suffered from extrasystoles for a few weeks two year ago while under considerable business strain developed a coronary attack on January 18, 1941. A second attack occurred a week later when he became aware of a disagreement between his physicians, and he reacted with anxiety to insecurity and with resentment to their letting him know of their doubts. He left the hospital on February 24th, feeling discouraged and worried about his future, fearing that his promising career was terminated, that he would have to accept marked financial curtailment, and become a semi-invalid. In this setting the patient had a mild attack of palpitation on February 27th.

When seen in consultation on March 2nd, the patient reviewed his illness and expressed anxiety about his future, and intense resentment to what he considered medical mismanagement. He was discouraged but there were no signs of an essential depression. I agreed with the internist that the emotional factors were important in the treatment. The psychiatric treatment would have to be cautious, and the emotional strain released during the interviews would have to be evaluated carefully from the point of view of his cardiac condition. It was agreed that the patient should continue in a convalescent state with gradually increasing activity.

On March 4th, treatment was started. The interviews were usually of an hour's duration, occurring every second day. In the first session, we reviewed the possibility of a successful life even if his career were terminated. In this, and the next few sessions, his personality development and his life were reviewed. He had always been very proud of his physique and strength, and despised weaklings. He believed in his will power and energy. In the last two years he had worked under great tension and had resented greatly public criticism of his work. A proud man who believed in himself, he was sensitive to the opinions of others about him. Any defeat was hard for him to bear, resulting in destructive self-analysis with unhappiness and resentment to those who had obstructed him. Until two years ago his sexual life had been satisfactory, but since then he had been uneasy about decreasing desires which might indicate early aging. A year ago his two children's adolescent problems had worried him, especially because of the anxiety of his overconscientious and socially ambitious wife. During these talks he became aware that he had drifted away from her and that he should renew the common interests which they had enjoyed in younger years. In adolescence, he had resolved that he would not become a financial burden like his father, who had quit his practice as a physician at an age of 50 because of gastrointestinal complaints. Both parents were still living and dependent on him financially. The mother was domineering but greatly admired by the patient and his sister, who was five years his senior. The father was considered gentle but inadequate. The patient revealed considerable conscious and repressed resentment to his father's inadequacy and a fear that he might become a similar failure. His wife was the opposite of his mother, and was protected by him. He had a great need to dominate her and had experienced great anxiety when his illness threatened to reverse their roles. (The mother-wife relationship became clear to him in the fifth session.) Through athletics he had developed social ease in a college where his family's financial limitations were considered a handicap. His brilliant intelligence and his ceaseless energy led to uninterrupted progress in a successful career, but his ultimate ambition had not been reached because of the war in Europe. In the last four years he felt unjustly treated by his superior whom he had idolized for years and who had helped him greatly but with a selfish interest. There was a definite lack of recognition which the patient had resented increasingly.

In the third session, March 8th, the patient's exaggerated loyalty to his superior was recognized. Through analysis he recognized the roots for this loyalty in the childhood and adolescent relationship to his mother and the transference of this loyalty to his wife, who had been his childhood sweetheart and in whom he had never been willing to recognize deficiencies. The next three sessions permitted him to obtain an objective picture of his mother's and wife's personalities. However, he did not gain a satisfactory understanding of the personality of his superior to whom he felt an increasing resentment.

On March 11th, when having an examination by the physician whose poor psychologic handling he had deeply resented, the patient reacted with mild apprehension. He recognized that fear of his physician's power and resentment of having to be dependent on him were due partly to his illness. In addition, the physician represented the type of successful man whom he disliked because social manners had won him his success, and because he was fat and unathletic.

After March 15th the discussions occurred once a week for a month, dealing primarily with a dynamic understanding of his role as father to his children, his ability to grow closer to his family, the planning and developing of possible physical and social recreation, and of cultivating an earlier interest in music. He made rapid progress during his physical convalescence and on May 1st he returned to work. Resentment to his superior had become largely resolved, but was still readily stimulated by criticism from him. He noticed that fatigue was the expression of emotional tension and learned to analyze the factors which contributed to it. Treatment was terminated on May 20th. The patient was seen for two interviews in September which were essentially a review of his present life and plans for the future in the light of his understanding of his past life. He has been in good physical health for five years, continuously active, and successful, and understanding himself much better than before his coronary attacks.

This patient demonstrates the influence of emotions, the significance of which could be understood only from a study of the individual life experiences. Interpersonal relationships gave rise to new emotional reactions and the reactivation of old ones. The patient cannot be treated without a full understanding of the family setting. The influence of other members of the family on the patient's illness must be studied as well as the influence of his illness on them. A constructive review of the illness with selected members of the family may prove to be essential psychotherapy for the patient.

One must investigate the significance of the illness to the patient with its personal, sociological, and economic implications. They may be real or dreaded exaggerations. Pain may cause intense apprehension, anger, or defeatism. The influence of an illness can be far-reaching and highly disturbing in many ways. During an illness the physician should be aware of the dynamic factors and realize that their importance may change with the progress of an illness. This submerging of some factors and emergence of new ones is readily seen in chronic illnesses but often less well recognized in those of short duration. This statement does not refer only to financial worries and changes in one's working potentialities but also to the personal dynamic factors of apprehension, hurt pride, and resentment of various kinds. An illness forces a patient to some kind of frustrating inactivity, to dependence on others, to philosophical acceptance and patience. It depends on the individual personality whether he can achieve these emotional adjustments, and how well, or whether he will react with open or suppressed emotions.

The type and duration of convalescence deserves much attention and special thought should be given to the factors which will be brought into activity with return to one's home or to part-time work.

The significance of insurance is usually impressed on the physician in accidents and in health problems where monetary factors seem to be retard the patient's urge to return to a completely self-reliant life. It is not the merely selfish motive of greed but more frequently insecurity. In such cases a discussion of the need for compensation and reassurance by the physician permits the patient to accept himself as being well. Resentment to inadequate compensation, to the unfairness involved in an accident, or to oneself for having been careless must be considered a problem which deserves the physician's full attention. It may save much time for a busy physician if he puts a few hours aside to study with the patient his personality reactions.

Acute and chronic illnesses must be considered differently with regard to their emotional implications on patient and family. To be sick in one's home in contrast to being in a hospital brings about quite different situations. Prolonged suffering may not only discourage a patient or his family but create situations which cause repetitious or persistent tension and resentment, often accompanied by guilt feelings, unhappiness, and defeatism.

The reactions to aging vary greatly and should be known to a physician so that he can help the patient to develop a constructive philosophy instead of a defeatist one. "Symptoms have different meanings, dependent on the individual's life and his cultural setting. Graying of the hair or increasing baldness may be a disturbing factor. The loss of teeth, and especially the need to use a dental plate, may be accepted only with great difficulty. Women especially are aware of skin changes. Decrease in muscular strength and declining ability for physical exertion may result in disappointment and fretting. Poor posture, which results from inability to make the increased muscular effort necessary to keep erect, may be an obvious sign of aging.

"The psychopathological reactions of aging are linked closely to the personality development. Personality reactions are designated pathological (that is, psychopathological) if they are unusual in degree or if they occur outside of the age period in which they normally occur. To illustrate: Loneliness is pathological if it prevents a person from leading a healthy life and obtaining satisfaction from his activities. A person also presents a pathological picture if at the age of 50 his outstanding traits and attitudes toward life correspond to those of a man of 65.

"The most frequent psychopathological reaction of aging is anxiety, which is due to various types of insecurity. Insecurity may shake a person's confidence in himself, in his body, in people, and in the attitudes of society. Anxiety may be expressed in general insecurity, in somatic symptoms and signs, and in an apprehensive attitude toward the future. Frequent depressive reactions are expressed in persistent or strong feelings of being lonely, discouraged, worried, defeated, depressed, or humiliated. Mild paranoid reactions are seen in strong envy and resentment, suspiciousness toward competitors, intense aversion to specific situations or persons, and jealousy. In some persons these convictions may assume the strength of delusions. The formation of incapacitating rut-like behavior may be recognized early in the habits of an individual. This behavior becomes a most serious problem when it reaches the degree of withdrawal from society and general activities, of apathy, or depressive moods. An increasing rigidity of personal standards may readily give rise to guilt feelings and dwelling on mistakes of the past, even those of youth and childhood. The loss of plasticity which characterizes every aging person may reach a pathological degree of rigidity with inability to adjust to people and life situations and with set modes of thinking, such as bias and prejudice."*

The treatment of these reactions to aging includes planning of an active life which offers as much satisfaction to the individual with his interests and ambitions as possible. It is a psychotherapeutic task which is interesting and frequently much more satisfactory than the average physician expects. The discussion of aging in Chapter I and in Chapter XIII may offer specific help.

In internal medicine the relationship of specific physical illnesses to personality reactions has attracted much attention. It seems to me important that one look for any possible factors which may explain emotions which affect health undesirably. A broad personality understanding as a basis for psychotherapy is especially important in many gastrointestinal and cardiovascular illnesses, allergic conditions, migraine, diabetes, anemia and nutritional disorders. In

---

* Diethelm, O.: *The Aging Person.* Reprinted from the *North Carolina Medical Journal,* 5, 1944.

many endocrine disorders the personality setting is characterized by immaturity and emotional instability.

It is important that patients recognize their physical constitutional tendencies and their limitations. After increased emotional strain, increased recreation is necessary. Such patients should know their resources and on what resources they can depend. Weekends should be carefully planned according to opportunities and personal inclination. Change of position, especially promotion, deserves careful review. A study of past successes may demonstrate what the patient is actually fitted for and what his potentialities are. Training along specific physical lines may be indicated. Some patients are benefited by climatic changes and by hydrotherapy and physiotherapy as these are carried out in certain health resorts. Even then a re-education of the whole person is necessary if more than temporary results are to be obtained.

The meaning of menarche and menopause is important. Medical and pseudomedical folklore has made menopause a dreaded event. It is of no greater psychologic importance than the beginning of menstruation and should not be accompanied by psychopathologic phenomena. Sexual decline is not associated with menopause.

A constructive psychologic attitude should be developed toward childbirth by physicians. This event is still dreaded to an extent which causes unnecessary anxiety and insecurity. The relaxation from tension on the second and third day after delivery is well known to obstetricians but is not sufficiently explained to the patient. This phase, and the time when a patient returns home, assumes responsibility for the infant, and is brought in close contact with members of her family are the periods when mild or marked postpartum psychopathologic reactions develop. Their occurrence proves the urgent need for obstetricians and pediatricians to use psychotherapy.

The physician must give advice in the physical and psychobiologic upbringing of the child. It is his obligation to create security in the parents and help them in all the many puzzling situations which will occur. Recognizing the dangers of strict discipline in early habit training and of suppression of the child's healthy spontaneity, his rules will serve the parents as a guide. His attention will be directed to the role the child plays in the family, with its rivalries, rejections, aggressions, and withdrawals. Prolonged enuresis or thumbsucking can be studied and helped by an analysis of the family situation and the particular child's reaction to it. Rejection by one or both parents may be seen in frank neglect, or resentment, or hidden in anxieties. The latter picture is seen in neurotic parents who may be in need of intensive psychotherapy. A physician should be prepared to recognize the point at which behavior in a child becomes pathologic, as indicated by the intensity or duration of the symptoms or their occurrence outside the average age limit. Early recognition should urge him to look for explanations, and through them, find means of adjustment. In children, modification of the psychotherapeutic approach to fit the child's personality with stress on healthy education, careful attention to environmental factors, and removal from undesirable settings are important.

The modern pediatrician is willing to learn the psychology and psychopathology of childhood and with it the means of treatment. He should be able to evaluate psychopathologic reactions so that he knows when he can treat the child and when he should refer the child to a psychiatric expert. In pediatric in- and out-patient services marked changes have been brought about by making consideration of the child's personality a routine procedure. The interpersonal relations in an in-patient service deserve much critical observation. Nurses must understand the nurse-patient relationship in every branch of medicine, but especially in pediatrics. Psychologists and social workers are indispensable in the study and treatment of children. Their importance, however, should also be recognized in the other medical and surgical divisions. The review of the problems of childhood and adolescence in Chapter I may serve as a basis of treatment.

In surgery, attention should be paid to psychologic pre- and postoperative care. There is little doubt that most postoperative excitements could be prevented if a careful physiologic and personality investigation preceded the operation. The anticipation of, and reaction to, anaesthesia and the individual patient's sensitivity to the drugs which are given to alleviate pain deserve study. Postoperative convalescence, especially mild depressive reactions, demand the surgeon's psychologic help. In recent years the psychologic importance of scars and of crippling conditions has been discussed constructively.

The role of the personality should be an obvious concern to the physician in industry and public health. The significance of personality factors in accidents is well known. Their importance in causing ill health and social maladjustment is increasingly appreciated. The need of psychobiologically oriented medicine for treatment and for maintenance of health is becoming generally accepted.

BIBLIOGRAPHY

1. RIPLEY, H. S.: Depressive Reactions in a General Hospital: A Study of 150 Cases. *Journal of Nervous and Mental Disease*, 105, 1947.
2. MITTELMANN, B.; WEIDER, A.; BRODMAN, K.; WECHSLER, D., and WOLFF, H. G.: Personality and Psychosomatic Disturbances in Patients on Medical and Surgical Wards. *Psychosomatic Medicine*, 7, 1945.
3. HUSCHKA, M.: A Psychiatric Consultation Service in a Pediatric Outpatient Department. *Journal of Pediatrics*, 24, 1944.
4. LINDEMANN, E.: Observations on Psychiatric Sequelae to Surgical Operations in Women. *American Journal of Psychiatry*, 98, 1941.
5. MUNCIE, W.: Postoperative States of Excitement. *Archives of Neurology and Psychiatry*, 43, 1934.
6. RUESCH, J.: Chronic Disease and Psychological Invalidism; a Psychosomatic Study. *American Society for Research in Psychosomatic Problems*, New York, 1946.
7. Convalescent Care. *The New York Academy of Medicine*, New York, 1940.
8. KAPLAN, O. J.: *Mental Disorders in Later Life*. Stanford University Press, 1945.

Chapter XX

TEACHING OF PSYCHIATRIC TREATMENT

SCIENTIFIC treatment must be based on a genetic-dynamic psycho-pathology which considers the somatic and environmental factors. The physician must therefore have a sound psychopathologic knowledge, and be well acquainted with the methods of psychopathologic study. In treatment he may use the aid of nurses and social workers. He must understand their procedures and their varying roles in his treatment of a patient over a prolonged period of time.

The teaching of psychiatric treatment must include a discussion of the initial interview and of the psychopathologic meaning of a psychiatric examination. The outline of examination offered must be inclusive if it is to elicit essential psychopathologic findings in any condition. It is imperative that one examine for all possible psychopathologic reactions, and avoid short-cuts. Furthermore, the initial examination can offer only a basis for the beginning of treatment. As one progresses, a check on various findings and a search for new findings are indicated. A detailed history of the development of the patient's complaints and of his present illness, of his previous health, of his personal life, including the family setting with its many personalities in his early life, is necessary to establish the basis for a psychopathologic study. Information obtained from members of the family about early life experiences and formative influences, or from others about important events in the patient's life may give dynamic leads to the physician. A review of the patient's outstanding personality features, although some of them may be proved superficial after treatment has progressed, gives the physician a psychodynamic formulation. This formulation, although it may be only preliminary, permits him to offer the advice needed or to attack the therapeutic problem in a planned, long-term way.

The teaching of psychiatric interviews has preoccupied teachers more and more with the progress of psychodynamic psychopathology. There is an obvious distinction between interviews which are primarily planned for orientation and those which are therapeutic.

An orientative interview should lay the basis for a well-conceived psychiatric examination and for the immediate therapeutic plan. It must be stressed that an orientative interview is also of therapeutic importance, bringing about an involved psychodynamic situation. It is therefore wise to be cautious in one's procedure. On the other hand, this interview will not serve its purpose if the necessary information is not obtained. Sound knowledge of dynamic psychopathology and the guidance of the teacher will help the beginner to determine what comprises "necessary information" in a given situation. The well-trained clinician is able to obtain an astonishing amount of information in his first interview, not only without disturbing the patient, but with considerable benefit to him.

The technique of therapeutic interviews in their narrower sense may vary greatly but should always be plastic, adjustable to any therapeutic demands and psychopathologic complications which may arise. Much latitude can be recommended to the therapeutically advanced graduate student whereas restrictions and methodical procedures should guide the beginner. Physicians who have not received special training in psychiatry should guard against a tendency to obtain too much dynamic material. Some teachers err by offering the student a rigid outline for interviews which does not permit the necessary freedom of action. Interviews should not be conducted on a question-answer basis. The physician should submit questions to the patient to elicit his responses in as complete a form as possible. The suitability of this therapeutic tool depends on the form of the question and on the way it is put to the patient. The recording of interviews by means of a concealed dictaphone, with subsequent review by the teacher, has advantages as well as disadvantages. Whenever one wishes to use this method, one should keep in mind its influence on the patient if he should become aware of the automatic recording. The knowledge that such recordings are carried out in a hospital may have an undesirable effect on some of the other patients. In the teaching in the Payne Whitney Clinic careful preparation and supervision of the student is preferred. Undesirable results can be prevented when the teachers know the patients well and participate as consultants in the treatment. The results in graduate and undergraduate teaching have been good for students and beneficial to patients.

The psychiatric examination must be of a type which is suitable to bring out the most essential psychopathologic findings in any kind of personality disorder, and which is adjustable to any situation with which a physician may be confronted. There is no fundamental difference in methods of examination and treatment in ambulatory and hospital practice. These same methods are used in obvious psychopathologic disorders, as well as in personality factors in physically ill patients, or in problems of how to obtain a satisfactory life. It is most important that a physician adjust his methods on a discriminatory basis without omitting any of the essential features.

A review of the commonly used psychiatric examination illustrates these points. Observation of the patient's appearance and behavior during one's whole contact with him, reveals underlying psychodynamic and psychopathologic factors in psychologic and physiologic reactions. His attitude to the physician and to the examination expresses his reaction to his symptoms and to his problems, and offers an indication of anticipated difficulties in the patient-physician relationship. His way of expressing himself, spontaneously or in response to questions, may indicate thinking disorders of varying types and intensity, and tendencies to substitutions and dissociations. The patient's subjective description of his emotions may bring out his own attitude to them, his degree of awareness of them, and the type of these emotions and their meaning. Emotions are the most valuable therapeutic indicators. The physician must try to understand and evaluate them by including in addition to the patient's subjective data, objective facts as observed in physiologic behavioristic and psychopathologic signs (attention, concentration, and thinking disorders), and significant psychodynamic factors.

A discussion of the patient's preoccupations reveals dynamic factors, either directly or in the form of projections, as well as his attitude to them of which the patient may be aware or which may be fully repressed. In evaluating the findings, the physician should consider whether or not they are linked to marked emotional reactions. If this relationship exists, one must determine whether the emotions are largely dependent on the preoccupations, or, on the contrary, causing them. Investigating the functions of orientations to time and place, to the present situation including persons present, and to the patient's own personality permits the physician to recognize clearness or disorders of consciousness and grasp. In these disorders, he will look for neurophysiologic factors which may be on a toxic or structural basis, or less frequently related to psychodynamic factors or intense emotions. Disorders in the recall of remote and recent past experiences and of immediate impressions are indicative of cortical disturbances. They may be of permanent nature or transient. The latter occur in various types of delirious disorders and in affective and schizophrenic thinking difficulties. All these symptoms may also be caused by intense emotional influences.

Knowledge of the span of attention, evaluated by the immediate repetition of digits, is important in order to know what to expect from a patient. The simple concentration test of serial subtraction of 7 from 100 orients the physician with regard to the patient's ability to cooperate in tasks and in psychotherapeutic discussion. Attention and concentration, and, to a less extent, general grasp and recall, may be affected for a brief or prolonged period by intense emotions. A general intellectual evaluation is necessary to reveal disorders of intellectual function. It is frequently overlooked that strong emotions, special preoccupations, and poorly defined schizophrenic illnesses may interfere with intellectual functions. In addition, disorders of attention or fatigue may aggravate the difficulties.

Judgment may be affected by any of these above disorders or by catathymic factors. Under "insight" the physician wishes to determine the patient's awareness of being ill, of the character of his illness, and of the special dynamic factors involved. The type of insight which the patient exhibits, offers the basis for the physician's therapeutic formulation. Most patients who lack insight feel sick, whether or not they are able to admit it. They are therefore willing to accept medical help if it is offered in some acceptable form.

This brief discussion demonstrates the need for a well-planned psychiatric examination before starting treatment. Anxiety and other emotions may be present or become activated during any personality disorder and its treatment. Their influences on the functions of the personality must be known to the physician who wishes to offer the best treatment indicated.

It should be stressed in the teaching of psychotherapy that the bringing forth of repressed material or confessions is not, as such, a sign of far-reaching or helpful analysis. The term "deep" therapy should be recognized as the individual teacher's expression of his psychologic concept and not be mistaken for an evaluation of psycho-therapeutic soundness. A teacher in psychotherapy as well as in psychiatric treatment in general should be well acquainted with current psychologic theories and their historical significance. It is a deplorable shortcoming of many teachers in psychiatry that they are unwilling to give up theories which at one time seemed valid and later proved to be futile. With the progress of medicine and the broader understanding of human beings, new facts became es-tablished, and new interrelationships which force the physician to new evaluations and theories became obvious.

No teacher should cling to the past and try to impress his stu-dents with dogmatic theories and the defense of a theoretical sys-tem. Progress in treatment during the last fifty years has been steady. Factual knowledge has increased and therapeutic techniques im-proved. Mistakes have been recognized and theories of the past have been supported by new facts or were discarded. There is in-creasing awareness on the part of teachers of the need to distinguish between facts and theories, to be acquainted with all outstanding current theories and therapeutic methods, and to present them in an objective form. A good teacher should offer a sound basis to his students and make it possible for them to use a critical curiosity which will permit them to develop steadily with the progress of medicine.

The undergraduate education which every physician should receive must include training in the methods of psychopathologic examination, of psychiatric treatment in general, and of psycho-therapy. In teaching general treatment, physical and environmental factors must be brought in constant relationship to the psychody-namic factors. The understanding of the well-functioning person-ality must be the basis for the student's approach to the sick person. Psychotherapy must be conceived in its broadest sense. Knowledge of dynamic factors should be broad enough to offer the physician not only possibilities for a sound guidance but also an awareness of his limitations. The student must be urged to investigate the patient's family, living and working conditions, and recreational facilities. The study of the social factors involved confronts him with the therapeutic task of the social worker and of social agencies. The intricate dynamics of the patient-physician relationship must be reviewed during all the years of clinical experience in any department of the hospital. The still unsatisfactory state of therapeutic indications and contraindications in psychiatry imposes on the teacher a most serious obligation to develop in his student a searching, critical attitude.

The undergraduate education of nurses must stress the importance of a broad dynamic psychopathology, the ability to recognize and describe the patient's behavior and how to deal with him correctly. The dynamic aspects of the nurse-patient relationship, of the physician's role in treatment, and of her relationship to the physician deserve much attention. It is obvious that in medical and nursing education, students can learn sound and broad psychiatric treatment only if their teachers stress the principles involved in patients in the in- and out-patient departments of psychiatric as well as general hospitals.

Graduate training in psychiatry should be planned for the whole period of residency in a way which insures the therapeutic responsibilities of the physician in accordance with his increase in knowledge and proficiency. Patients should be selected carefully in accordance with this program. The teacher must share fully in the treatment and carry the ultimate responsibility. His guidance should be firm but not interfering in the patient-physician relationship. He should play the role of a consultant and be accepted as such by the patient. A transference relationship will develop between patient and consultant, but every effort should be made by the consultant to prevent this relationship from developing into a type which will interfere with the transference relationship to the treating physician. A consultant must be willing to give up his personal interest in patients whom he may have seen or treated previously. It is important that he examine the patients only in the presence of the treating physician in order to prevent misunderstandings and therapeutic interference. In his personal contact with the patient, the consultant should check on the psychopathologic findings through observation and discussion. He may demonstrate how the psychotherapeutic technique of the interview might be modified in this individual or suggestion or reassurance might be offered. The psychodynamic relationship of consultant to patient permits strengthening of previously offered therapeutic formulations by the treating physician. Much time must be devoted to constant review of the physician's reaction to his patient. Such a review must be carried out on a personal basis which is best established if the physician undergoes a study of his own personality by the consultant. It is a debatable point whether or not the administrative position of the consultant may be a hinderance to such a study. The young psychiatrist must learn to become increasingly aware of the patient's relationship to him and of his reaction to the patient. The recognition of one's own counter-transference is a long and arduous task which starts in training and will improve during all one's years in psychotherapeutic activity.

The most careful teaching of psychiatric treatment is offered in a well-planned in-patient department which comprises all types of personality disorders, from adolescence to old age and includes somatic disorders. Training must include specific methods in psychotherapy (e.g., hypnosis) and in somatic procedures (insulin and convulsive therapy, intravenous administration of barbiturates for psychotherapeutic use). Treatment in the out-patient service is important because it imposes a greater amount of responsibility on the young physician than a well-organized in-patient department. In addition, he has to learn to use a less intensive treatment and may learn the value of brief psychotherapeutic interviews and group psychotherapy. In many problems, he must rely on the help of the social worker and make use of community resources through means of social agencies. For all these reasons, it is desirable that treatment in the psychiatric out-patient department and in the in- and out-patient departments of the general hospital be reserved for the time allocated to the second and especially the third year of training.

Didactic courses may be an important adjunct in the teaching of treatment. However, treatment of patients, under a careful supervision which will guide the physician and protect the patient, must be carried out by the young psychiatrist if he wishes to acquire mastery. A well-trained psychiatrist should have the opportuinty to study and practice all the various types of treatment which have been discussed in the preceding chapters.

Training in psychoanalytic treatment has received careful attention. The principles of a thorough analysis of the physician and of supervised treatment are generally accepted.

The development of graduate training of nurses has not been parallel to that of physicians. The same principles which have proved their worth in the resident training of physicians might well be applied. It is important that nurses be familiar with the treatment of all types and degrees of psychopathologic disorders. It is undesirable to let the same nurse take care of a patient over a long period of time. One should also avoid keeping a nurse (or a physician) for years in charge of disturbed or essentially chronic patients. This policy will lead to a highly undesirable attitude which will affect the treatment detrimentally.

Every hospital should aim to be a teaching center. The philosophy of teaching forces the practice of the most critical and progressive treatment. The teaching attitude will make itself felt in the behavior of every hospital employee and will lead to a progressive administration of hospitals.

BIBLIOGRAPHY

1. DIETHELM, O., and JONES, M. R.: The Influence of Anxiety on Attention, Learning, Retention, and Thinking. *Archives of Neurology and Psychiatry,* 58, 1947.
2. RENNIE, T. A. C.: Psychotherapy for the General Practitioner: A Program for Training. *American Journal of Psychiatry,* 103, 1947.
3. WHITEHORN, J. C.: Guide to Interviewing and Clinical Personality Study. *Archives of Neurology and Psychiatry,* 52. 1944.

Chapter XXI

EVALUATION OF CURRENT PROGRESS AND TRENDS

LOOKING OVER a long period of years, progress in treatment is steady and continuous although frequently more rapid at one time or along certain lines than others. There may be periods of quiet but never of stagnation. Sometimes theoretical knowledge is ahead of practical applications; then again, surprising practical results along unorthodox lines may challenge our theoretical foundations. It is most hazardous, however, if one proposes for a new therapeutic procedure a theoretical basis which is at complete variance with established facts in medical sciences but which seems to answer critical objections which may be raised against the therapeutic procedure.

Through his training and his philosophy of aiding the suffering patient and of preventing any harm, a physician is inclined to become conservative. It is essential that he keep informed of advances in treatment and that he view new procedures and offered explanations with critical openmindedness. He should be willing to accept therapeutic results if the data are clearly presented so that he can form his own opinion. Criticism should not lead to a denial of the results presented, but should be directed at the interpretation of the facts and against unwarranted generalizations.

This chapter permits a review of recent progress and of therapeutic procedures which are not well established as yet. Some may sooner or later become fully recognized as proven progress, while others may be discarded. Arriving at a sound judgment of the justifiability and applicability of a proposed procedure may have to be postponed considerably. This may occur when the main interest is directed at improvement of the technique used and not enough effort is directed at establishing the physiological, psychological, and environmental dynamic factors in the treatment and the therapeutic indications and contraindications.

A good therapist will always be impatiently waiting for further advances in treatment which will permit him to be helpful in the many clinical situations in which he has not succeeded in the past. He will, however, also recognize his many minor and major successes and keep in mind which aspects and procedures have been found fundamentally sound. It is for this reason that a considerable number of patients treated 15 to 20 years ago are offered as illustrations in this book. They illustrate well the features of treatment which are still important. These cases also emphasize the fact that a physician should not look for perfect goals. In all these patients some psychotherapeutic aspects might now be handled differently, or physical agents might be used. The results obtained, however, should make us consider critically the theories and procedures of today in the ever-changing progress of treatment. They also warn us not to believe that psychiatric treatment has changed completely just because marked advances have been made along certain lines and for some psychopathological conditions.

Many valuable points are stressed by the authors of a symposium on the evaluation of therapeutic results.[1] Pertinent is the observation that in child psychoanalysis equally good results are achieved by Melanie Klein's and Anna Freud's approaches, although their theories and techniques vary greatly. The author suggests, therefore, that it might be the physician's personality and manner of application rather than the theory which is therapeutically essential. This point illustrates well, in psychoanalytic treatment as well as in psychotherapy in general, the trend to be guided less by strict adherence to theories than by factual results, with an increasing obligation to analyze them for the factors involved.

There are several therapeutic procedures as well as general trends in treatment which deserve special attention.

Use of Indirect Methods: Despite the large number of psychological tests, especially of the projective type, which have been in use in recent years, their usefulness in therapy is most limited. A good clinician will usually obtain in the course of a careful investigation the dynamic material which is indicated in the tests. There may be some justification for their use in an out-patient service where pressure of time forces curtailment of optimal therapeutic attention to individual cases. On the other hand, the important fact may be overlooked that every diagnostic psychiatric study has therapeutic implications. A careful life history and evaluations of the patient's own personality and of personality features of persons who are or have been important in his life are obviously psychotherapy. Therapeutic factors are also at work when a physician or, if necessary, a social worker obtains detailed facts from relatives, friends, or employers. These therapeutic gains cannot be obtained if the physician relies on tests and questionnaires.

A test which has been found therapeutically valuable is Murray's Thematic Apperception Test.[2] This test may reveal much dynamic material in patients who are unable to express themselves; for example, adolescents and chronic alcoholics. Through the test the psychiatrist may see leads which may permit him to direct therapeutic efforts in a better planned way. The full therapeutic usefulness of this test cannot be evaluated until further critical studies have been published.

Group Psychotherapy: Progress seems to have developed from increased experience with this therapeutic procedure, while the theoretical understanding has advanced little. The present trend seems to favor the active participation of the group in the treatment rather than offering orientation and guidance through discussion by the psychiatrist. One trend is to strengthen the individual personality through group association and to make him develop sound standards through becoming concerned about the group reaction to his behavior and ideas. Emphasis is therefore placed on individual participation in discussion.[3] Another trend considers the essential function of the therapist to help the patient express himself, if necessary through appropriate questions to facilitate overcoming of resistances. The goal is then to make this patient and the other patients in the group understand unconscious emotional conflicts.[4] Little is as yet known about termination of treatment in patients who do not seem to be able to function satisfactorily if the group support is withdrawn. Increasing attention is becoming directed to group psychotherapy for chronic cases. A striking and unexplained observation is the unsatisfactory cohesiveness of the female group, in which one finds a persistent tendency to receive help through the therapeutic relationship with the group leader rather than with all members of the group. The same observation has been made on floors limited to psychoneurotic patients in the Payne Whitney Clinic. Group psychotherapy, while of value in the treatment of chronic psychoneurotic conditions, of psychosomatic reactions, and of alcoholism, has not proven as economical a procedure as has been hoped.

Convulsive Therapy: The therapeutic use of convulsions has widened constantly through a better understanding of indications and a refinement in the technique of inducing convulsions and preventing complications. While for reasons not understood permanent memory defects may result, this occurrence is so rare that it cannot justify hesitation in advising convulsive therapy. Well understood nursing care and the use of curare are now preventing most fractures. Ambulatory treatment is therefore feasible. Indications for ambulatory treatment have not been well considered as yet. There may be cases where such procedures are indicated if the depressed patient does not present suicidal dangers and if the convulsive treatment is accompanied and followed by well-planned psychotherapy. In other depressed patients with suicidal dangers a relatively short stay in the hospital for convulsive treatment may be followed by ambulatory psychotherapy.

The importance of psychotherapy if one wishes more than temporary improvement seems to be now generally accepted. (Case 11, Chapter IX, illustrates this procedure.) At times it may be desirable to give enough convulsions to obtain a limited improvement, then follow this by a period of psychotherapy, and finally terminate the depression by an additional brief series of convulsions. This procedure would be indicated if the lack of need for treatment should cause the patient to terminate treatment after marked symptomatic improvement has occurred. The trend has been to increase the number of convulsions to twenty or thirty in patients who do not show satisfactory results. It seems that physicians frequently try to force unobtainable improvement. Better results may eventually be obtained from a variation in the frequency of the convulsions as well as their total number based on increased physiological knowledge. Postconvulsive electroencephalographic changes last longer with each succeeding convulsion. Shortening the interval between convulsions intensifies and lengthens the postconvulsive changes. Some authors therefore recommend several convulsions a day in marked paranoid and catatonic excitements or daily convulsions five times a week until twenty convulsions have been administered. This latter procedure has been advised for schizophrenic disorders in childhood and early adolescence.

Electronarcosis is an electrically induced state of unconsciousness which has been recommended for the treatment of paranoid schizophrenia.[5] Through the application of an alternating current to the brain, a convulsion is produced and then a state of prolonged unconsciousness which can be terminated readily. The patient is usually kept in an unconscious state for seven minutes. Treatments are administered three times and later twice and then once a week until a total of twenty treatments has been reached. The value of electronarcosis in schizophrenia is still disputed. The results seem to be less satisfactory than with insulin therapy.[6]

Insulin Treatment: There has not been any essential change in recent years and there is still considerable difference of opinion with regard to the superiority of this method which induces a comatose or a subcomatose state. The present trend seems to favor subcomatose treatment combined with intensive psychotherapy. (See Case 7, Chapter VIII.)

Combined insulin-convulsive therapy is recommended in patients in whom either treatment gave unsatisfactory results, especially in prolonged schizophrenic excitements and paranoid reactions. Others prefer to have a course of thirty effective insulin treatments immediately followed by fifteen or twenty convulsions, administered two or three times weekly.

Surgical Procedures on the Brain: In recent years new surgical procedures as well as modifications of the previously published methods have been recommended, with the purpose of obtaining more satisfactory results or of decreasing infections, hemorrhages, and other complications. On the whole, all the current methods offer a considerable degree of safety, although unfortunate accidents including death remain possibilities. Theoretical knowledge has increased little, while practical results have become impressive.[7]

It is still unclear what specific results are obtained with the various types of operative procedures. The many theories which have been offered have not advanced or even changed our conception of psychiatric disorders. The success of other psychiatric treatments should not be disregarded. On the other hand, beneficial results have been obtained in cases where other treatments had previously failed; for example, in chronic schizophrenic excitement, persistent and highly disturbing delusional and hallucinatory reactions, and in markedly incapacitating compulsive disorders. It seems probable that anxiety, and possibly other emotions, is decreased or abolished, and thus hallucinations, delusions, and aggressiveness are diminished. The therapeutic effect might be similar to insulin treatment but is more far-reaching and lasting. Good results are also obtained in the alleviation of intractable pain and in phantom limb. In either condition the patient may not be aware of his symptoms any longer, or he may notice them but not experience pain or unpleasant sensations. Actual decrease of pain is the exception. Occasionally pain may return but will be helped by a second lobotomy.

The development of symptoms attributable to brain damage has remained unclear. Unsatisfactory interest in self and environment, blunting of emotional reactions, temper outbursts, decreased spontaneous activities and low goals of achievement, increased and often apparently uncontrollable food intake are frequently observed after successful operative treatment of chronic excitements and paranoic reactions. These same symptoms have, however, been observed in many spontaneous improvements of similar cases. It is at present impossible to state whether in these operated patients one deals with schizophrenic, paranoid, or other reactions of withdrawal of interests from the outer world, or with actual brain damage. Although considerable psychological testing has been carried out, the results remain unclear. Frequently the studies were done without satisfactory pre-operative studies, or the tests were not well enough conceived to elicit defects. It is also still unknown what damages might become obvious after the lapse of several years. There is therefore a reluctance to consider any but the above mentioned indications for surgical procedure. On the other hand, psychiatrists increasingly urge brain surgery in acute and subacute paranoid and other schizophrenic conditions if they have not yielded satisfactorily to insulin and convulsive treatment and to psychotherapy.

The significance of moderate cerebral atrophies is unclear. In a few patients porencephalic cysts have been noticed, supposedly caused by degenerative changes, minor hematomata, or lesions of the ventricular wall. Although these findings were considered insignificant, the question of the influence of aging on these changes was raised.[8] In the postoperative phase confusion and urinary incontinence may be troublesome but usually clear up after several days. In about 10 per cent epileptic seizures are said to occur and necessitate sustained administration of phenobarbital.

Techniques which are currently advocated and performed bilaterally include (1) cutting of the fronto-thalamic or fronto-temporal fibers (lobotomy, leucotomy); (2) extirpation of a circumscribed area of cortex of the frontal lobe with secondary degeneration of fibers (for example, topectomy); and (3) interference of connections between the frontal lobe and the dorsomedial nucleus of the thalamus (thalamotomy). From a psychiatric point of view there is little therapeutic superiority of any of these methods recognizable as yet.

Surgical procedures are only a part of a successful treatment. Psychotherapy in general and along specific lines, including planned re-education, is important. Rehabilitation to life outside the hospital after several years of hospitalization may present grave and even insurmountable obstacles. Many changes may have taken place in the patient's family and in the social setting. Much planning and effort may be needed to achieve desirable modifications. In the case which is presented below some of these difficulties were not overcome until a year after discharge from the hospital. Another chronic schizophrenic patient in whom all disturbing psychopathological symptoms had disappeared after lobotomy asked for readmission to the state hospital. Life in the hospital seemed to promise her more ease and contentment than she could find in a home and in a community which had become strange to her during a separation of seven years.

Case 44:

Lobotomy was performed in a chronic paranoid schizophrenic illness. The record is offered in detail to demonstrate the ineffectiveness of insulin and electric convulsive therapy as well as of intensive psychotherapy in this chronic condition. There is no doubt that the present improvement is related to the surgical procedure.

A 40 year old married woman reacted with prolonged mild depression, restlessness, and dissatisfaction to the death of both parents which had occurred within a few months. After about a year (in May 1941) she developed an acute depressive paranoid reaction, and after two weeks was admitted to the Payne Whitney Psychiatric Clinic.

The patient had a normal development in childhood. She was a quiet, reserved child who in college became a recognized leader socially. Although intelligent, her scholastic achievements were mediocre. After having worked with social agencies for two years, she married at 24. Her main interests were social activities, but she remained reserved and never developed close friendships. She was cold to her children and little interested in her husband's professional activities. He was of her age, idealistic and sociable, and never aware of how little he and his wife had in common. As long as servants were available, the household ran smoothly. When financial reverses in 1931 forced upon her the full household activities, she carried them out willingly but never well. There was always considerable untidiness, and her husband had to help continuously. She felt above most people socially, although this attitude was not wholly justified by her background, but resented openly their economic superiority. Both the patient and her husband were stubborn and opinionated. She was resentful to his behavior but suppressed these emotional expressions. At times she became self-assertive and showed a tendency to suspiciousness. From 31 to 33 she lived a secluded life with her children in a small village in France under the vague pretext of a need to live in such a culture. Her sexual life seemed adequate, but she never expressed sexual interests spontaneously and it is not known whether or not she obtained orgasm frequently. Her self-centered and aloof attitude with inadequate attention to practical life remained the same from 31 until her acute illness at 41. Her domineering parents who had spoiled her in childhood lived in her house from 1934 till their death in 1940. She resented this burden greatly and was intolerant to them and to her children. She kept aloof from an unmarried brother and sister who were both seclusive and unsuccessful in their work.

In the hospital the patient was frequently in a state of constant agitation, often depressed, but more frequently resentful and angry. Her delusions were that she was going to be tortured and that she would have to remake the universe. The world seemed changed and she had been changed physically, but she would not say in what way. She often urinated on the floor. While under the influence of cold wet packs and prolonged baths she was usually quiet. Barbiturates given three or four times daily also seemed to decrease her restlessness and agitation, but her delusions persisted. Her physician was able to establish a friendly relationship with the patient after about three weeks of treatment and to reassure her when she was fearful.

In September she became negativistic, refused food, and frequently had to be tube fed; at times she assaulted nurses. These attacks seemed to be the expression of general anger and not provoked by any special situation or person. Fear, anxiety, and resentment were the leading emotions. In the middle of October insulin treatment was started and mild coma was obtained with 70 units. During the next few weeks she became quiet, participated in occupational therapy and group activities, and was able to have her husband and children visit her twice a week. Her delusions persisted, but she was able to discuss them with her physician. After forty successful treatments she began to revert to her previous behavior, and insulin therapy was discontinued the beginning of December. (Fifty successful treatments had been given.) She stated she would like to talk to her physician but was unable to do so. Under the influence of intravenously administered sodium amytal she expressed resentment against the personnel and her illness. During repeated sodium amytal treatments she expressed herself less well.

In January 1942 electrically induced convulsions were administered twice a week. The treatment was discontinued after seven convulsions because she had developed marked confusion. Another thirteen convulsions were administered in March and April. There was little change in her behavior. Additional delusions were mentioned — people thought she was not married and considered her children illegitimate. In July 1942 she was transferred to a state hospital. Her condition changed little except that at times she seemed more depressed, and she made several suicidal attempts. In 1945 her daughter was admitted to another psychiatric hospital in an acute catatonic illness. The patient seemed to react little to the news of her daughter's illness. In spring, 1946, when informed of her daughter's recovery, she became quiet although still resentful and occasionally assaultive. After several therapeutic interviews while under the influence of intravenously administered sodium amytal the patient improved. She expressed resentment to the personnel, blamed herself for her daughter's illness and expressed a wish to be discharged. Her husband took her home in July 1946. During a seven-month period with her family the patient stayed mostly in her room, refused to dress, and demanded constant attention. She was disorderly and untidy. She expressed freely the delusions that her husband and her children were persecuting her and at times denied violently the identity of her husband.

In January and February 1946 she became assaultive, fearful, angry, and negativistic, and she was returned to the hospital the beginning of March. In the hospital her behavior and delusions were similar to those before discharge.

In October 1947 the patient was transferred to the Payne Whitney Clinic for lobotomy. Following our customary policy the patient was studied in an eight-week preoperative phase. During this period intensive psychotherapeutic efforts were made to influence the patient's psychopathological reactions but with little effect. The patient was untidy, dishevelled, and suspicious. At times she appeared fearful. She refused to participate in activities and soon became negativistic. Her delusions were that the nurses mixed up her thinking, that they tried to make her appear sick. At other times she mimicked people and her behavior was silly. Her memory for remote and recent events seemed poor. She had difficulty in grasping questions and concentrated poorly. In conversations she showed much blocking and perseveration. There were daily outbursts of anger and assaultiveness. At other times she was erotic, exposed herself freely, and insisted that she was her physician's wife.

A bilateral frontal lobotomy was performed on December 11, 1947. One-inch trephines were made on each side, the posterior margin of which lay one cm. anterior to the coronal suture. An incision was made in the right cortex and carried down to the white matter of the frontal lobe. All the white fibres were divided, the line of incision passing just anterior to the tip of the frontal horn of the ventricle and inferiorly exposing the sphenoidal ridge. The same procedure was carried out on the left side.

For about 18 hours after operation the patient was well oriented, read and described a newspaper story, talked spontaneously, and described herself as "cheerful." However, on her husband's visit she doubted his identity. From her second post-operative day there was a rapidly progressive return of her negativistic resistance, and tube feeding became necessary on December 22, 1947. She was easily angered, cursed the nurses, and at other times mimicked them. She smeared her wall with feces. Following operation her temperature rose and remained elevated with daily spiking to about 38.8° until December 27th. When fever subsided, the patient began to eat well. At times she was pleasant, but more frequently angry or petulant, striking nurses readily when urged to do things. She mimicked others and was childlishly playful and soon again resentful and suspicious. Occasionally she expressed the delusion of having died. This behavior lasted till the middle of January. During this period she reviewed some parts of her illness and expressed intense resentment of her husband's rigidity and lack of thoughtfulness. Interviews were frequently followed by prolonged diatribes of obscenity and cursing of other patients and nurses.

During the latter half of January and in February and March, the patient showed progressive improvement. She became more cooperative. When tense, she relaxed well in prolonged baths. Her sudden, superficial, and quickly evaporating mood changes (anger, anxiety, self-blame, and depression) became less frequent. The patient joined the group and worked in occupational therapy, but tended to resist and resent changes in the activities which had been started. There was little interest in personal appearance, but she accepted suggestions for improving it without resentment. Her appetite was good and she slept well without sedation. In bi-weekly interviews with her physician her past life was reviewed, as was her rejection of her daughter and her ambivalent attitude to her son.

During the month of April psychotherapeutic efforts were directed at achieving more interest in her personal appearance and in her relationship with other patients and the nurses. She delighted in making embarrassing remarks, was vague and inattentive. Her examination revealed satisfactory concentration and good memory for remote and recent events, and she was now reacting well to her husband and children's visits.

Since her discharge on May 1, 1948, the patient has shown steady improvement. She saw her psychiatrist regularly once a month for about a year, and since then has seen him once in two or three months. In the beginning she did not dress well and paid insufficient attention to her household and family. This changed during the fall of 1948. She also became friendly with her daughter and her social activities increased. The most distressing symptom to her husband is her tendency to overeat, which has lead to a weight of 180 pounds (before 1940 she weighed about 135 pounds). The last examination in October 1949 and the reports of her husband indicate that she can now be gracious and friendly. She is well dressed but shows signs of being untidy or slightly dishevelled. Although aware when she is blunt in her expression, she does not feel that it is worthwhile to repress her reaction to people. She is overtalkative, somewhat euphoric and silly, and often irritable. There is a lack of evaluating spontaneously in a conversation that which is appropriate and essential. She makes witty remarks which she repeats frequently. All behavior abnormalities, especially occasional temper outbursts, are minimized by her. There is a lack of sustained interest in work and in her friends and a definite tendency to apathy. She is more affectionate to her husband and children than before her illness, but her emotions lack depth and persistence. Psychological testing revealed no pathology in intellectual performance. The patient is taking phenobarbital twice daily because she had two convulsions in the fall of 1948.

It is obvious that lobotomy has lead to a remarkable improvement in this paranoid schizophrenic patient which permits her to live a fairly normal life outside the hospital. The pathological symptoms may be the expression of her schizophrenic illness or related to brain damage. There is, however, no way by which the latter assumption could be substantiated.

Pharmacologic Treatment of Anxiety: It has been found that Dibenamine (N N-dibenzyl-beta-chloro-ethylamine) decreases anxiety.[9] The drug is administered orally in the amount of 240 mg. three times daily, taken immediately after meals. In an exceptional patient mild toxic symptoms (nausea) may occur, and only 120 mg. three times daily may be indicated. This drug has been found efficacious in symptomatic control of intense anxiety in neurotic conditions but less so in depressive and schizophrenic reactions. In panic reactions insulin therapy is to be preferred, except when the mild degree of the panic reaction justifies ambulatory treatment. The drug may be a useful adjunct to psychotherapy in patients in whom the anxiety interferes with carrying out desirable activities.

Treatment of Alcoholism: The two main trends which have developed in the treatment of alcoholism are pharmacologic therapy and treatment in the out-patient departments of general hospitals.

Pharmacologic treatment has been tried for twenty years. The goal was to establish a conditioned reflex aversion to alcohol. By administering apomorphine while the patient was drinking alcoholic beverages, an associative link was established between the alcoholic beverage and nausea and vomiting. This resulted in nausea and even vomiting when the patient saw, smelled, or tasted alcoholic beverages without drinking the beverage. Whether or not one establishes a conditioned reflex response in Pavlov's sense is disputed. In the last 10 years Voegtlin [11] and others have refined the method and the results have improved. It is considered important for the exhibition of the alcoholic beverage to precede and overlap the nausea and vomiting, which is induced by a hypodermic injection of emetine hydrochloride. The treatment is briefly formulated to the patient before the emetine solution is administered (6 minims of a 40 cc. sterile aqueous solution containing 3.25 gm. of emetine hydrochloride, 1.65 gm. of pilocarpine hydrochloride, and 1.5 gm. of ephedrine sulfate). After the injection the patient drinks one ounce of whiskey in lukewarm water. After a second drink the patient will vomit. Whiskey may be offered to induce two to three vomitings during the first treatment, which lasts about 20 minutes. The subsequent daily treatments are essentially the same except that dosage of emetine will be increased. It is necessary to use different kinds of liquor in order to achieve aversion to the alcohol and not to a specific liquor. The aversion can be established in five to eight treatments, administered on successive days. The success of this type of treatment depends not only on the careful carrying out of the conditioning procedure but also on the use of psychotherapy. The treatment is carried out in a well-planned hospital setting. The general atmosphere and the suggestive influence of physician and nurses are important factors. An analysis of personality factors with explanation and advice from the physician are contributory to the final adjustment. The success also depends on the selection of suitable patients; that is, patients who are eager for help and who are willing to undergo the unpleasantness of the treatment. Alcoholic patients who suffer from severe psychopathological maladjustments are usually excluded, as are patients with active peptic ulcer, coronary and myocardial disease, active tuberculosis, and hernia. Often authors have proposed more drastic procedures, which have, however, attracted less attention and are being discarded.

Based on observations in various industries it has been known that certain chemicals may induce sensitivity to small amounts of alcohol, resulting in nausea, tachycardia, and headaches. In recent years the use of tetraethylthiuram disulfide, under the trade name of antabuse, has been advocated.[11] The toxic effect occurs only when the patient drinks alcoholic beverages and it is claimed to be due to accumulation of acetaldehyde resulting from metabolism of the alcohol. The symptoms are first palpitation and tachycardia, then nausea with a marked drop in blood pressure. The drug has not been sufficiently studied as yet and its use involves definite dangers. The therapeutic principle is partly to establish an aversion reaction to alcohol and to have the patient protect himself by the daily use of the drug with its known effect in case alcoholic beverages are consumed. Through the regular administration of the drug over a period of two weeks, the patient's sensitivity to the drug increases, so that finally a small daily protective dosage is sufficient. The procedure is not well worked out and various modifications are tried. Indications and contraindications are still unclear and the results therefore cannot be evaluated at present.

The Belgian method of injecting alcohol intravenously (Curéthyl treatment) for establishing sensitivity to alcohol has been abandoned after a few years of enthusiastic use in some European countries, but this procedure is used in general hopsitals for the treatment of delirium tremens. No satisfactory theoretical basis for this method has been offered and the results have never been reviewed scientifically.

Through the efforts of lay organizations physicians have become increasingly interested in out-patient treatment of chronic alcoholism and in brief in-patient treatment of acute and chronic alcoholism. Alcoholics Anonymous has brought forth a much needed impetus for treatment as well as a place of security to many of these patients. Similar movements have been most influential in several European countries since the turn of the century. Any physician who wishes to treat alcoholic patients must be aware of all resources in his community and cooperate with such groups whenever it will be of help to his individual patient. For the permanent adjustment of a recovered alcoholic patient, a sound social life is essential but often exceedingly difficult to achieve. Our present day society makes total abstinence a difficult problem by promulgating the right to drink but not considering equally the privilege of not drinking.

Whether an out-patient service for alcoholic patients should be part of a general or a psychiatric hospital is less important than the fact that each patient must be studied physically, psychologically, and socially. The European experience argues against establishing special hospitals for alcoholics, but excellent results have been obtained in several places by the use of farms or special types of colonies for such patients. The results seem to depend on careful selection of suitable patients and on an organization of well regulated daily activities. The morale of the group, created and maintained by the lay and professional therapist, exerts a strong suggestive influence and offers security and stability.

Treatment of Drug Addiction: The leading trend in the treatment of drug addiction has remained abrupt withdrawal. On the other hand, there have been several publications which urged a gradual reduction and a substitution of morphine by another drug which can be withdrawn abruptly with relatively minor withdrawal symptoms.[12] The drug methadon (6-dimethylamino-4-4-diphenyl-3-

hepatone) is substituted for morphine by starting in doses of 10 to 20 mg. (⅙ to ⅓ grains) three times daily twenty-four hours before morphine is discontinued. After morphine has been withdrawn abruptly, methadon is reduced and withdrawn in the course of the following ten days. The withdrawal symptoms of methadon are not very marked.

There is no doubt that in some patients the substitution of morphine by methadon in order to achieve withdrawal with mild symptoms is highly desirable; for example, addicts with serious cardiac conditions. On the other hand, methadon presents a marked addiction liability, and its euphoric effect is equal to that of morphine. In past years psychiatrists with much experience in the treatment of drug addiction have warned strongly against substitution of one drug by another addiction forming drug. Experience has shown that such treatment resulted frequently in new or combined addiction.

Insulin treatment for withdrawal symptoms has not received favorable comments in recent years and has been considered useless in a thorough study of treatment of drug addiction.[13] There seems to be considerable discrepancy among various authors with regard to withdrawal symptoms in morphine addiction. At the United States Public Health Service Hospital at Lexington, Kentucky, very marked and highly disturbing symptoms are observed, while in our experience the symptoms were not marked and certainly never unbearable. Only in a minor group can the difference of the amount used explain these divergent observations. It may be that the intensity of the withdrawal symptoms depends to a considerable extent on the personality organization. The patient who seeks help from a private practitioner, especially a patient who is still leading a successful life, may suffer from less serious psychopathology than those in government institutions. The knowledge that abrupt withdrawal is practiced may also act as a screening factor.

Rehabilitation in Convalescence and in Chronic Cases: As part of a broad medical trend to develop sound principles of rehabilitation, considerable thought has been given to rehabilitation in psychiatrically disabled persons.[14] Sound rehabilitation of a physically handicapped person must include attention to psychological factors and treatment of each patient as an individual. Aptitude and other psychological testing may be indicated; the use of State and Federal Agencies as well as of private employment agencies may be necessary. Social workers will be helpful in making adjustment to the home after discharge from a hospital, during a period of convalescence or partial or marked invalidism. These workers may also modify attitudes of members of the family, of the community, and of employers and co-workers. They should not only be helpful in finding work or opportunities for education but also in pointing out suitable recreation and opportunity for socialization.

These same principles apply to the rehabilitation of psychiatrically handicapped and disabled patients. Efforts at rehabilitation should start before discharge from the hospital and should be part of the psychotherapeutic process in hospital and ambulatory practice. A special aspect of psychiatric rehabilitation is the frequent need to help in the adjustment of patients who have little or no previous experience in work. To this group belong young schizophrenic and psychopathic patients. Among well-to-do or wealthy patients, especially women, chronic psychoneurotic conditions may have led to invalidism or ill-planned leisure and idleness. Chronic alcoholism will always necessitate well-planned efforts at rehabilitation. The aging person may be saved from permanent hospital treatment. Epileptic patients can be fitted into a normal life. Many feebleminded persons can be made useful and self-supporting members of the community. Through the efforts of psychiatrists and psychologists many aspects of mental health have become accepted. Professional advice is sought in industry by management and labor. Concern about the personality of the child has spread to a large number of schools. Public health departments in cities and states and in medical schools recognize the need of investigating and fostering mental health. This concept is also becoming progressively part of medical practice in our complex modern hospital.[15] Opportunities are becoming recognized and utilized in the treatment of patients in medical and surgical departments, in children's and women's hospitals, in the personnel health departments and in administrative planning. Hospitals recognize increasingly their obligation to be the center for promoting good physical and mental health in the community.

BIBLIOGRAPHY

1. OBERNDORF, C. P.; GREENACRE, P.; and KUBIE, L.: Symposium on the evaluation of therapeutic results. *Internat. J. Psycho-Analysis, 29:* 1948.

2. MURRAY, H. A.: *Thematic Apperception Test.* Cambridge, Harvard, 1943.

3. COTTON, J. M.: Group psychotherapy: An appraisal. In: *Failures in Psychiatric Treatment.* (Edited by Paul H. Hoch.) New York, Grune & Stratton, 1948.

4. WENDER, L., and STEIN, A.: Group psychotherapy as an aid to out-patient treatment in a psychiatric clinic. *Psychiatric Quart., 23:* 1949.

5. TIETZ, E. B.; THOMSON, G. N.; VAN HARREVELD, A.; and WIERSMA, C. A. G.: Electronarcosis, its application and therapeutic effect in schizophrenia. *J. Nerv. & Ment. Dis., 103:* 1946.

6. REES, L.: Electronarcosis in the treatment of schizophrenia. *J. Ment. Sc., 95:* 1949.

7. MOORE, B. E.; SIMON, B.; FRIEDMAN, S.; and RANGER, C. O.: Successes and failures following frontal lobotomy. *New York State J. Med., 49:* 1949.

8. STJERNBERG, F.: Pneumoencephalographic findings in some cases of leucotomy. *Acta psychiat. et neurol., 47:* 1947.

9. ROCKWELL, F. V.: Dibenamine therapy in certain psychopathologic syndromes. *Psychosom. Med., 10:* 1948.

10. LEMERE, F.; VOEGTLIN, W. L.; BROZ, W. R.; O'HALLORAN, P.; and TUPPER, W. E.: Conditioned reflex treatment of chronic alcoholism: VII, technique. *Dis. Nerv. System, 3:* 1942. Review in *Quart. J. Stud. on Alcohol, 3:* 1942-43. (The review contains a detailed description of the technique.)

11. JACOBSEN, E., and MARTENSEN-LARSEN, O.: Treatment of alcoholism with tetraethylthiuram disulfide (Antabus). *J.A.M.A., 139:* 1949.

12. VOGEL, V. H.; ISBELL, H.; and CHAPMAN, K. W.: Present status of narcotic addiction. *J.A.M.A., 138:* 1948.

13. WIEDER, H.: Objective evaluation of insulin therapy of the morphine abstinence syndrome. *J. Nerv. & Ment. Dis., 110:* 1949.

14. RENNIE, T. A. C.; BURLING, T.; and WOODWARD, L. E.: Vocational rehabilitation of the psychiatrically disabled. *Ment. Hyg., 33:* 1949.

15. DIETHELM, O.; BINGER, C.; DANIELLS, H. E.; DUNN, W. H.; FRASER, A. W.; KOHL, R. N.; LHAMON, W. T.; RIPLEY, H. S.; ROBBINS, H. C.; WOODWARD, W. D.; and WOLF, S.: Mental hygiene in a general hospital. *Psychosom. Med., 11:* 1949.

INDEX

This Book

TREATMENT IN PSYCHIATRY

By

OSKAR DIETHELM, M.D.

was set, printed, and bound by the Pantagraph Printing and Stationery Company of Bloomington, Illinois. The type face is Intertype Garamond, set 12 point on 13 point. The page size is 6 x 9 inches. The type-page size is 26 x 43 picas. The text paper is 70 lb. white Warren's Olde Style. The cover is Bancroft, Arrestox Buckram, T.

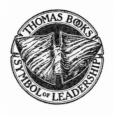

2nd (Cornell) Division
Neurological Service
Bellevue Hospital